THE CANADIAN TYPE 2
DIABETES
SOURCEBOOK

3ʳᴰ EDITION

M. SARA ROSENTHAL, PH.D.

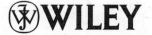

WILEY

John Wiley & Sons Canada, Ltd.

This book is available for bulk purchases by your group or organizations for sales promotions, premiums, fundraising, and seminars. For details, contact: John Wiley & Sons Canada, Ltd., 6045 Freemont Blvd., Mississauga, ON L5R 4J3. Tel: 416-236-4433. Toll-free: 1-800-567-4797. Fax: 416-236-4448. Website: www.wiley.ca

Author and Publisher have used their best efforts in preparing this book. John Wiley & Sons Canada, Ltd., the sponsor, and the author make no representations or warranties with respect to the accuracy or completeness of the contents of this book and specifically disclaim any implied warranties of merchantability or fitness for a particular purpose. There are no warranties that extend beyond the descriptions contained in this paragraph. No warranty may be created or extended by sales representatives or written sales materials. The accuracy and completeness of the information provided herein and the opinions stated herein are not guaranteed or warranted to produce any specific results, and the advice and strategies contained herein may not be suitable for every individual. Neither John Wiley & Sons Canada, Ltd., the sponsor, nor the author shall be liable for any loss of profit or any other commercial damages including but not limited to special, incidental, consequential, or other damages.

Although every effort has been made to ensure that permissions for all material were obtained, those sources not formally acknowledged should contact the publisher for inclusion in future editions of this book.

Library and Archives Canada Cataloguing in Publication Data

Rosenthal, M. Sara
  The Canadian type 2 diabetes sourcebook / M. Sara
Rosenthal. — 3rd ed.

Includes bibliographical references and index.
Issued also in electronic format.
ISBN 978-0-470-15702-2

  1. Non-insulin-dependent diabetes—Popular works. I. Title.

RC662.18.R667 2009   616.4'62   C2009-900712-6

Production Credits
Cover and interior design: Adrian So
Typesetting: Thomson Digital
Author photo by Captured Moments
Printer: Friesens

John Wiley & Sons Canada, Ltd.
6045 Freemont Blvd.
Mississauga, Ontario
L5R 4J3

Printed in Canada

1 2 3 4 5 FP 13 12 11 10 09

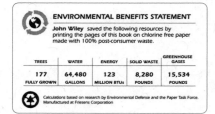

ENVIRONMENTAL BENEFITS STATEMENT
John Wiley saved the following resources by printing the pages of this book on chlorine free paper made with 100% post-consumer waste.

TREES	WATER	ENERGY	SOLID WASTE	GREENHOUSE GASES
177 FULLY GROWN	64,480 GALLONS	123 MILLION BTUs	8,280 POUNDS	15,534 POUNDS

Calculations based on research by Environmental Defense and the Paper Task Force.
Manufactured at Friesens Corporation

ACKNOWLEDGEMENTS

This third edition would not have been possible without the meticulous research assistance of medical librarian, Ellen Tulchinsky. I wish to especially thank Professor Nadir Farid, MD, for his assistance with respect to the low glycemic index content, as well as colleagues from The Endocrine Society, who were helpful with suggestions and comments.

I also wish to thank the following people (listed alphabetically) for their commitment, hard work, and guidance on previous editions of this text:

Irwin Antone, MD, CCFP; Brenda Cook, RD; Tasha Hamilton, BaSc, RD; Stuart Harris, MD, MPH, CCFP, ABPM; Dennis Karounos, MD; Ann Kenshole, MD; Anne Levin, BScPT, MCPA; Gary May, MD, FRCP; Barbara McIntosh, RN, BScN, CDE; the late James McSherry, MB, ChB, FCFP (1943–2002); Judy Nesbitt; Mark Nesbitt; Robert Panchyson, BScN, RN; Diana Phayre; and Robert Silver, MD, FRCPC.

CONTENTS

FOREWORD

When I started to examine Type 2 diabetes, it all seemed so simple; all you had to do was control your blood sugar. You could do this by losing some weight or taking one or two pills. I was certain that this would make sense to patients and they would comply. Now, after a few years of delving into what happens in the "real world," I have a very different view.

I think the medical community's usual approach to people with diabetes or, for that matter, with any chronic disease, is somewhat flawed. The typical model is the following: the doctor diagnoses, the doctor prescribes, and the patient then complies. This can work for acute medicine, but not for chronic diseases. For chronic diseases, there should be an exchange of roles. Instead of the doctor or clinic being the central character in diabetes care, it should be you, the health care consumer—with clinic, nurse, doctor, pharmacist, nutritionist, etc., as the supporting actors. We need to shift from the doctor-management approach to one of self-management. Books like this one play a vital role in a self-management approach.

Some of the themes of this new pathway are as follows:

We need to move from a fixed *table d'hôte* menu to an *à la carte* menu of information, knowledge, and solutions. We tend not to individualize information, but rather to send out generic information that is often overwhelming or not specific enough for an individual's health care needs. The Internet has helped to change some of these problems, but the quality of that information remains a concern.

We need to consider barriers to care beyond basic information. We all know we should eat well and exercise, but how do I help you identify your unique barriers and the characteristics that enable you to actually do it? Do I bring in your partner? Put the information on your hand-held computer? Talk to your peers?

We need to reframe the risks and benefits, putting them in the consumer's perspective. As health care professionals, we spend a lot of time looking at long-term trials that show "significant" gains in risk reduction. These gains may be evident in the literature, but are often cold comfort to patients. For example, when I see patients for arthritis or asthma and I give them pills or puffers, they usually feel better immediately. However, people with diabetes are often taking many medications, but do not actually feel better—in fact, they often feel worse—and the incentives for good control are very different and certainly less obvious.

We need to redefine our conception of diabetes. Diabetes is not a disease as much as it is a risk factor. Heart disease is our most common foe and diabetes is a major risk factor for heart problems. Treating diabetes is like making a contribution to your RRSP; you don't get the benefit until much further down the road. The contribution can take many forms: lowering blood pressure and/or cholesterol, stopping smoking, maintaining good glucose control, and getting active.

We need to remember the basics. In medicine we have come up with many fancy interventions, but at the end of the day, good health still rests on a few core principles: healthy eating, being active, and having a positive attitude. For people who suffer from a chronic condition such as diabetes, I would add self-empowerment to the list. When individuals take charge of their lifestyle, emotional well-being, and role as health care consumers, there is greater opportunity to improve their health.

Enabling self-management is what M. Sara Rosenthal's *Canadian Type 2 Diabetes Sourcebook* (3rd ed.) is all about. This book is not meant to be read all at one sitting. It is not meant to convert you from a fast-food junkie to a never-make-a-mistake eater. Rather, it is meant to be a comprehensive resource that is there for you when you need the right information at the right time. There is no perfect pathway to optimum diabetes care—only *your* pathway. Health care professionals and diabetes experts can only try to make it easier for you to do the right thing. Certainly, this book gives you all the information you need to make those choices. The next step is up to you. Good luck!

Michael Evans, MD, CCFP

Principal Investigator Knowledge Translation Program, Continuing Education Research Scholar, Family Healthcare Research Unit Assistant Professor, Department of Family and Community Medicine, University of Toronto Staff Physician, Toronto Western Hospital, University Health Network

INTRODUCTION
ALL IN THE FAMILY

Let me tell you a little bit about my family, which will tell you why I'm interested in the subject of Type 2 diabetes.

In 1978, my grandmother, obese and physically inactive, who had Type 2 diabetes, dropped dead from a massive heart attack at the age of 62. She was survived by her own mother by a full decade. I have still never quite recovered from the loss because it was such an untimely death. To this day, I dream of her. In a recurring dream, she is alive and well, but I know that her heart will give out at any moment. The feeling that she will "die again" always interferes with my dream visits; even in the dream world, my time with her is limited. My grandfather, a family physician who died in 1989, used to say that my grandmother "ate herself to death." And the more I research Type 2 diabetes, the more I understand what he meant by this comment.

According to the US National Institute of Diabetes and Digestive and Kidney Diseases (NIDDK), more than 85 percent of people with Type 2 diabetes are overweight. My grandmother was a textbook case. In her mid-forties, she developed "late-onset diabetes mellitus," known today as Type 2 diabetes. (I explain all the labels of this disease in Chapter 1.) My grandmother was an out-of-control diabetic who outlived her baby sister, who also died from complications of Type 2 diabetes. (My aunt, too, was obese.) Despite the fate of her little sister, my grandmother never made any effort to adjust her own eating habits.

My mother, who has spent most of her adult life battling obesity, used to be coaxed into eating rich desserts by my grandmother with comments such as "It's a sin not to eat it."

Indeed, my grandmother's great character flaw was her appetite. She could never pass up rich and tasty foods, and part of the reason is attributed to the hard times she experienced coming of age in the Prairies during the Depression. She went on to develop heart disease and apparently had spent most of her forties and fifties as a very unwell woman, continuously plagued with one health problem after another. Given this information, probably no one is surprised that she died. After all, the woman was a "walking time bomb." The funny thing is, everyone who loved her was shocked by her death. My great-grandmother bore the terrible fate of outliving almost all of her children, who were all obese; most of them died from complications related to Type 2 diabetes.

This is the book I wish my grandmother and her siblings had read. I want to give you the information my grandmother should have had, and might have used, if it had been available to her.

According to the 2008 Canadian Diabetes Association (CDA) Guidelines, 1.8 million adult Canadians, or 5.5 percent of the population, were diagnosed with Type 2 diabetes in 2005. This is a significant increase from 1998, when those already diagnosed with Type 2 diabetes in Canada was 4.8 percent (or 1,054,000 adult Canadians). This means that if we count only those already diagnosed with Type 2 diabetes in Canada, there has been a 70 percent increase since the publication of the 1998 Canadian Diabetes Association clinical practice guidelines, which coincided with the first edition of this book. This number will continue to grow given Canada's demographic trends. An aging population, increasing immigration from high-risk populations, and a growth in the Aboriginal population will increase the burden of diabetes over the next 10 years. Researchers project that by 2016, Canadians diagnosed with Type 2 diabetes will grow to 2.4 million.

My grandmother was one of the original founders of the Winnipeg Art Gallery, and was particularly drawn to Aboriginal artwork. The irony is that she did not know how much she had in common with Aboriginal Canadians, whose rates of Type 2 diabetes have been soaring out of control since the 1940s. Today the rate of diabetes among Aboriginal Canadians is five times that of non-Natives—one of the highest rates of diabetes worldwide. In fact, the artists my grandmother loved the most probably suffered from the same disease she did. For this reason, I urge you to read Chapter 10.

Unless you live in a large Canadian city, you may not have immediate (or any!) access to the right health care professionals. Take heart—there are other ways to get the information you need to manage your disease. The Canadian Diabetes Association (CDA) website (www.diabetes.ca) is the first place you should visit once you're diagnosed. As I'll stress again and again in this book, Type 2 diabetes is a genetic disease, but by modifying your lifestyle and diet, you may be able to delay the onset of the disease.

If you have any of these signs or symptoms of Type 2 diabetes, as outlined by the CDA, this book can help:

- Unusual thirst
- Frequent urination
- Weight change (gain or loss)
- Extreme fatigue or lack of energy
- Blurred vision
- Frequent or recurring infections
- Cuts and bruises that are slow to heal
- Tingling or numbness in the hands or feet
- Trouble getting or maintaining an erection

It is important to recognize, however, that many people who have Type 2 diabetes may display no symptoms.

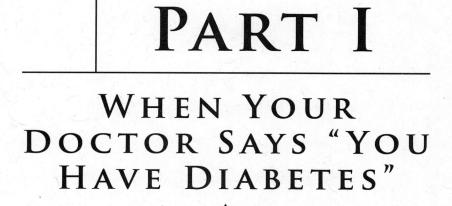

PART I

WHEN YOUR DOCTOR SAYS "YOU HAVE DIABETES"

1

WHAT IS TYPE 2 DIABETES?

You've just come home from your doctor's office. You can't remember anything he or she said other than those three horrible words: "You have diabetes." What does this mean? How will your life change? You've never been any good at diets, meal plans, or exercising. And since you can't stand the sight of blood, how can you be expected to prick your finger every day to monitor your blood sugar? As of 2008, in addition to the more than 2.4 million Canadians currently affected by Type 2 diabetes, up to 6 million more have "pre-diabetes," putting them at an increased risk for developing Type 2 diabetes and its complications. If left untreated, approximately 25 percent of people with pre-diabetes will progress to Type 2 diabetes within three to five years. Whether you've just been diagnosed with Type 2 diabetes, are told you're at risk, or have been living with it for years, this is a difficult disease to understand.

NAMES, NAME CHANGES, AND DEFINITIONS

Over the years, the names for different types of diabetes have changed, creating a lot of confusion for people who are newly diagnosed with Type 2 diabetes. Other names for this disease were used when our parents or grandparents were diagnosed, and a lot of people over 40 still remember them. When Canada's Dr. Frederick G. Banting first got the idea for developing a therapy for diabetes in 1921 (see Appendix 1), "diabetes," like the world war, wasn't yet numbered. It was long known, however, that there was a "milder" diabetes and a more severe form, but diabetes wasn't officially labelled Type 1 and Type 2 until 1979.

When you see the word "diabetes," it refers to *diabetes mellitus,* which means, according to the Canadian Diabetes Association's *Diabetes Dictionary,* "a condition in which the body either cannot produce insulin or cannot effectively use the insulin it produces," causing, in turn, high blood sugar (hyperglycemia). But the literal meaning of the word "diabetes" is from the Greek *siphon.* The word *mellitus* is Latin for "sweet." That doesn't mean much today, but it does make sense: In Ancient Greece, diabetes used to be diagnosed by "urine tasters" since the urine becomes sweet when blood sugar is dangerously high. The Greeks noticed that when people with sweet urine drank fluids, the fluids came out in the form of urine immediately, like a siphon. Hence the term "diabetes mellitus" was coined and has stuck to this day.

Confusing Type 2 with Type 1

Many people confuse Type 2 diabetes with Type 1 diabetes, a misunderstanding that interferes with getting accurate information about Type 2 diabetes, so here's what you need to understand: Type 2 diabetes can be managed, reversed, or even prevented by modifying your lifestyle; managing Type 2 diabetes does not necessarily require insulin. Most diabetes experts agree that it is poor diet, combined with a sedentary lifestyle, that triggers the Type 2 gene for those of us who are genetically predisposed to it. In other words, a combination of environment and genes is at work with Type 2 diabetes.

Type 1 diabetes is *completely different.* It cannot be reversed or prevented through lifestyle modification. The working theory, believed by most diabetes experts, is that Type 1 diabetes is an *autoimmune* disease that just strikes without warning. Here, the immune system attacks the beta cells in the pancreas, effectively destroying them. The result is that no insulin is produced by the pancreas at all. Type 1 diabetes is usually diagnosed before age 30, often in childhood. For this reason, Type 1 diabetes was once known as *juvenile diabetes,* or *juvenile-onset diabetes.* Because of organizations such as the Juvenile Diabetes Foundation, we will still see "juvenile diabetes" widely used in the literature on diabetes, even though it is technically an outdated term. It is also misleading, since we are now diagnosing Type 2 diabetes in young children, especially in Aboriginal Canadians or children who are obese.

Because people with Type 1 diabetes depend on insulin injections to survive, it was also once called *insulin-dependent diabetes mellitus* (IDDM). Only 10 percent of all people with diabetes have Type 1 diabetes.

The Many Names for Type 2 Diabetes

Most people with diabetes have Type 2 diabetes. Since Type 2 diabetes is a disease of resistance to, rather than an absence of, insulin, it often can be managed through diet and exercise without insulin injections. For this reason, Type 2 diabetes was once called *non-insulin-dependent diabetes mellitus* (NIDDM). But since many people with Type 2 diabetes may require insulin down the road (see Chapter 6), NIDDM is an inaccurate and misleading name and is not used any more. In fact, about one-third of all people with Type 2 diabetes will eventually need to begin insulin therapy.

When people with Type 2 diabetes require insulin, they can mistakenly believe that their diabetes has "turned into" Type 1 diabetes, but this isn't so. In the same way that an apple cannot turn into a banana, Type 2 diabetes cannot turn into Type 1 diabetes. For reasons I will discuss later in this book, Type 2 diabetes can progress and become more severe over the years, requiring insulin therapy. That's why the terms "NIDDM" and "IDDM" were dropped; they are both inaccurate and misleading. Nonetheless, you may still see these terms widely used in diabetes literature currently circulating.

Since Type 2 diabetes doesn't usually develop until after age 45, before it was named NIDDM, it had even earlier names: *mature-onset diabetes* or *adult-onset diabetes*. *Mature-onset diabetes in the young* (MODY) referred to Type 2 diabetes in people under 30 years old. None of these terms is used any more. The term "latent autoimmune diabetes" (LADA) has been used more often to describe the small number of people who are diagnosed with Type 2 diabetes, who actually have Type 1 diabetes—the autoimmune form of diabetes. The most important thing to remember is that currently "Type 2 diabetes" is the most commonly used name for the disease, and is the term most likely to be used in the medical literature.

"Type I and Type II" versus "Type 1 and Type 2"

It's worth noting that since 1979, when the types of diabetes were numbered, most literature used Roman numerals (I and II) instead of the commonly used Arabic numerals (1 and 2). As a result, many people remain confused over whether "Type I and Type II" diabetes were the same thing as "Type 1 and Type 2" diabetes. *Yes, Type I and Type II diabetes mean the same thing as Type 1 and Type 2 diabetes.* In the late 1990s, consensus in the diabetes medical community was reached over finally dropping the Roman numerals, and using only "1" and "2" in the literature to distinguish between the two types of diabetes.

WHAT HAPPENS IN TYPE 2 DIABETES?

Diabetes is a disease in which your blood glucose, or sugar, levels are too high. Glucose comes from the foods you eat. Insulin is a hormone that helps the glucose get into your cells to give them energy. Insulin is made by your *beta cells,* the insulin-producing cells within the *islets of Langerhans*—small islands of cells afloat in your pancreas. The *pancreas* is a bird beak-shaped gland situated behind the stomach.

With Type 1 diabetes, your body does not make insulin. With Type 2 diabetes, the more common type, and the subject of this book, your body does not make or use insulin well; in the latter case, you may be making too much insulin, in fact, but your body doesn't seem to be able to recognize it. Without enough insulin, the glucose stays in your blood. Over time, having too much glucose in your blood can cause serious problems. It can damage your eyes, kidneys, and nerves. Diabetes can also cause heart disease, stroke, and even lead to the amputation of a limb. So if you have Type 2 diabetes, your pancreas is functioning. You are probably making plenty of insulin, but your body just isn't using it well. This is called "insulin resistance."

Insulin Resistance

If you have insulin resistance, your muscle, fat, and liver cells do not use insulin properly. The pancreas tries to keep up with the demand for insulin by producing more. Eventually, the pancreas cannot keep up with the body's need for insulin, and excess glucose builds up in the bloodstream. Many people with insulin resistance have high levels of blood glucose and high levels of insulin circulating in their blood at the same time.

Insulin resistance tends to run in families, and therefore there is a genetic predisposition to it. Excess weight (especially around the waist, known as "adiposity") also contributes to insulin resistance because too much fat interferes with the muscles' ability to use insulin. Meanwhile, a lack of exercise further reduces the muscles' ability to use insulin.

People with insulin resistance tend to have too much weight around their abdominal areas, high LDL (low-density lipids or "bad cholesterol") cholesterol levels, and low HDL (high-density lipids or "good cholesterol"), as well as high triglyceride levels and high blood pressure. When you have this combination of problems, it's known as the metabolic syndrome (once called Syndrome X). People with metabolic syndrome are also at risk for heart attack and stroke (see Part 3).

High Blood Sugar

The high blood sugar that results from insulin resistance can lead to a number of other diseases, including cardiovascular disease (heart disease and stroke) and peripheral vascular disease (PVD), a condition in which the blood doesn't flow properly to other parts of your body. This can create a number of problems, discussed in Part 3. Many people who suffer a heart attack or stroke have Type 2 diabetes. High blood sugar can also become aggravated by glycogen, a form of glucose that is stored in the liver and muscles, which is released when you need energy. Insulin enables your cells to store glucose as glycogen. But when your cells are resisting insulin, glycogen can be released in a confused response because it appears to the cells that there is no sugar in the blood.

When You Have Type 2 Diabetes but Require Insulin

Insulin resistance, characterized by the body's inability to use insulin, sometimes leads to a condition in which the pancreas stops making insulin altogether. The cells' resistance to insulin causes the pancreas to work harder, causing too much insulin in the system (aka hyperinsulinemia) until it just plumb tuckers out, as the saying goes. Your pancreas is making the insulin and knocking on the door, but the cells aren't answering. Your pancreas will eventually say, "Okay, fine! I'll shut down production, since you obviously aren't using what I'm making." But this isn't always the reason that you need insulin.

Often the problem is that your body becomes increasingly more resistant to the insulin your pancreas is producing. This is sometimes exacerbated by medications or by the progression of the disease over time. Controlling your blood sugar becomes harder and harder until, ultimately, you need to inject insulin.

You may also require insulin if you go for long periods with high blood sugar levels. In this case, the high blood sugar can put you at very high risk for other health complications, discussed in Part 3. It is not unusual to be diagnosed with Type 2 diabetes in a later stage and be prescribed insulin.

CONDITIONS THAT CAN LEAD TO TYPE 2 DIABETES

There are a variety of risk factors for Type 2 diabetes, such as high cholesterol or obesity, which I discuss in Chapter 2. The following conditions, however, are said to be definite precursors to Type 2 diabetes, meaning that if you have any of the following conditions, you are at very high risk of developing Type 2 diabetes.

Pre-diabetes: Impaired Fasting Glucose (IFG) and Impaired Glucose Tolerance (IGT)

Pre-diabetes is dangerous because it not only increases your risk of developing full-blown Type 2 diabetes, but of developing cardiovascular disease. According to the CDA, you have "pre-diabetes" if you have a fasting plasma glucose (FPG) level of 6.1–6.9 mmol/L or are found to have impaired glucose tolerance on a 75 g oral glucose-tolerance test (OGTT).

Who gets an OGTT? Well, if you have an FPG level between 5.6 and 6.0 mmol/L and one or more risk factors for Type 2 diabetes, the CDA recommends that you have an OGTT. Risk factors for Type 2 diabetes are discussed in the next chapter. The advantage of knowing that you have pre-diabetes is that you can make the necessary lifestyle changes to prevent developing full-blown Type 2 diabetes, or start on certain preventative medications. Studies have consistently shown that through lifestyle changes, including moderate weight loss and regular exercise, the onset of Type 2 diabetes can be delayed by up to 58 percent.

Table 1.1: What Your Readings Mean

Suggested Screening Age: 40 or over		
Fasting Plasma Glucose Test FPG (fasting for eight hours)		
Normal	**IFG**	**Diabetes**
<6.1 mmol/L	≤6.1 mmol/L–6.9 mml/L	≥7.0
Two hours after an oral glucose-tolerance test (drinking a special sweet drink)		
Normal	**IGT**	**Diabetes**
<7.8 mmol/L	7.8 mmol/L–11.0 mmol/L	≥11.1 mmol/L
IFG = impaired fasting glucose		
IGT = impaired glucose tolerance, referring to test results two hours after an oral glucose-tolerance test		
≥ = equal to, or greater than		
< = less than		

Source: Canadian Diabetes Association, 2008 Clinical Practice Guidelines: S11, 2008.

Metabolic Syndrome

Metabolic syndrome describes insulin resistance and impaired fasting glucose levels and a distinct collection of other health problems that include abdominal obesity, hypertension, and dyslipidemia. People with metabolic syndrome do not yet have Type 2 diabetes, but are at a much higher risk of developing it, along with cardiovascular disease. According to the CDA, if you have three or more of the following conditions, you are considered to have metabolic syndrome:

- High fasting blood glucose levels (5.6 mmol/L or higher)
- High blood pressure (130/85 or higher)

- High level of triglycerides, a type of fat in your blood (1.7 mmol/L or higher)
- Low levels of HDL, the "good" blood cholesterol (lower than 1.0 mmol/L in men or 1.3 mmol/L in women)
- Abdominal obesity or too much fat around your waist (a waist circumference of greater than 102 cm [40 inches] in men and greater than 88 cm [35 inches] in women)

The more of these conditions you have, the higher your risks of developing Type 2 diabetes and heart disease.

Gestational Diabetes Mellitus (GDM)

Gestational diabetes refers to diabetes first diagnosed during any stage of pregnancy. If you developed (or will develop) gestational diabetes during pregnancy, consider yourself put on alert. In a new 2008 study published in the *Canadian Medical Association Journal*, researchers found that nearly 19 percent of women who develop gestational diabetes during pregnancy are likely to develop Type 2 diabetes after pregnancy. If you are genetically predisposed to Type 2 diabetes, a history of gestational diabetes can raise your risk of eventually developing the disease. Gestational diabetes develops more often in women who were overweight prior to pregnancy and women who are over 35; gestational diabetes increases with maternal age. If your mother had gestational diabetes, you are also more likely to develop it. For a more detailed discussion, see Chapter 12.

If you had diabetes prior to your pregnancy (Type 1 or Type 2), this is known in the medical literature as *pre-existing diabetes,* which is a completely different story and not at all the same thing as gestational diabetes.

Pancreatitis

Diabetes can be caused by a condition known as pancreatitis, which means inflammation of the pancreas. This occurs when the pancreas's digestive enzymes turn on you and attack your own pancreas. This can cause the gland to bleed and can cause serious tissue damage, infection, and cysts. (Other organs, such as your heart, lungs, and kidneys, could be affected in severe cases.) Pancreatitis is most often chronic, as opposed to acute (sudden), caused by years of alcohol abuse. More men than women have chronic pancreatitis. In rare cases, chronic pancreatitis is inherited, but experts are not sure why this is. People with chronic pancreatitis tend to have three main symptoms: pain, weight loss (due to poor food absorption and digestion), and diabetes (the type depends on how much damage was done to your islet, or insulin-producing, cells).

The treatment is to first stop drinking. Then you will need to be managed like any other diabetes patient: blood glucose monitoring, meal planning, and possibly insulin injections.

SECONDARY DIABETES ("SIDE-EFFECT" DIABETES)

This occurs when your diabetes is a *side effect* of a particular drug or surgical procedure.

A number of prescription medications, including steroids or Dilantin, can raise your blood sugar levels, which would affect the outcome of a blood sugar test, for example. Make sure you tell your doctor about all medications you're on prior to having your blood sugar checked.

If you've had your pancreas removed (a pancreatectomy), diabetes will definitely develop. It may also develop if you've experienced severe injury to your pancreas, liver disease, or iron overload.

As you can see, this is a complicated disease to understand, and a disease that has gone through many name changes in recent years, making things even more confusing. By now, you should have a good understanding of what Type 2 diabetes is and how it is different from other types of diabetes you may have heard about. The next chapter is about who is most likely to develop Type 2 diabetes. The good news is that some lifestyle changes can reduce risk.

2

WHO GETS TYPE 2 DIABETES?

Screening studies show that Type 2 diabetes is prevalent all over the world, particularly in countries that are becoming Westernized. The most recent statistics from 2008 show a dramatic increase in the prevalence of Type 2 diabetes in Canada and around the world. In Canada, 5.5 percent of the population were already diagnosed with Type 2 diabetes as of 2005. Diagnosed diabetes has now grown 70 percent since the publication of the 1998 Canadian Diabetes clinical practice guidelines (this edition reflects the 2008 Canadian Diabetes clinical practice guidelines). This number will continue to grow given the aging population (the first baby boomers reached 60 in 2006), increasing immigration from high-risk populations, and growth in the Aboriginal population. Researchers project an increase of diagnosed diabetes in Canada to 2.4 million by the year 2016.

Many people won't realize they have Type 2 diabetes until they develop a complication of Type 2 diabetes, such as eye problems, nerve problems, cardiovascular disease, or peripheral vascular disease—all discussed in Part 3. This is why screening is so important, and why understanding who is at risk is critical. There are many things that you can do to prevent or delay the onset of Type 2 diabetes; if you can do that, you'll benefit from a lower risk of health problems associated with Type 2 diabetes. Approximately 30–60 percent of Type 2 diabetes may be prevented through lifestyle or medication intervention. The Diabetes Prevention program found that people at risk of developing

Type 2 diabetes were able to cut their risk by 58 percent with moderate physical activity (30 minutes a day) and weight loss (5–7 percent of body weight, or about 7 kg [15 lb]). For people over 60, the risk was cut by almost 71 percent.

If you are aged 40 or over, you are at risk for Type 2 diabetes and should be tested at least every three years. In addition, if any of the following risks factors apply to you, you should be tested earlier and/ or more often.

- You are a member of a high-risk group (Aboriginal, Hispanic, Asian, South Asian, or African descent).
- You are overweight with a BMI over 25, especially if you carry most of your weight around your middle.
- You have immediate family members with Type 2 diabetes.
- You already have health complications that are associated with diabetes.
- You have given birth to a baby that weighed more than 4 kg (9 lbs).
- You had gestational diabetes (diabetes during pregnancy).
- You have impaired glucose tolerance or impaired fasting glucose.
- You have high blood pressure.
- You have high cholesterol or other fats in the blood.
- You've been diagnosed with polycystic ovarian syndrome, acanthosis nigricans (darkened patches of skin), or schizophrenia.

Several cofactors contribute to your risk profile and can change your risk from higher to lower. The purpose of this chapter is to give you a clear idea of where you fit into this risk puzzle. That way, you'll be more aware of early warning signs of the disease, which will make it easier for you to get an accurate diagnosis. If you've already been diagnosed with Type 2 diabetes, this chapter will help you understand *why* you developed the disease and what you can do today to eliminate some of the factors that may be aggravating your condition. For example, you can significantly lower your risk of developing diabetes by changing your lifestyle or diet.

RISK FACTORS YOU CAN CHANGE

Clearly, Type 2 diabetes more than meets the requirements of an epidemic. The World Health Organization reported in 2008 its global estimate. Currently, more than 180 million people worldwide have diabetes, and that number is likely to double by the year 2030. Type 2 diabetes comprises 90 percent of people with diabetes around the world. In 2005, an estimated 1.1 million people died from diabetes; almost 80 percent of diabetes deaths occur in low- and middle-income countries; almost half of diabetes deaths occur in people under the age of 70; and 55 percent of diabetes deaths are in women. Furthermore, the WHO projects that diabetes deaths will increase by more than 50 percent in the next 10 years without urgent action. China will soon be catching up: Between 2006 and 2015, China will lose $558 billion in forgone national income due to heart disease, stroke, and diabetes alone.

Calculating your risk of getting a particular disease is a very tricky business. To simplify matters, I've divided this chapter into two sections: modifiable risk factors (risk factors you can change), and risk markers (risk factors you cannot change, such as your age or genes). It's also crucial to understand that risk estimates are only guesses that are not based on you personally, but on people *like* you, who share your physical characteristics or lifestyle patterns. It's like betting on a horse. You look at the age of the horse, its vigour and shape, its breeding, its training, and where the race is being run. Then you come up with odds. If you own the horse, you can't change your horse's colour or breeding, but you can change its training, its diet, its jockey, and, ultimately, where it's being raced, when, and how often. Chance, of course, plays a role in horse racing. You can't control acts of God. But you can decide whether you're going to tempt fate by racing your horse during a thunderstorm.

The following are modifiable risk factors. You can remove the risk if you make the change.

High Cholesterol

Cholesterol is a whitish, waxy fat made in vast quantities by the liver. It is also known as a lipid, the umbrella name for the many different fats found in the body. That's why liver or other organ meats are high in cholesterol! Cholesterol is needed to make hormones as well as cell membranes. Dietary cholesterol is found only in foods from animals and fish. If you have high cholesterol, the excess cholesterol in your blood can lead to narrowed arteries, which in turn can lead to a heart attack. Saturated fat, discussed in detail in Chapter 8, is often a culprit when it comes to high cholesterol, but the highest levels of cholesterol are due to a genetic defect in the liver. Since people with diabetes are four times more likely to develop heart disease and five times more likely to suffer a stroke, lowering your cholesterol, especially if you're already at risk for Type 2 diabetes, is a good idea. The usual pattern in Type 2 diabetes is to have high triglycerides, lower than optimal levels of "good cholesterol" or HDL, and normal levels of "bad cholesterol" or LDL.

Insulin's Role in Lipid Control

Insulin not only keeps blood sugar in check, it also keeps the levels of "good cholesterol" (HDL, high-density lipoproteins), "bad cholesterol" (LDL, low-density lipoproteins), and triglycerides in check. When you're not making enough insulin or your body isn't using insulin efficiently, your LDL levels and your triglycerides rise, but, more important, *your HDL levels fall,* which can lead to heart disease. When diabetes is under control, cholesterol levels will return to normal, which will cut your risk of heart disease and stroke as well.

Checking Your Cholesterol

In Canada, total blood cholesterol levels are measured in millimoles per litre. If you're over 30, cholesterol levels of less than 5.2 mmol/L are considered healthy. If your cholesterol levels are between 5.2 and 6.2 mmol/L, discuss with your doctor lifestyle changes that can lower cholesterol levels. If your levels are greater than 6.2 mmol/L, your doctor may recommend cholesterol-lowering drugs if your lifestyle changes were not successful.

For people 18–29 years of age, a cholesterol level less than 4.7 mmol/L is considered healthy, while a level ranging between 4.7 and 5.7 mmol/L is considered too high, warranting some lifestyle and dietary changes. In this age group, a reading greater than 5.7 may even warrant cholesterol-lowering drugs. High cholesterol is also called hypercholesterolemia. Another term used in conjunction with high cholesterol is hyperlipidemia, which refers to an elevation of lipids (fats) in the bloodstream; lipids include cholesterol and triglycerides (the most common form of fat from food sources in our bodies). There are no specific targets for triglyceride levels because there are no studies that support one specific target. However, a triglyceride level of less than 1.5 mmol/L is considered optimal.

Total blood cholesterol levels do have targets, but they are meant as guidelines only. You also have to look at the relative proportion of high-density lipoprotein (HDL) or "good cholesterol" to low-density lipoprotein (LDL) or "bad cholesterol" in the blood. If you're over 30, an LDL reading of less than 3.4 mmol/L and an HDL reading of more than 0.9 mmol/L is considered healthy; if you're 18–29, an LDL reading of less than 3.0 mmol/L and an HDL reading of more than 0.9 is considered healthy.

International guidelines advise that optimal LDL should be 2.5 mmol/L or less, and optimal HDL should be 1.1 mmol/L or more. The Canadian Diabetes Association also recommends that if the total cholesterol/HDL ratio is ≥4.0, it's too high. Getting it below 4 in this case would be achieved through better blood sugar control, weight loss, physical activity, and quitting smoking. Medication would also be an option in this case.

Cholesterol-Lowering Drugs

For many, losing weight and modifying fat intake simply aren't enough to bring cholesterol levels down to optimal levels. You may be a candidate for one of the numerous cholesterol-lowering drugs. These medications, when combined with a low-fat, low-cholesterol diet, target the intestine, blocking food absorption, and/or the liver, where they interfere with the processing of cholesterol. These are strong drugs, however, and ought to be a last resort after really giving a low-fat, low-cholesterol diet a chance. You might be given a combination of cholesterol-lowering medications to try with a low-cholesterol diet. It's important to ask about all side effects accompanying your medication because they can include gastrointestinal problems, allergic reactions, blood disorders, and depression. One study looking at male patients taking cholesterol-lowering drugs found an unusually high rate of suicide and accidental trauma. There have not been enough studies on women taking these drugs to know for certain how they interact with women's health conditions. As of this writing, the following therapies are recommended to lower your bad cholesterol (LDL), and improve your total cholesterol and good cholesterol. The drug you'll be offered will vary depending on your cholesterol level and overall health. All these drugs will have some side effects or interactions that must be discussed with your doctor and pharmacist.

Statins (e.g, Atorvastatin [Lipitor]; Fluvastatin [Lescol]; Lovastatin [Mevacor and generic]; Pravastatin [Pravachol and generic]; Rosuvastatin [Crestor]; Simvastatin [Zocor and generic]: Statins hinder the liver's ability to produce cholesterol, keeping LDL levels to a minimum while increasing levels of HDL. They are designed to get your LDL to 2.0 or lower.

Fibrates (e.g., gemfibrozil or Lopid, fenofibrate or Lipidil Micro/Lipidil Supra, Lipidil EZ, bezafibrate or Bezalip): These lower total cholesterol and triglyceride levels in the blood with a variable effect on LDL and HDL.

Nicotinic acid (e.g., niacin or Niaspan): Niacin, a water-soluble B vitamin, can lower LDL and triglyceride levels, and also increases HDL.

Bile acid sequestrants (e.g., cholestyramine resin or Questran; colestipol HCl, or Colestid): These drugs help lower LDL by helping the body eliminate cholesterol through the gut.

Cholesterol absorption inhibitor (e.g., ezetimibe [Ezetrol]: This lowers LDL.

Hypertension (High Blood Pressure)

Five million Canadian adults currently have high blood pressure, representing 22 percent of the adult population. But of those with high blood pressure, 42 percent are unaware of their condition, and only 16 percent have it treated and under control. Nine out of 10 Canadians will develop high blood pressure or hypertension during their lives. One in three with hypertension can normalize their blood pressure through diet. (See the DASH diet guidelines further on.)

One in three Canadians who have hypertension would have normal blood pressure if they consumed less sodium in their diets. Studies show that First Nations, Inuit, and Métis people, as well as people of African heritage or South Asian descent, are more likely to have high blood pressure than the general population.

What is blood pressure? The blood flows from the heart into the arteries (blood vessels), pressing against the artery walls. The simplest way to explain this is to think about a liquid-soap dispenser. When you want soap, you need to pump it out by pressing down on the little dispenser pump, the "heart" of the dispenser. The liquid soap is the "blood" and the little tube, through which the soap flows, is the "artery." The pressure that's exerted on the wall of the tube is therefore the "blood pressure."

When the tube is hollow and clean, you needn't pump very hard to get the soap; it comes out easily. But when the tubing in your dispenser gets narrower as a result of old, hardened, gunky liquid soap blocking the tube, you have to pump much harder to get any soap, while the force the soap exerts against the tube is increased. Obviously, this is a simplistic explanation of a very complex problem, but essentially, the narrowing of the arteries forces your heart to work harder to pump the blood: high blood pressure. If this goes on for too long, your heart muscle enlarges and becomes weaker, which can lead to a heart attack. Higher pressure can also weaken the walls of your blood vessels, which can cause a stroke.

The term "hypertension" refers to the tension or force exerted on your artery walls. (*Hyper* means "too much," as in "too much tension.") Blood pressure is measured in two readings: X over Y. The X is the systolic pressure, which is the pressure that occurs during the heart's contraction. The Y is the diastolic pressure, which is the pressure that occurs when the heart rests between contractions. In "liquid soap" terms, the systolic pressure occurs when you press the pump down; the diastolic pressure occurs when you release your hand from the pump and allow it to rise back to its resting position.

In the general population, target blood pressure readings are less than 130 over 80 (<130/80). Readings greater than 130/80 are considered by diabetes educators to be too high for people with di-abetes, or people with kidney disease, and in the general population, readings of 140/90 or higher are generally considered to be high blood pressure/hypertension by the Heart and Stroke Foundation. For the general population, 140/90 is definitely "lecture time," when your doctor will begin to counsel you about dietary and lifestyle habits. By 160/100, many people are prescribed a hypertensive drug, which is designed to lower blood pressure.

Let's examine some of the causes of hypertension. The same factors that put you at risk for Type 2 diabetes, such as obesity, can also put you at risk for hypertension. Hypertension is also exacerbated by tobacco and alcohol consumption and too much sodium or salt in the diet. (People of African descent tend to be more salt-sensitive.)

If high blood pressure runs in the family, you're considered at greater risk of developing hypertension. High blood pressure can also be caused by kidney disorders (which may be initially caused by diabetes) or pregnancy (known as pregnancy-induced hypertension). Medications are also common culprits. Estrogen-containing medications (such as oral contraceptives) and non-steroidal anti-inflammatory drugs (NSAIDs)—such as ibuprofen, nasal decongestants, cold remedies, appetite suppressants, certain anti-depressants, and other drugs—can all increase blood pressure. Be sure to check with your pharmacist or doctor.

How to Lower Your Blood Pressure without Drugs

- Change your diet and begin exercising (see chapters 7, 8, and 11).
- Limit alcohol consumption to no more than 60 mL (2 oz) of liquor or 250 mL (8 oz) of wine or 750 mL (24 oz) of beer per day and even less for liver health.
- Limit your salt intake by cutting out all foods high in sodium, such as canned soups, pickles, soy sauce, convenience and snack foods, canned meats, and canned fish.
- Increase your intake of calcium or dairy products and potassium, which is found in bananas, cantaloupes, oranges, melons, potatoes, prunes, and molasses.
- Stop smoking.

- Lower your stress levels. Studies show that by lowering your stress, your blood pressure decreases.

The DASH Diet

DASH stands for "Dietary Approaches to Stop Hypertension," an eating plan known to lower hypertension. To follow the DASH diet:

- Reduce sodium intake to 1,500 mg per day. If you find this too difficult to manage, aim for 2,400 mg per day instead, but make sure it's no higher (and do try to reduce this amount over time).
- Lower saturated fat, cholesterol, and total fat (you'll do this by following the guidelines in Chapter 8).
- Reduce red meat, sweets, and sugar-containing beverages (see chapters 7 and 8).
- Include whole-grain products, fish, poultry, and nuts; this is low glycemic eating as well as "good fats" eating (see chapters 7 and 8).
- Emphasize fruits, vegetables, and low-fat dairy foods (see chapters 7 and 8).

Table 2.1: 8 Ways to Reduce Sodium

1. Wherever possible, use reduced-sodium or no-salt-added products. These days, even cereal manufacturers often offer a reduced-sodium alternative.

2. With vegetables, choose fresh as often as you can, otherwise look for canned or frozen vegetables that don't contain salt.

3. Rinse canned foods, such as tuna, to get rid of excess salt.

4. Don't use salt when you cook rice, pasta, and hot cereals like oatmeal. Also, avoid the instant or flavoured varieties, as these usually have added salt.

5. Look for other ways of adding zest to your food. Natural flavour enhancers like lemon and garlic are tasty, *healthy* alternatives to salt.

6. Opt for fresh poultry, fish, and lean meat rather than their canned, smoked, processed, or cured (as in bacon or ham) alternatives.

7. On those days when convenience is a must, check the labels of ready-made pizzas, canned soups, salad dressings, and so on. Most contain a lot of sodium but, again, there *are* alternatives.

8. Recognize the language of sodium: pickled or cured, soy sauce, or broth.

Blood Pressure-Lowering Drugs

If you can't lower your blood pressure through lifestyle changes, you may be a candidate for some of the following blood pressure-lowering drugs (listed in alphabetical order):

- *Ace-inhibitors:* Ace-inhibitors lower blood pressure by preventing the formation of a hormone called angiotensin II, which causes the blood vessels to narrow. Ace-inhibitors are also used to treat heart failure. Possible side effects include a cough and swelling of the face and tongue.
- *Alpha-blocking agents:* Alpha-blocking agents block the effects of noradrenaline, a stress hormone, allowing the blood vessels to relax. Blood pressure decreases with treatment, as does cholesterol. You may also notice an increase in HDL, or "good cholesterol." A possible side effect is blood pressure variation when standing versus reclining.
- *Angiotensin receptor blockers (ARBs):* Similar to Ace-inhibitors, ARBs block the effects of angiotensin II on the cells of the blood vessel wall. Essentially ARBs act farther down the angiotensin pathway. They're popular because they tend to have fewer side effects than Ace-inhibitors, but appear to be equally effective in terms of blood pressure control.
- *Beta-blockers:* Beta-blockers alter the way hormones like adrenaline control blood pressure. They slow the heart rate by decreasing the strength of its contractions. Beta-blockers are most often used by young people and/or people with coronary artery disease. Possible side effects include fatigue and an increase in blood sugar and cholesterol levels. Another major problem with beta-blockers is that because they block adrenaline, they can mask signs of hypoglycemia (see Chapter 14), which could be dangerous if your blood sugar levels are not well controlled.
- *Calcium-channel blockers:* Calcium-channel blockers limit the amount of calcium entering the cells, allowing the muscles in the blood vessels to relax. Possible side effects include ankle swelling, flushing, constipation, and indigestion.

- *Centrally acting agents:* These drugs act through centres in the brain to slow the heart rate and relax the blood vessels. Possible side effects include stuffy nose, dry mouth, and drowsiness.
- *Diuretics:* Also known as water pills, diuretics work by flushing excess water and salt (often 1–2 kg [2–4 lbs] worth!) out of your system. But diuretics may actually increase the risk of heart attack by leaching potassium salts needed by the heart, and the heart may respond to blocked nerve signals by trying harder and harder until it fails. Another common side effect of diuretic therapy is low potassium. Levels of potassium tend to drop when diuretics replace the low-fat diet you've worked so hard to maintain. If you make sure not to substitute one therapy for another, diuretics will not affect your potassium levels. Other side effects include increased blood sugar and cholesterol levels.
- *Direct renin inhibitors:* These lower blood pressure to a similar extent as other anti-hypertensive drugs, but studies showing the effectiveness of the drug in preventing heart disease and strokes have not been completed yet.
- *Vasodilators:* Vasodilators dilate or relax the blood vessels, thereby reducing blood pressure.

Obesity

Obesity is the strongest risk factor for developing Type 2 diabetes. Basically, the longer you've been obese, the more you are at risk. I am not referring to people who need to lose weight for cosmetic reasons; I'm referring to people whose BMI is above 25, making them overweight or obese, depending on the BMI. (See Chapter 11.) Instead of aiming to lose 5 kg (11 lbs), just aim for 2 kg (4 lbs). Even 2 kg (4 lbs) will allow your body to use insulin more effectively.

Sedentary Lifestyle

If you don't exercise and are not active, you're sedentary. (See Chapter 9 for more information.)

Sleep Deprivation or Sleep Disorders

There are studies linking obesity, and hence Type 2 diabetes, to lack of sleep, snoring, loss of rapid eye movement (REM) sleep, and a range of other sleep disorders. When you don't sleep well or get enough sleep—particularly REM sleep, which occurs in deep sleep—you will be irritable and drowsy during the day. That means you'll eat more and will likely crave fast-energy foods high in sugar or starch. By visiting a sleep-disorder clinic or, in some cases, by going to a time-management seminar, you should be able to get your ZZZs. A 2006 study noted that men who reported they slept between five and six hours per night were twice as likely to develop diabetes, and men who slept more than eight hours per night were three times as likely to develop diabetes.

The hormonal and metabolic implications of too little sleep have a huge impact. Lack of sleep can lead to problems with metabolic and endocrine function, including decreased carbohydrate tolerance, insulin resistance, and lower levels of the hormone leptin, leading to obesity.

Smoking

Smoking not only increases your risk for lung cancer, heart attack, and stroke, but it is a catastrophic habit when combined with diabetes. Each year, 45,000 Canadians die of smoking-related illnesses. But people with diabetes face an even greater risk from smoking: Just like high blood glucose levels, the noxious chemicals in cigarette smoke attack blood vessels, accelerating atherosclerosis (hardening of the arteries) and impairing the blood's ability to carry oxygen to the tissues. Together, the deadly combination of high blood glucose and smoking dramatically increases damage to the blood vessels that feed the heart, brain, eyes, kidneys, and peripheral nerves, speeding up the long-term complications of diabetes. People with diabetes are already at increased risk for heart disease; however, if they smoke, they face three times the risk for heart attack than a person with diabetes who does not smoke. As of this writing, here is a summary of the types of methods people use for quitting smoking:

- *Behavioural counselling:* Behavioural counselling, either group or individual, can raise the rate of abstinence from 20–25 percent. This approach to smoking cessation aims to change the mental processes of smoking, reinforce the benefits of not smoking, and teach skills to help the smoker avoid the urge to smoke.
- *Nicotine replacement:* The FDA has approved five types of nicotine-replacement therapy: nicotine gum, patch, inhalers, nasal spray, and lozenges. There are several types of products available, and your doctor or pharmacist can guide you.
- *Bupropion:* Bupropion (Zyban) and a newer novel drug, Varenicline (only the second nicotine-free smoking-cessation drug to gain FDA approval in 2006), are appropriate for patients who have been unsuccessful using nicotine replacement. Your doctor can assess whether you are an appropriate candidate for this drug.
- *Alternative therapies:* Hypnosis, meditation, and acupuncture have helped some smokers quit. In the case of hypnosis and meditation, sessions may be private or part of a group smoking-cessation program.

RISK FACTORS YOU CAN'T CHANGE

By *modifying* any of the modifiable risk factors above, you can help to offset your risk of developing Type 2 diabetes if you have any of the following risk markers. While you can't change your genetic make-up, medical history, or age, you can significantly reduce the odds of these factors predisposing you to Type 2 diabetes.

Age

The risk of developing Type 2 diabetes increases with age. Screening by age 40 is the current recommendation. Perhaps at no other time in history have we seen so many people over age 40—the so-called baby boom generation. This may, in part, account for the increase we're seeing in Type 2 diabetes, as well as other age-related diseases. However, the lifestyle and dietary habits you practise before age 40 count—either against you or for you. So, by changing your diet and becoming more active before age 40, you may not necessarily be able to prevent your genetic fate, but you may certainly be able to delay it. And in the event that you develop Type 2 diabetes, a healthy diet and active lifestyle will go a long way in controlling the disease.

It's crucial to keep in mind that studies regarding diet, lifestyle, and Type 2 diabetes are still unclear, although experts certainly agree that there is a strong relationship between genetic markers for diabetes and environmental factors, such as activity levels, weight, and diet.

Menopause

When women reach menopause, estrogen loss can lead to some well-documented problems, such as osteoporosis (estrogen helps to maintain calcium levels) and heart disease (estrogen raises HDL levels, or "good cholesterol," which protects pre-menopausal women from heart disease). Estrogen also helps to protect against insulin resistance. Even if you decide against hormone therapy, diet and lifestyle changes can lower your risks of heart disease, osteoporosis, and Type 2 diabetes substantially. (See Chapter 13 for more details.)

Genes

Most diabetes experts believe that Type 2 diabetes is a genetic disease, which means you have the "wiring" installed for Type 2 diabetes at birth. Fortunately, we do understand some of the outside factors that can trip the Type 2 switch. Body shapes, diet, and activity levels are strong switch-trippers. On the other hand, if you don't have any Type 2 diabetes genes (in other words, you're not "wired" for this disease), these outside factors cannot, by themselves, cause you to develop Type 2 diabetes. For instance, there are plenty of obese and sedentary people walking around who do not have Type 2 diabetes, nor will they develop the disease in the future.

When underdeveloped populations become urbanized and adopt a Western lifestyle, there is an explosion in Type 2 diabetes, but the genes must be present in order to allow for the disease in the first place.

This is more proof that there is a genetic-environmental combo platter at work when it comes to this disease. What aspect of Westernization triggers Type 2 diabetes in these regions? "Western" means many things, including a higher-fat diet, less physical activity, as well as access to medical care, which means populations are living longer.

What Are the Odds?

Type 2 diabetes is caused by multiple factors. The odds of developing it have to do with some genes interacting with some environmental factors. Obesity, excess calories, deficient calorie expenditure, and aging can all lead to a resistance to insulin. If you remove the environmental risks, however, you can probably modify the risk of Type 2 diabetes.

Your Ethnic Background

As discussed earlier, Aboriginal cultures develop Type 2 diabetes at far higher rates than other Canadians. Type 2 diabetes has reached epidemic proportions among Aboriginal peoples in Canada, with the national age-adjusted prevalence three to five times higher than that of the general population and as high as 26 percent in individual communities. (See Chapter 10 for more details.)

One explanation for this involves the "thrifty gene theory," so named because it is believed to have evolved out of biological efficiency, or thriftiness. It is thought to be responsible for the higher rates of Type 2 diabetes in the Aboriginal and African-North American populations. This means that the more recently your culture has lived indigenously or nomadically (that is, living off the land you came from and eating seasonally), the more efficient your metabolism is. This explanation dominated the thinking of genetic predisposition to insulin resistance and Type 2 diabetes for many years, but several researchers reject this explanation. For now, there are as many scientists supporting the theory as there are rejecting it. It remains, according to many scientists, to be the only plausible theory that explains why certain groups get sick from nutrient excess. If you're an Aboriginal North American, only about

100 years have passed since your ancestors lived indigenously. This is an exceedingly short amount of time to ask thousands of years of hunter-gatherer genes to adjust to a Western diet. If you're African-North American, your ancestors did not live here any longer than about 400 years; prior to that, they were living a tribal, nomadic lifestyle. Again, 400 years is *not* a long time.

As for Hispanic populations or other immigrant populations, many come from families who have spent generations in poverty. Their metabolisms adjusted to long periods of famine and are often overloaded by Western foods. The other problem is poverty in North America. Aboriginal, African, and Hispanic populations tend to have much lower incomes and are therefore eating lower-quality food, which, when introduced to the "thrifty gene," can trigger Type 2 diabetes.

Type 2 diabetes seems to occur in South-East Asian populations at Western rates even when the diet is Eastern. East Indians, in particular, have very high rates of heart disease. In fact, the prevalence of Type 2 diabetes in India is among the highest in the world, with more than 28 million cases in 2007. Prevalence will grow more rapidly in India than in any other developing or developed nation, climbing to more than 60 million cases by 2017.

Your risk of developing Type 2 diabetes depends on your mix of genes and your current and past lifestyle and diet. If you are part Aboriginal and part European, for example, you will probably need to be more conscientious about your diet than if you were part Asian and part European. Studying your family tree and family history of Type 2 diabetes is the best way to assess the damage and make the necessary changes in your own diet and lifestyle to repair it.

Other Medical Conditions

There are genetic diseases, endocrine diseases, medical conditions, and medications that can affect insulin action and lead to insulin resistance and/or Type 2 diabetes. Any disease that affects the pancreas, such as pancreatic cancer or conditions leading to removal of the pancreas, would also lead to diabetes or cystic fibrosis. (See Table 2.2 for more information.)

Table 2.2: Rare Diseases or Conditions Causing Insulin Resistance*

Note: This table lists some extremely unusual or rare diseases that could result in insulin resistance or affect insulin action in the body. Most primary care doctors would not see most of these diseases in a lifetime of practice. For more information about any of the diseases listed in this table, please contact the National Organization for Rare Disorders (NORD) at 1-800-999-6673 (voice mail only), or 203-744-0100, or visit www.rare diseases.org. For genetic patterns of some of these diseases, you can write to genetic_counselor@rarediseases.org

Other Genetic Syndromes Sometimes Associated with Diabetes

Down syndrome
Friedreich's ataxia
Huntington's chorea
Klinefelter syndrome
Laurence-Moon Bardet-Beidl syndrome
Myotonic dystrophy
Porphyria
Prader-willi syndrome
Turner's syndrome
Wolfram's syndrome

Endocrine Disorders or Diseases Affecting Insulin Production or Action

Acromegaly
Aldosteronoma
Cushing's syndrome or Cushing disease
Gluconoma
Hyperthyroidism
Pheochromocyoma
Somatostatinoma

Diseases of the Pancreas

Cystic fibrosis
Fibrocalculous pancreatopathy
Hemochromatosis
Neoplasia
Pancreatitis
Trauma/pancreatectomy

Source: Adapted from American Diabetes Association, "Diagnosis and Classification of Diabetes Mellitus," Diabetes Care, 2007, 30 (suppl. 1):S42–S47.

SIGNS AND SYMPTOMS

These are the signs of Type 2 diabetes:

- Weight gain. When you're not using your insulin properly, you may suffer from excess insulin, which can increase your appetite. This is a classic Type 2 symptom.
- Blurred vision or any change in sight.
- Drowsiness or *extreme* fatigue at times when you shouldn't be drowsy or tired.
- Frequent infections that are slow to heal. (Women should be on the alert for recurring vaginal yeast infections.)
- Tingling or numbness in the hands and feet.
- Gum disease. High blood sugar affects the blood vessels in your mouth, causing inflamed gums; the sugar content can get into your saliva, causing cavities in your teeth.

Managing Type 2 diabetes is a 24-hour, seven-day-a-week job. Despite this, a great many people with Type 2 diabetes never receive any diabetes education whatsoever. Even when diabetes education is made available, educating people about diabetes will just get more challenging in the future, since increasing numbers of Canadians do not speak English as their first language or come from completely different cultures. Clearly, diabetes is taking its toll on our health care system. It is likely that as more people age and are diagnosed with Type 2 diabetes, which is clearly the trend in Canada and around the world, less education will be available as doctors and diabetes educators become overburdened with patients. The next chapter focuses on pediatric Type 2 diabetes, now a major epidemic among obese children, in particular.

3

PEDIATRIC TYPE 2 DIABETES

Pediatric Type 2 diabetes generally refers to Type 2 diabetes diagnosed in individuals under 18, and includes adolescents. Before 1997, virtually all diabetes in young individuals was thought to be Type 1 diabetes (what used to be called juvenile diabetes). Now, Type 2 diabetes in children has gone from extremely rare to not uncommon. It may jump to "common" in a population that never experienced this disease prior to the 1990s. All experts agree that this is extremely alarming.

THE MAIN CAUSE: THE EPIDEMIC OF CHILDHOOD OBESITY

According to the Children's Exercise and Nutrition Centre at McMaster University in Hamilton, childhood obesity is considered an epidemic. The major cause of the rise of Type 2 diabetes in children is obesity. Fifteen to 20 percent of the pediatric population is now obese. By 2010, almost 50 percent of children in North America will be overweight. Since the late 1970s, the prevalence of overweight has doubled among children six to 11, and tripled among those 12–17. The problem falls disproportionately on Aboriginal children, children of colour, and Hispanic children. Type 2 diabetes in children is a consequence. In the recent National Health and Nutrition Examination Survey III data on the prevalence of the metabolic syndrome (see Chapter 1), roughly 4 percent of all adolescents and nearly 30 percent of overweight children had metabolic syndrome. If current obesity rates continue, one in three babies born in 2000 will eventually develop Type 2 diabetes before they are adults.

The current theory is there appears to be a latency period between obesity and Type 2 diabetes. Type 2 diabetes may be on the rise in young adults and adolescents who were obese as children.

How We Got Here

North American children are considered the worst examples of child-hood obesity. Children are now developing obesity-related diseases that were once diagnosed only in adults. In addition to Type 2 dia-betes, it is not unusual for obese children to be diagnosed with high cholesterol. Most countries look at North American children as the examples of "what not to become." Children today spend about 22 hours per week in front of the television, consuming high-fat snacks while they're watching the advertising of more high-fat snacks. If you count computer time, text messaging, and other types of screen use, children spend 38 hours a week in front of some type of screen; that almost equals the hours spent on the average full-time job. Children watch more than 30,000 commercials per year, and roughly 25 percent of North American children between the ages of two and five actually have a TV in their room.

Between the late 1970s and the early 1990s, when the prevalence of childhood obesity had doubled (from 8–14 percent in children aged six to 11, and from 6–12 percent in children in their teens), other countries began to take action regarding food advertising to children. For example, as early as 1992, Sweden banned all television advertis-ing directed at children younger than 12. Ads have been banned from children's television programming in Norway, Belgium, Ireland, and Holland.

Advertising Junk Foods and the Diets of Childhood Obesity

Since the 1980s, we have seen an explosion in advertising to children. Food is advertised more than any other product. In 1987 researchers who surveyed advertising on Saturday morning network television counted 225 commercials; 71 percent were junk food ads. The number of commercials increased to 997 in 1994; the majority of the ads, again, were for junk foods: sweet cereal, candy, fast foods, soft drinks, cookies, and salty snacks. The researchers did not count any commercials for fruits, vegetables, bread, or other real foods.

There is a direct connection between obesity and television commercials. The more commercials children watch, the fatter they get. Several studies have documented that children who watch television are fatter. Nearly 70 percent of all foods advertised are fast foods; only about 2 percent of food advertising describes real foods, such as fruits, vegetables, grains, or beans. Of all foods advertised to children in North America, 95 percent of the commercials describe foods high in sugar, salt, and fat. Most US children now get about 25 percent of their total vegetable servings in the form of potato chips or french fries.

The connection between watching television and becoming obese is being studied at the University of Alberta. Researchers have designed a three-month program to teach children about the benefits of exercise, watching less TV, and sticking to a healthier diet. Genetic factors play only a small role in this problem. Although 40 percent of children may have a tendency to become overweight, sedentary living and high-fat snacking are the switches that trip the obesity gene.

Limiting television time does not stop children from being sedentary, nor does it prevent their exposure to advertising. Children now spend hours at their computers, on the Internet, and other screens. Many consumer and parent groups have sought to ban advertising to children under seven, who frequently think the ads are part of the movie or computer game. This confusion makes them the most gullible targets.

The Soft Drink Link

One of the largest contributors to childhood obesity is the soft drink industry. Soft drink manufacturers have spent money to increase the amount of soft drinks North American children consume. They have forged relationships with schools, providing school supplies with product logos in exchange for exclusive rights to vending in the school district.

(In the United States, such relationships are known as "pouring rights" contracts.) Regular soft drinks are made of carbonated water, some flavouring, and about 50 mL (10 tsps) of sugar. A 360 mL (12 oz) can contains about 160 calories, and caffeine levels can exceed 100 mg—equal to a cup of coffee. There is no nutritional value in soft drinks; they are junk food, or what The Center for Science in the Public Interest refers to as "liquid candy." Nutritionists advise that any other beverage would be better than a regular soft drink, including sweet juices, which at least have vitamins. Between 1985 and 1997, schools purchased 30 percent less milk, and increased their purchases of soft drinks by 1,100 percent.

In 1981, teens drank twice as much milk as soft drinks; today this figure has been reversed. Worse, about one-fifth of North American toddlers (one- and two-year-olds) now are given soft drinks in their bottles or no-spill cups.

OTHER CAUSES OF PEDIATRIC TYPE 2 DIABETES

Obesity alone is not the only factor contributing to this rise. It seems that children of certain ethnicities are more at risk, such as children of Aboriginal, Hispanic, South Asian, Asian, or African descent. In most cases, obesity is still a contributing factor.

The best snapshot of the future we have comes from the SEARCH for Diabetes in Youth Study, published in *JAMA* in 2007. This study looked at diabetes risk for US children and teenagers in 2002–2003. The risk of diabetes before age 20 was 24.3 percent per 100,000 with a higher risk seen in Aboriginal children and children of African, Asian, or Hispanic descent. Among children diagnosed with Type 2 diabetes, it's estimated that boys will lose about 18 years of life and 31 years of quality of life, while girls will lose about 19 years of life, and 32 years of quality of life. Children will suffer the same complications of Type 2 diabetes, with the exception of diabetes eye problems.

For reasons discussed in Chapter 2, in Canada, children of First Nations origin are at particular risk. For example, roughly 1 percent of First Nations children have Type 2 diabetes. The College of Physicians and Surgeons of Manitoba recommends that First Nations children six years and older who are obese or who have a strong family history of diabetes be screened for diabetes on an annual basis. In the US, the prevalence of Type 2 diabetes among Pima Indian youth doubled between 1977 and 1986, while Type 2 diabetes incidence in Pima Indian children was 5.7 times higher in 1991–2003 compared with 1965–1977. The Chicago Diabetes Registry reported alarming increases in Type 2 diabetes among African-American and Hispanic children between 1985 and 2001.

Children on Psychiatric Drugs

There are a range of drugs used on children who have various psychiatric disorders. Although the CDA has specifically identified anti-psychotic drugs or "atypical neuroleptic" drugs, the range of drugs used on children diagnosed with various forms of autism, mood disorders, ADHD, and so forth, can alter children's appetites, leading to obesity and obesity-related diseases. If your child's obesity is presumed to be a side effect of another drug, then it's critical to reassess your child's medication if your child is at risk for Type 2 diabetes. In cases such as these, dietary modification or lifestyle intervention may not be the answer to weight loss in your child.

Exposure in Utero

While obesity and ethnicity (usually both) appear to be the main cause of Type 2 diabetes in children, there also appears to be a link between pediatric Type 2 diabetes and gestational diabetes (meaning exposure to diabetes in utero). The offspring of women who had gestational diabetes may be more at risk for pediatric Type 2 diabetes. Women with gestational diabetes should consider breastfeeding for at least six months, which is shown to offer some protection against diabetes in some populations.

PREVENTION AND SCREENING

The CDA recommends biannual screening for diabetes in children 10 years and older with any two of the following risk factors:

- Obesity
- High-risk ethnicity
- Family history
- Hypertension
- Polycystic Ovarian Syndrome
- Acanthosis nigricans (dark patches of skin on the back and shoulders; is associated with high insulin resistance)
- Children on anti-psychotic or neuroleptic medications

With regular and earlier screening of at-risk children, the opportunity to find pre-diabetes (see Chapter 1) can lead to interventions that can prevent the development of full-blown Type 2 diabetes. Since in almost all cases, obesity precedes Type 2 diabetes, the recommended intervention for reducing a child's risk of developing Type 2 diabetes is to treat the initial problem of obesity. Treating obesity requires all of the following:

- Dietary modification (see chapters 7 and 8). In particular, pediatric obesity specialists recommend a low glycemic index diet for the whole family, and a "don't bring junk or fake food into the home" rule. An emphasis on real foods and no packaged foods is considered key to changing the family's diet. A terrific resource is: *Ending the Food Fight: Guide Your Child to a Healthy Weight in a Fast Food/Fake Food World* by David Ludwig, MD, PhD, an expert in childhood obesity.
- Intensive family counselling and involvement in dietary modification are critical.
- Limit all screen time to two hours daily.
- Exercise interventions (see Table 3.1, page 41) are crucial.

Programs that solely involve dietary counselling and pediatric clinic visits apparently don't show the same results. It is recognized in all literature on pediatric obesity that obese children are creatures of habit, a habit that is set by the family. If the entire family changes its habits, the children will benefit. The focus must therefore be on the family, and not just on the child.

Table 3.1: Recommended Activities for Obese Children and Teenagers

- Perform household chores (cleaning, mowing, washing dishes, taking out the trash)
- Take the stairs instead of elevators or escalators
- Avoid sitting; stand when talking on the telephone
- Walk to school instead of being driven
- Use a rocking chair when watching television
- Play outside
- Don't stand still: walk back and forth when waiting
- Wash the family car
- When doing homework, stop every 15–30 minutes for a brief walk

Source: T. Rowland, Obesity Management (August 2008):186.

Screening for Diabetes Type

If your child is screened for diabetes and is diagnosed with it, it's critical to ask your doctor "What type?" or "Are you sure it's Type 2 diabetes and not Type 1?" Since in the past, most children with diabetes had the autoimmune form of the disease that was not related to obesity, ethnicity, or lifestyle (called Type 1 diabetes, discussed in Chapter 1), it's important that you rule out Type 1 diabetes. One way to confirm this is to test for the *absence of islet autoantibodies*; islet autoantibodies would be present in Type 1 diabetes, but not in Type 2. There are also diagnostic tests for genetic defects in beta cell function (the cells that make insulin). If there are genetic defects present, then this suggests more of a genetic cause for diabetes, rather than a lifestyle-related cause, such as obesity or diet.

TREATING PEDIATRIC TYPE 2 DIABETES

It's believed that Type 2 diabetes may have an earlier and more aggressive course in children, meaning that complications will be seen earlier. The debate over aggressive treatment for Type 2 diabetes in children rages as a result, since the only medications that can be used are medications not tested in children.

In some children, the risk of cardiovascular complications is so alarming that debate over putting children on adult medications, such as cholesterol-lowering drugs, is ongoing. Many pediatric researchers find this solution unacceptable, as there is no information about what the side effects of these drugs would be in children, or what would happen if someone were to stay on these drugs for 40–50 years. Some data do show that cholesterol-lowering drugs will slow the progression of heart disease in children. Most experts agree that the treatment for pediatric diabetes needs to be the same as preventing it in the first place: treating obesity. Some obesity drugs, such as Orlistat (see Chapter 11), may play a role, but most doctors are skeptical about using these drugs in children. The consensus in all pediatric literature is to start with lifestyle modification and intervention, and resort to medication only in extreme cases. This should be combined with routine screening and monitoring of glucose levels, cholesterol, blood pressure, and so forth.

Annual screening for the same diabetes complications one would expect in adults must be done in children as well. Children should be checked for nerve damage (numbness), eye problems, kidney problems, cavities or tooth decay, and so forth.

Cases in Which Medication Is Necessary

There are certainly cases when medication is necessary. For example, in children with Type 2 diabetes who are morbidly obese, with a BMI over 40 (or 50, as several case reports show), bariatric surgery may be a consideration (see Chapter 11). In some cases, Metformin (see Chapter 6) may be necessary. In some cases in which children are at great risk for cardiovascular problems, cholesterol-lowering drugs or other medications may need to be added. The general rule is to treat a severe case of Type 2 diabetes in a child as one would an adult; however, unless it's severe, lifestyle interventions and modifications are the rule to avoid using drugs not tested in children.

The rise in Type 2 diabetes in children is thought to be caused by our toxic diet and sedentary society. The children reflect the health of our society at large. All pediatric literature on this subject emphasizes that changes must be made at the policy and public health level to create healthier diets and environments for our children. For example, in many public schools, physical education is minimal. Parents' fear of children's safety has limited outdoor play that is not strictly supervised. Sports activities are often cost-prohibitive for many parents. Ultimately, by eliminating activity from children's lives, we've created terrible states of health for them. Returning to real foods and simpler activities is generally advocated for children's health, and the primary prevention of obesity and obesity-related diseases such as Type 2 diabetes.

4

YOUR DIABETES HEALTH CARE TEAM

Diabetes is a major problem for the North American health care system. According to the Canadian Diabetes Association, by 2010, it's estimated that diabetes will cost the Canadian health care system $15.6 billion a year, and that number will rise to $19.2 billion by 2020. Furthermore, a person with diabetes can potentially face direct costs for medication and supplies ranging from $1,000–$15,000 a year. As a result, there is really no such thing as one "diabetes doctor" who manages the disease completely. Your primary care physician often acts as overall supervisor of your condition, but ideally, this doctor should be working with a team of health care professionals, which includes the following:

- *A certified diabetes educator (CDE):* CDEs come from a variety of backgrounds. They can be dietitians, nurses, physicians, or social workers. Each of these professionals must write a CDE exam in Canada and practise within the scope of his or her own discipline and relevant legislation. CDEs are absolutely vital to managing diabetes. They will help you gain control of your disease by teaching you how to adjust your diet, incorporate physical activity into your routine, test your blood and record the results, as well as manage any medication or insulin that's been prescribed. You should also be able to find a CDE via the Canadian Diabetes Education Certification Board (www.cdecb.ca).

- *A dietitian:* In addition to a CDE, you should see a dietitian regularly during your first year with diabetes. If you learn to plan meals accordingly, you may be able to control your diabetes without taking any medications.
- *An exercise/fitness instructor or trainer:* This is any professional who can tailor a fitness program that suits your lifestyle and level of ability. Check with your CDE, the Canadian Diabetes Association, the YMCA/YWCA, or your local community centre for lists of fitness instructors. You do not need a referral to one; you can simply make an appointment independent of your doctor.
- *Community health representative (CHR):* This is someone from your community who works with you and your family, as well as with other health care professionals, to educate you about diabetes. CHRs are usually found in rural areas where access to doctors is poor. CHRs attend a four-day training session and complete a skills test, but skills training and experience vary widely, although CHRs are required to review and update their skills annually. CHRs are common in Aboriginal Canadian communities.
- *An endocrinologist and other specialists:* This is discussed further on page 52.
- *A pharmacist:* Since you may be expected to do home glucose tests, your pharmacist will recommend the right glucose meter for you and will become a valuable source of information on drug interactions and their effects on your blood sugar. A diabetes care centre in your neighbourhood is an ideal place to purchase your diabetes products and consult with a pharmacist.

While clearly there is treatment for Type 2 diabetes, it is a complex disease that can be managed only through a multilayered approach. The goal of treatment is not just to relieve symptoms, but to prevent a range of other diseases in the future. Self-managing your disease while maintaining your quality of life can happen only if you're willing to learn and change your lifestyle. That means asking questions and participating in your treatment.

There are various stops along this treatment highway. How many times you stop depends on how well you can control your blood sugar. Some of you may be able to control diabetes solely through diet and exercise (see chapters 7–9). Some of you may need to combine diet and lifestyle modification with diabetes pills, while some of you may need to use insulin to control your disease.

This chapter will guide you through the maze of treatments and health care professionals you'll encounter. It will also give you the right questions to ask so you can get the right answers. Only then can you be expected to participate more fully in decisions that affect your diabetes and the rest of your life.

THE RIGHT PRIMARY CARE DOCTOR

A primary care doctor is the doctor you see all the time. For example, you would see this doctor for a cold, flu, or an annual physical; this is the doctor who refers you to specialists.

In Canada, primary care doctors today are *general practitioners* (four years of medical school and one year of internship), *family practitioners* (four years of medical school and a two-year residency in family medicine), or *internists* (four years of medical school and a four-year residency in internal medicine). During medical training, rotations are done in a variety of specialties, such as psychiatry, endocrinology, obstetrics and gynecology, emergency medicine, and so on. During a residency, the years are spent in a teaching hospital under the supervision of teaching faculty (assistant, associate, or full professors of medicine) who teach one specialty. The number of years spent in a residency program after four years of medical school varies depending on the university and specialty. To qualify as a specialist, such as an endocrinologist, a doctor must do a residency in endocrinology. A fellowship year is required after that, and the doctor must be eligible to write exams for the Fellowship of the Royal College of Physicians of Canada. The letters FRCP stand for Fellow Royal College of Physicians. (FRCS stands for Fellow Royal College of Surgeons.) In the United States, the *R* is replaced with *A* for American (College of Physicians/Surgeons).

The majority of people with Type 2 diabetes are cared for by their primary care doctors, but the quality of care may vary. What you'll find today is that most primary care doctors in Canada become very good at treating a few conditions. Some see a lot of patients with diabetes; others see more pregnant women; still others see more elderly patients requiring palliative care. It all depends on the magic phrase "patient population." *Where is* the doctor's practice located? *Who are* the people in that neighbourhood?

The CDA has a position statement available on its website (www. diabetes.ca) on access to health services for diabetes patients, and it is something to keep in mind when you're pondering the best care possible for your disease management. "People with diabetes have a right to timely, affordable, and ongoing diabetes and comprehensive treatment services provided by qualified professionals, including a Diabetes Healthcare Team and other specialists.... Upon diagnosis, physicians should refer patients with diabetes to a diabetes education program, with waiting periods not to exceed those specified by the Canadian Diabetes Association's guidelines with respect to diabetes education.

Therefore, a primary care physician may not be the best doctor to manage your diabetes if that doctor doesn't see many diabetes patients. Some doctors are also behind the times when it comes to diabetes and do not immediately recognize early warning signs or high-risk groups. Nor do all primary care doctors counsel their patients about newer approaches to therapy, namely, self-monitoring of blood glucose levels, which, though optional in Type 2 diabetes, may not be discussed as an option. (See Chapter 5.)

Each province may differ when it comes to its individual health care system helping you to manage your diabetes. The Government of British Columbia's Ministry of Health Services (www.health.gov.bc.ca) offers fairly detailed guidelines on diabetes care, and how it should be managed. This site offers a great list of tips for working with your doctor, such as making sure that you have a regular family doctor, being your own advocate, and working with your doctor to set goals for blood glucose levels. The types of specialists and other medical professionals that you may see may vary from province to province. You can discuss the referral options (if necessary) with your family doctor. See page 55.

When you're diagnosed with diabetes, ask your doctor the following questions. It will help determine whether you should stay with your doctor or look for another one:

1. *What is your philosophy about blood sugar monitoring?* Any doctor who does not discuss the option of your purchasing a glucose meter and self-monitoring your blood sugar levels may not be up to date. The Canadian Diabetes Association recommends that people with Type 2 diabetes get into the habit of self-testing their blood sugar. A discussion about it with your doctor is warranted, even though self-testing remains optional pending more convincing data. A good family doctor should present the facts to date: "Here's what some people think; here's what I think; here are my recommendations." (Ultimately, the decision is yours.)

2. *How often will you be checking my glycosylated hemoglobin or glycohemoglobin levels?* If your doctor says, "Huh?" get out of there and find another doctor! This is a blood test known as the A1C (formerly known as the HbA1c).

3. *Will you be referring me to a specialist?* The answer should be "Yes!" If you've been diagnosed with diabetes, you need to see other health care professionals as soon as possible, such as an endocrinologist who specializes in diabetes, a certified diabetes educator, a dietitian, and an ophthalmologist (or optometrist if the former isn't available). If your doctor says, "I can manage your condition without referring you elsewhere," get out of that office and go elsewhere.

4. *Where can I go for more information?* Any doctor who does not tell you to call the Canadian Diabetes Association as soon as you're diagnosed with diabetes is not worth seeing.

The Alarm Bells

If you hear the following words come out of your doctor's mouth, go elsewhere:

- *"You have borderline diabetes or just a touch of sugar."* (There's no such thing. There is such a thing as impaired fasting glucose and impaired glucose tolerance, discussed in Chapter 1.)
- *"You don't need to change your diet; I'll just give you a pill."* (In general, no medication should be prescribed until you've been sent to a dietitian, who will work with you to modify your diet and lifestyle. In cases where medication is warranted immediately, you must still see a dietitian.)
- *"You don't need to see a specialist."* (You *do* need to see a specialist.)
- *"You have a recurrent yeast infection. This is perfectly normal."* (Chronic vaginal yeast infections are a classic sign of diabetes in post-menopausal women.)

Patients' Rights Specific to Diabetes

Applying your rights as a patient to diabetes specifically, here are some things you should expect from your health care provider:

- *As much information about your diabetes as you want:* Any doctor who is reluctant to refer you to other sources of information (books, Internet sites, etc.) and a referral to a diabetes educator and dietitian is not giving you proper care.
- *Answers to your questions about diabetes:* If there isn't time during an exam or checkup, make another appointment that serves as a question-and-answer period.
- *Regular assessments:* When you have diabetes, you should be seen at least every three months for a checkup or at regular intervals. It's important to ask how much advance booking time you need to get an appointment.
- *Participation in treatment plans:* You'll need to educate yourself about your diabetes before you can participate, but you have many options in treatment.

- *Decent emergency care and an opportunity to meet your doctor's substitute:* Who looks after you when your doctor is on holidays or sick?
- *Privacy and confidentiality:* Diabetes often taints relationships with employers, co-workers, and insurance companies. Find out what your doctor's legal obligations are with respect to health records, and what are *yours?*
- Information about fees and costs: What is covered by the province and what is not? How much of your medication and equipment is covered by your drug plan? Your doctor should be able to give you an estimate for your diabetes care products in case you are not covered. He or she should also be able to give you cheaper products if you cannot afford what is being prescribed. Pharmacists and the Canadian Diabetes Association are also helpful.
- A change to another doctor: If you're unhappy with your current doctor, or simply need a change, you have every right to switch. Make sure you arrange for your records to be transferred. Some costs may be involved, however.
- A second opinion or a consultation with a specialist: No family doctor should deny you a referral to a specialist.

Your Doctor's Rights

Your doctor has the right to expect the following from you:

- *Honesty:* If you're not being truthful about how often you're checking your blood sugar levels or about what you're eating, or if you are not being honest in recording your log to avoid a lecture, your doctor can't be blamed if your health deteriorates.
- *Courtesy and respect:* Treat your doctor like a business associate. If you make an appointment, show up; if you need to cancel, give 24 hours' notice. If you have a problem, go through reasonable channels; dial the after-hours emergency number the doctor leaves with the answering service, or call your doctor's office during business hours.

- *Good reporting:* Don't tell your doctor that you're not feeling well and expect a diagnosis. Tell your doctor what your *specific symptoms are.* Better yet, write them down before you visit your doctor.
- *Questions:* If you don't ask a particular question, you can't blame your doctor for not answering it.
- *Follow-through:* If you don't follow your doctor's advice, you can't blame the doctor if you experience side effects to medications or worsening symptoms. If you don't think your doctor's advice is reasonable, say so and discuss it. Maybe your doctor doesn't have a full understanding of your condition; maybe you don't have a full understanding of your doctor's suggestions.
- *Self-management:* Don't call your doctor 10 times a day with every little change in your blood sugar levels. You should be able to monitor your blood sugar levels and adjust your diet and medication regimen accordingly. Emergencies or illness are different situations, however, and your doctor should be notified since even a common virus will elevate your blood sugar level.

YOUR DIABETES SPECIALIST

A diabetes specialist is an endocrinologist who subspecializes in diabetes. Sometimes they're called "diabetologists." Endocrinologists are hormone specialists. Some see more thyroid patients than diabetes patients. Others specialize in reproductive endocrinology (male and female hormones). Therefore, it's important that you consult with someone who almost exclusively manages diabetes patients. The shortest route to a diabetes specialist is to ask your primary care doctor for a referral. If your primary care doctor refuses to refer you (this, by the way, is not unusual), call the Canadian Diabetes Association and ask them for a list of endocrinologists in your area.

If you live in an underserviced area (there are several of these in Canada!), ask people you know if they know someone with diabetes, and then call them! Who are *they* seeing? You may need to go outside your area to a larger city, but it's worth the trip to avoid being mismanaged.

Your primary care doctor can continue to manage the rest of your referrals to ophthalmologists (for diabetes eye disease), podiatrists for foot care, and so on. (See Part 3 for more details.)

Questions to Ask Your Specialist

To maximize time with your diabetes specialist, here are few good questions to get you started:

1. How severe is my diabetes? (If you are experiencing other health problems as a result of your diabetes, the disease is likely more advanced.)
2. Does my hospital or treatment centre have a multidisciplinary diabetes education care team? (This means that a number of health care professionals—certified diabetes educators, clinical nurse specialists, dietitians, endocrinologists, and other relevant specialists—discuss your case together and recommend treatment options.)
3. What treatment do you recommend, and why? (For example, if insulin therapy is being recommended over oral hypoglycemic agents, find out why. And find out how this particular treatment will reduce the odds of complications.)
4. How will my treatment help the risks and side effects associated with diabetes, and who will help me adjust my medications or insulin?
5. How long do you recommend this particular treatment? (Lifelong? On a wait-and-see basis?)
6. What if I forget to take a pill or insulin shot? What are the consequences?
7. What other health problems should I look out for? (You'll want to watch for symptoms of high or low blood sugar, as well as symptoms of long-term complications, such as eye problems or numbness in your feet.)
8. How can I contact you between visits?
9. Can I take other medications? Or how will my pills or insulin affect other medications I'm taking?

10. What about alcohol? How will alcohol consumption affect any pills or insulin I'm on? How do I compensate for it?
11. Will I be able to participate in new studies or clinical trials using new drugs or therapies?
12. Are there any holistic approaches I can turn to as a complement to diabetes pills or insulin therapy?

OTHER SPECIALISTS

Since diabetes can involve a variety of complications in the future, you may need to consult some or all of the following specialists:

- *Internist:* This is a doctor who specializes in non-surgical treatment of a variety of medical problems, including diabetes. Often internists serve as primary care doctors.
- *Ophthalmologist:* This is an eye specialist who will monitor your eyes and make sure that you're showing no symptoms of diabetes eye disease (see Chapter 17). If you are, this is the specialist who will treat your condition.
- *Cardiologist:* This is a heart specialist. People with Type 2 diabetes are four times more likely to suffer from heart attacks. You may be sent here if you are experiencing symptoms of heart disease or angina.
- *Nephrologist:* This is a kidney specialist. Since kidney disease is a common complication of diabetes, you may be sent here if you're showing symptoms of kidney disease (protein in your urine).
- *Gastroenterologist:* This is a GI (gastrointestinal) specialist. Diabetes often results in a number of chronic gastrointestinal ailments. You may be sent here if you have symptoms of chronic heartburn, reflux, and other gastric aches and pains.
- *Neurologist:* This is a nerve specialist who will see you if you're experiencing nerve damage as a result of your diabetes.
- *Gerontologist:* This is a doctor who specializes in diseases of the elderly. If you are over 65 and have a number of other health

problems, this doctor will help you balance your various medications and conditions, in conjunction with your diabetes.

- *Obstetrician/gynecologist:* If you develop diabetes during pregnancy, you'll need to be under the care of an obstetrician for the remainder of your pregnancy. All women should see a gynecologist regularly for Pap smears, breast health, and consultation regarding sexual health, contraception, and hormone-replacement therapy after menopause.
- *Urologist:* This is a doctor who specializes in male reproductive problems. Impotence is often a complication with diabetes, and this is the doctor who will be able to determine the cause of your impotence.
- *Podiatrist:* This is a foot doctor who can help you monitor foot health. If you're experiencing severe problems with your feet (see Chapter 20), your family doctor will likely send you here.

Other specialists or programs that you may be referred to include: Diabetes nurse educator, nutritionist/dietician, physiotherapist, a cardiac rehabilitation centre, healthy heart program, community health nurse, social worker, diabetes support group, or a stop-smoking program.

When You Want a Second Opinion

Getting a second opinion means that you see two separate doctors about the same set of symptoms. If you answer *yes* to one of the questions below, you're probably justified in seeking a second opinion.

1. *Is the diagnosis uncertain?* If your doctor can't give you a straight answer about what's going on, you're justified in seeing someone else.
2. *Is the diagnosis life-threatening?* In this case, hearing the same news from someone else may help you cope better with your illness or come to terms with the diagnosis.
3. *Is the treatment controversial, experimental, or risky?* You might not question the diagnosis but have problems with the

recommended treatment. For example, if you're not comfortable with treatment approach A, perhaps another doctor can recommend treatment approach B.

4. *Is the treatment not working?* If your oral hypoglycemic agents can't seem to control your blood sugar levels, maybe it's time for insulin. In this case, getting a second opinion may help to clear up the problem.

5. *Are risky tests or procedures being recommended?* If you find a particular test or procedure frightening, a second opinion will either help confirm your suspicions, or confirm your original doctor's recommendations.

6. *Do you want another approach?* If you have poor control over your diabetes, your doctor may want you to begin taking insulin, while another doctor may prescribe dietary changes along with anti-diabetic medication.

7. *Is the doctor's competence in question?* If you suspect that your doctor doesn't know what he or she is doing, go somewhere else to either reaffirm your faith in your doctor or confirm your original suspicions.

WHAT THE DOCTOR ORDERS

Throughout the year, your managing doctor (primary care physician or endocrinologist) should order a variety of blood tests to make sure that your blood sugar levels are as controlled as they can be, and that no complications from diabetes are setting in.

The A1C Test

The most important test is one that checks your glycolsylated hemoglobin levels, known as the A1C test (formerly the HbAlc test). Hemoglobin is a large molecule that carries oxygen to your bloodstream. When the glucose in your blood comes in contact with the hemoglobin molecule, it conveniently sticks to it. The more glucose stuck to your hemoglobin, the higher your blood sugar is. The AlC test actually measures the amount of glucose stuck to hemoglobin. And since each hemoglobin molecule stays in your blood about three to four months before it is replaced, this test can show you the average blood sugar level over the last three to four months. If you have cardiovascular problems, you will need to have the A1C test more often.

What's a Good A1C Result?

Just like your glucose monitor at home, the goal of the A1C test is to make sure that your blood sugar average is as close to normal as possible. Again, the closer to normal it is, the less likely you are to experience long-term diabetes complications. The 2008 CDA Guidelines recommend that for most people with diabetes, A1C should be measured every three months to ensure that glycemic goals are being met or maintained. Once your diabetes is under control, testing at least every six months is fine.

Table 4.1: Recommended Blood Glucose Targets for People with Diabetes*

	A1C**	Fasting Blood Glucose/ Blood Glucose before Meals (mmol/L)	Blood Glucose Two Hours after Eating (mmol/L)
Target for most patients with diabetes	≤7.0%	4.0–7.0	5.0–10
Normal range	≤6.0%	4.0–6.0	5.0–8.0

* This information is based on the Canadian Diabetes Association's 2008 Clinical Practice Guidelines for the Prevention and Management of Diabetes in Canada and is a guide. Talk to your doctor about your blood glucose target ranges.

** A1C is a blood test that indicates an average of your overall blood glucose levels over the past 120 days. A1C targets for pregnant women and children 12 years of age and under are different.

Problems with the A1C Test

If your child comes home with a report card showing a B average, it doesn't mean your child is getting a B in every course; it means that he or she could have received a D in one course and an A+ in another. Similarly, the A1C test is just an "average mark." You could have a decent result, even though your blood sugar levels may be dangerously low one day and dangerously high the next.

If you suffer from sickle cell disease or other blood disorders, the A1C results will not be accurate either. In this case, you may wind up with either false high or low readings.

And at any time, if your home blood sugar tests (if you've opted for self-testing) over the past two or three months do not seem to match the results of the A1C test, be sure to check the accuracy of your meter, and perhaps show your doctor or certified diabetes educator how you are using the meter in case your technique needs some refining.

Other Important Tests

It's important to have the following routine tests done at least once a year and more often if you are at high risk for complications.

Blood Pressure

As discussed in Chapter 2, high blood pressure can put you at greater risk for cardiovascular problems. Diabetes can also cause high blood pressure. That's why it's important to have your blood pressure checked every four to six months.

Cholesterol

As discussed in Chapter 2, high cholesterol is a problem for people with diabetes, while diabetes can also trigger high cholesterol. Your cholesterol is checked through a simple blood test that should be done once upon diagnosis, and once a year thereafter. If you have Type 2 diabetes, you should have your cholesterol tested every one to three years. More frequent testing may be necessary if you're taking medications.

Table 4.2: Target Lipid Ranges for the General Population*

Total Cholesterol	LDL	HDL	Total/HDL Ratio	Triglycerides
<5.2	<3.5	>1.0 (men)	<5.0	<1.7
	>1.3 (women)			
LDL = low-density lipids, or "bad cholesterol"				
HDL = high-density lipids or "good cholesterol"				

*Note: All values are expressed in millimoles per litre (mmol/L)

Source: www.heartandstroke.ca, 2008.

Table 4.3: Target Lipid Ranges for People with Diabetes at Risk for Cardiovascular Disease

LDL: ≤ 2.2
Total/HDL: <4.0

Source: Canadian Diabetes Association, 2008 Clinical Practice Guidelines for the Prevention and Management of Diabetes in Canada: S109.

Eye Exam

Since diabetes can cause what's known as diabetes eye disease or diabetic retinopathy (damage to the back of your eye), annual eye exams are crucial. Your eye exam should also rule out cataracts and glaucoma.

Foot Exam

When you have diabetes, nerve damage and poor circulation can wreak havoc on your feet. Be sure to have a thorough foot exam each year to check for reduced sensation, feeling, or circulation, and evidence of calluses or sores. See Chapter 20 for more details.

Glucose Meter Checkup

If you've opted to test your own blood sugar, it's important to compare your home glucose meter's test results to a laboratory blood glucose test. In fact, it's a good idea to do this every six months. All you do is bring your meter to the lab when you're having a blood glucose test done. After the lab technician takes your blood, do your own test within about five minutes and record the result. Your meter is working perfectly so long as your result is within 15 percent of the lab test (if your meter is testing whole blood, as opposed to plasma).

Kidney Tests

One of the most common complications of diabetes is kidney disease, known in this case as *diabetic nephropathy* (diabetic kidney disease). This condition develops slowly over the course of many years, but there are usually few symptoms or warning signs. To make sure no damage to the kidneys has occurred, it's important to have your urine tested regularly to check the health of your kidneys. See Chapter 19 on kidney health in Part 3.

When you have diabetes, you are the most important part of your diabetes health care team. The next chapter will show you all the things you can do to maximize your health and stay in control of your diabetes. By helping yourself, you will help your health care providers do their job a little better: the job of taking care of you.

5

DIABETES SELF-CARE

Diabetes self-care is all about eliminating your diabetes symptoms, and then remaining as symptom-free as possible. Diet (chapters 7 and 8), combined with exercise (Chapter 9), is the best way to remain symptom-free. This will help you lose weight if you need to, as well as distribute an even amount of calories to your body throughout the day. By not putting any unusual strain on your body's metabolism, you will likely *not* experience any surprises when it comes to your blood sugar levels. Exercise makes insulin much more available to your cells, while your muscles use sugar as fuel.

The CDA recommends the following targets for glycemic control for people with Type 2 diabetes:

- A1C: ≤ 7.0 percent
- Fasting plasma glucose or pre-prandial (pre-meal) plasma glucose: 4.0–7.0 (mmol/L)
- Two-hour post-prandial (post-meal) plasma glucose: 5.0–10.0 (5.0–8.0 if A1C targets are not being met)

TESTING YOUR OWN BLOOD SUGAR

In order to plan your meals and activities properly, you have to know what your blood sugar levels are throughout the day. One of the most important research projects ever undertaken was the Diabetes Control and

Complications Trial (DCCT). This trial proved beyond a doubt that when people with Type 1 diabetes kept their blood sugar levels as normal as possible, as often as possible, they could dramatically reduce the odds of developing small blood-vessel diseases related to diabetes, such as kidney disease, eye problems, and nerve disease, all discussed in Part 3.

The evidence is somewhat conflicting on how often it is necessary to self monitor, if at all, and it points to the real need for good communication on this matter with your health care provider in order to tailor your regimen to your specific needs. Data from the Fremantle Diabetes Study (FDS) reported in 2006 and 2007, in the journals *Diabetes Care* and *Diabetologia* respectively, concluded that neither self-monitoring of blood glucose (SMBG) testing nor its frequency was associated with much benefit in Type 2 diabetic patients regardless of treatment. It was also noted that SMBG was not independently associated with improved survival. Painting a different picture in another 2006 study, researchers looking at data from the ROSSO (RetrOlective Study of Self-monitoring of blood glucose and Outcome) trial concluded that SMBG was associated with decreased complications and death; the ROSSO trial concluded that SMBG was associated with a healthier lifestyle and/or better disease management.

Glucose meters were first introduced in 1982. They allow people with diabetes to test their own blood sugar any time they want without having to rely on doctors. When your parents or grandparents struggled with diabetes in the past, there was no such thing as a glucose meter. They had to go to the doctor to get their blood sugar tested regularly. There are still people who rely on the doctor to test their blood sugar. If you are still going to your doctor for a blood sugar test, purchase a glucose meter before your next doctor's visit and ask your doctor to show you how it works. There is no reason to continue to rely on a doctor to test your blood sugar. That said, you should have laboratory blood tests done at least once a year to make sure your meter results are accurate.

How Frequently Should You Test?

Even the latest Guidelines from the CDA offer somewhat conflicting advice on how often to test your blood sugar, just as the recent studies noted above. Most physicians feel that the more involved you become in managing your blood sugar, the better off you'll be in the long run and therefore they support frequent self-testing of blood sugar in their Type 2 patients. The Canadian Diabetes Association, as noted below, also recommends that people with Type 2 diabetes frequently self-test their blood sugar. In fact, in a newly diagnosed person with Type 2 diabetes, frequent daily testing will show *individual patterns* of glucose rises and dips. This information may help your health care team tailor your meal plans, exercise routines, and medication regimens. And if you do have to take insulin in the future, you will need to get into the habit of testing your own blood sugar anyway. According to the CDA's 2008 Guidelines, frequency should be individualized to your needs, but for those who are using insulin, who have Type 2 diabetes, frequent testing, such as 3 times a day, is associated with improved glycemic control.

Not all physicians agree with this policy, however. Some physicians have told me that for some of their patients with Type 2 diabetes, the struggle to make necessary diet and activity changes is hard enough, and the frequent blood sugar testing can complicate that goal. In other words, for some people, it's too much to handle; the blood sugar testing interferes with more crucial goals, such as losing weight.

You have to be able to find a plan that works for you and put together realistic goals with your diabetes health care team. The CDA does acknowledge that SMBG in people who are recently diagnosed with Type 2 diabetes will see a benefit. Regardless of your doctor's approach to frequent self-testing of blood sugar, there are a host of easy-to-use home blood sugar monitors that give you more choice in diabetes self-care than ever before, so you should take advantage of them. Your doctor, pharmacist, or diabetes educator can recommend the right glucose meter for you. When you get your glucose monitor, experts suggest you compare your results to one regular laboratory test to make sure you've purchased a reliable and accurate machine.

Use the information in the boxed text below as a general guideline for testing times, and take it to your health care provider to help design a reasonable plan that works for you. Testing schedules are usually tailored for each individual.

When to Test Your Blood Sugar

In the days when diabetes patients went to their doctors' offices for blood sugar testing, they were usually tested first thing in the morning before eating (called a fasting blood sugar level) or immediately after eating (known as a post-prandial blood sugar level). It was believed that if either the fasting or post-prandial levels were normal, the patient was stable. This is now known to be completely false. In fact, your blood sugar levels can bounce around all day long. Because your blood sugar is constantly changing, a blood sugar test in a doctor's office is pretty useless because it measures what your blood sugar is only for that nanosecond. In other words, what your blood sugar is at 2:15 p.m. is not what it might be at 3:05 p.m.

It makes the most sense to test yourself before each meal, so you know what your levels are before you eat anything, as well as about two hours after meals. Immediately after eating, blood sugar is normally high, so this is not the ideal time to test anybody. In a person without diabetes, blood sugar levels will drop about two hours after eating in response to the natural insulin the body makes. Similarly, test yourself two hours after eating to make sure that you are able to mimic a normal blood sugar pattern, too. Ideally, this translates into at least four blood tests daily:

- When you wake up
- After breakfast/before lunch (i.e., two hours after breakfast)
- After lunch/before dinner (i.e., two hours after lunch)
- After dinner/or at bedtime (i.e., two hours after dinner)

The most revealing information about your blood sugar control is in the answers to the following questions:

1. What is your blood sugar level as soon as you wake up? (In people with Type 2 diabetes, it is often at its highest point in the morning.)
2. What is your blood sugar level two hours after a meal? (It should be much lower two hours after eating than one hour after eating.)

3. What is your blood sugar level when you feel ill? (You need to avoid dipping too low or high since your routine is changing.)

Variations on the theme:

- Test yourself four times a day (times indicated above) two to three times a week, and then test yourself two times a day (before breakfast and before bedtime) for the remainder of the week.
- Test yourself twice a day three to four days a week in a rotating pattern (before breakfast and dinner one day; before lunch and bedtime the next).
- Test yourself once a day every day, but rotate your pattern (day 1 before breakfast; day 2 after dinner; day 3 before bedtime, and so on).
- Test yourself four times a day (times indicated above) two days a month.

A Brief History of Blood Sugar Tests

At one time, the only way you could test your blood sugar level yourself was by testing your urine for sugar; if the result showed that sugar was in your urine, you had already reached your renal threshold (kidney limit). Renal thresholds vary between about 6 and 11 mmol/L, but the limitations of urine testing were that it could only test for *really* high blood sugar levels and the results were delayed, meaning that you could be getting readings on urine that had been in the bladder for hours versus fresh urine (urine that has been in the bladder for less than an hour). Urine testing is also useless for checking low blood sugar. Far more accurate home blood sugar testing became available with the development of glucose meters in 1982, but the first meters were very expensive—about $600. Thankfully, meters today are quite affordable.

The first models measured glucose levels in whole blood, while laboratories were still measuring glucose levels in blood plasma. The difference is technical and not important to you personally. What you need to know, however, is that the readings vary. This meant that doctors needed to add about 12 percent to the glucose meter's recordings in order to get an accurate picture. This standard has changed. Today, all glucose meters measure glucose levels in plasma. If you're using an older glucose meter, don't panic when your next glucose meter suddenly gives you readings that are 10–15 percent higher than your last meter. It doesn't mean that you are losing control of your diabetes; rather, your meter is measuring glucose levels in your plasma instead of whole blood. Some diabetes literature recommends that you ask the pharmacist if the meter is a whole blood test or a plasma test, but most diabetes educators will tell you that this question is pretty redundant these days as all glucose meters are now plasma tests. Some blood sugar monitors allow blood to be tested from the forearm or other parts, in place of the fingertip. The Canadian Diabetes Association states that fingertip blood appears to result in more accurate readings overall, especially in people who have fluctuations in blood sugar or who may be hypoglycemic.

Choosing and Using Your Glucose Meter

As in the computer industry, glucose meter manufacturers tend to come out with technological upgrades every year. The information can help you gauge whether your diet and exercise routine is working, or whether you need to adjust your medications or insulin. The following is a list of features to keep in mind when choosing a glucose meter for yourself:

- Overall size of the meter
- Testing speed: time to deliver the reading
- Amount of blood needed for each test
- Ability to store results in the meter's memory
- Cost of the meter
- Cost of the strips
- Ease in reading the display

The directions for using a glucose meter vary according to manufacturer. Be sure to read the directions carefully, and to ask your pharmacist for guidance if there's something you don't understand. You could also get training from a diabetes educator in your community. Any pharmacist, nurse, doctor, or diabetes educator that you consult could also watch you test to make sure that you are using your meter correctly. It's a good idea to record your results in a logbook. *For example, a target reading before meals ranges from 4–7 mmol/L; a target reading after meals ranges from 5–10 mmol/L. In non-diabetic people, blood sugar readings before meals range from 4–6 mmol/L, and after meals, 5–8 mmol/L.*

Factors That Can Taint Your Test Results

Keep in mind that the following outside factors may interfere with your meter's performance.

- *Hematocrit:* Amount of red blood cells in the blood. Patients with higher hematocrit values will usually test lower for blood glucose than patients with normal hematocrit. If you know that your hematocrit levels are abnormal, you should speak with your health care provider about the possible effects on glucose testing.
- *Third-party test strips:* There are many test strips available that are developed as a less expensive option to the strips sold with a particular meter. Be sure that the test strip you use is compatible with your meter. If you are unsure whether or not a certain strip will work with your meter, call the manufacturer.
- *Other substances:* Many substances already present in the blood could interfere with the testing process. These can include uric acid, glutathione, and vitamin C (ascorbic acid). Discuss any concerns with your health care provider.
- *Other medications you're taking:* Studies show that some meters can be inaccurate if you're taking acetaminophen, salicylate, ascorbic acid, dopamine, or levodopa. As a rule, if you're taking any medications, check with your doctor, pharmacist, and glucose meter manufacturer (call their 1-800 number) about whether your medications can affect the meter's accuracy.
- *Altitude, temperature, and humidity:* The worst place to keep your meter and strips is in the bathroom, where humidity can

ruin your strips unless they're individually wrapped in foil. Keep your strips in a sealed container away from extreme temperatures. Don't store your meter and strips, for example, in a hot glove compartment; don't keep them in the freezer either. Also, room temperature and altitude can potentially cause unpredictable effects on glucose readings. Always follow instructions for the storage and handling of both the meter and test strips.

- *Bright light:* Ever tried to use a calculator or portable computer in bright sunlight? It's not possible because the light interferes with the screen. Some meters are photometric, which means they are affected by bright light. If you plan to test in sunlight, get a biosenser meter that is unaffected by bright light (there are several).
- *Touching the test strip:* Many glucose meters come with test strips that cannot be touched with your fingers or a second drop of blood. If you're all thumbs, purchase a meter that is unaffected by touch and/or allows a second drop of blood.
- *Wet hands:* Before you test, thoroughly dry your hands. Water can dilute your blood sample.
- *Motion:* It's always best to test yourself when you're standing still. Testing on planes, trains, automobiles, buses, and subways may affect your results, depending on the brand of glucose meter.
- *Dirt, lint, and blood:* Particles of dirt, lint, and old blood can sometimes affect the accuracy of a meter, depending on the brand. Make sure you clean the meter regularly (follow the manufacturer's cleaning directions) to remove buildup. If your meter requires battery changes, make sure you change them! There are meters on the market that do not require cleaning and are unaffected by dirt, but they may cost a little more.

Glycosylated Hemoglobin

The most detailed blood sugar test cannot be done at home yet. This is a blood test that checks for glycosylated hemoglobin (glucose attached to the protein in your red blood cells), known as *glycohemoglobin* or A1C levels. This test can tell you how well your blood sugar has been controlled over a period of two to three months by showing what percentage of it is too high. It's recommended that you get an A1C test every three months. This test is discussed in more detail in Chapter 4.

OTHER WAYS TO SELF-CARE

Diabetes self-care is also about managing your overall health, which has an impact on your diabetes.

Losing Excess Weight

Statistics from 2004 from the Canadian Community Health Survey (CCHS) noted that 23.1 percent of Canadians aged 18 or older, an estimated 5.5 million adults, had a body mass index (BMI) of 30 or more, indicating that they were obese. Excess weight in a diabetic can further complicate his or her health in numerous ways, and losing the weight is very important. If you adjust the carbohydrates and fats you're eating according to the guidance provided in chapters 7 and 8, and incorporate exercise into your routine, you'll lose weight. Weight loss can greatly improve your body's ability to use insulin. There is no need to start a crash diet or panic about your weight, however. Eating the right foods at the right times will result in weight loss. Weight loss will become a fringe benefit. As you lose weight, your blood sugar levels will drop, which may affect any diabetes medication you're on. For example, if you're taking pills that stimulate your body to make insulin and if you don't adjust your dosage to your weight loss, you may experience hypoglycemia (low blood sugar, discussed in Chapter 14). Weight loss will also decrease the odds of developing complications from diabetes, such as heart disease. Studies show that a target weight loss of just 5 percent of your body weight can dramatically reduce the odds of developing diabetes complications. For more information on weight loss, see chapters 7, 8, and 11. For more on complications, see Part 3.

Watching Highs and Lows

Once you begin meal planning and exercising, your body will operate more efficiently, which could mean that your blood sugar levels might be too low, especially if you're taking an oral hypoglycemic agent.

A blood sugar level less than 3.5 mmol/L is too low. Immediately ingesting sugar in the form of juice, candy, or a sweet soft drink will raise your sugar to normal levels again. In addition, if you're taking insulin, it will be some time before you get good at it, and you may also suffer from a low. For this reason, I devote all of Chapter 14 to hypoglycemia, which will explain what happens during a low, what to do when it occurs, and how to avoid it in the future.

Management errors can cause high blood sugar (hyperglycemia) as well, which will cause all the classic diabetes symptoms discussed in Chapter 2. Early signs of high blood sugar are extreme thirst, dry and flushed skin, mood swings, or unusual fatigue, but many people notice no symptoms at all.

Common reasons for a change in blood sugar levels are:

- overeating, or eating more than usual
- eating less than is in your usual meal plan
- a change in exercise routine
- missing a medication dose or an insulin shot (if you're taking insulin)
- an out-of-the-ordinary event (illness, stress, upset, excitement)
- a sudden mood change (extreme fright, anger, or sadness)
- pregnancy

In response to unusual strains or stress, your body taps into its stored glucose supplies for extra energy. This will raise your blood sugar level as more glucose than usual is released into your system. Whether you're fighting off a flu or fighting with your mother, digesting all that food you ate at that all-you-can-eat buffet, or running away from a black bear, your body will try to give you the extra boost of energy you need to get through your immediate stress.

A Word about Ketones

When blood sugar levels are excessively high, the body tries to get energy from other things: fat and muscle. Ketones (ketoic acid) are the by-product when the body breaks down fat or muscle. The body tries to get rid of them through the kidneys by flushing them into the urine. High ketones, along with high blood glucose, cause *diabetic ketoacidosis* (DKA), which results in an emergency.

Symptoms of DKA can include:

- Frequent urination or frequent thirst for a day or more
- Fatigue
- Nausea and vomiting
- Muscular stiffness or aching
- Mental stupor that may progress to coma
- Rapid breathing
- Fruity breath odour

Additional symptoms that may be associated with DKA are: headache, decreased consciousness, breathing difficulty while lying down, and low blood pressure.

It's rare for people with Type 2 diabetes to develop ketoacidosis unless they are under severe stress. However, the Guidelines do recommend ketone testing for individuals with Type 2 diabetes during periods of acute illness accompanied by elevated blood glucose (BG) when pre-prandial BG levels remain elevated (>14.0 mmol/L) or when DKA symptoms, such as those listed above, are present.

Just be aware of the signs of DKA, and if you're concerned about your risk for DKA, discuss it with your doctor.

Adjusting Your Routine When You're Sick

If you have Type 2 diabetes, it's important to call your doctor whenever you're sick with even just a cold or flu. Fighting off even the common viruses will elevate your blood sugar levels and will require some juggling of your regular routine until you get the hang of it yourself.

Until you can get in to see your doctor, stay on your meal plan. If that's not possible, drink about a half a cup of calorie-free fluid (could be water or calorie-free diet soda), alternating with half a cup of calorie-containing fluid (such as juice or broth) every hour you are awake. Over-the-counter medications may alter your blood sugar levels unless they are sugar-free. You should also test your blood sugar every four hours when you're ill to accommodate higher blood sugar levels, especially if there is vomiting or diarrhea. If you're taking any medication, stick to your usual plan and take it as prescribed at the usual times.

You may need to go on insulin temporarily if your blood sugar levels remain high. This would not be the case with a cold, but may be necessary if you have a flu. The Canadian Diabetes Association advises that anyone with diabetes consider having a flu shot once a year, as well as being immunized for pneumococcus. (This bacterial infection can cause both meningitis and pneumonia.)

When you're not ill, but you have an unusually high blood sugar reading at any time of day (over 11 mmol/L), it's time to see your doctor, too.

YOUR DIABETES HEALTH DIARY

One of the best ways to care for yourself is to keep a health diary, in which you record any unusual symptoms, and the times and dates those symptoms occur. Without your diary or health record, your doctors could be working in the dark and may not be able to design the right therapy program for you.

What Your Health Diary Should Record

The most important information your health diary will contain is the pattern of your blood sugar's peaks and valleys. Dates and times of these peaks and valleys may be important clues to establish the pattern. Your meal plan, exercise routine, and medication regimen should be tailored to anticipate these peaks and valleys. You may need to incorporate a snack to prevent a low, or go for a 20-minute walk after dinner to prevent a high. Since there are a variety of factors that can affect your blood sugar levels, your diary should also record the following:

- any medication you're taking
- unusually high or low readings that fall outside your pattern

- stressful life events or situations
- illness
- out-of-the-ordinary events (no matter how insignificant)
- changes in your health insurance or status
- severe insulin reactions (if you're taking insulin)
- general medical history (surgeries, tests you've had done, allergies, past drug reactions)

Know Your Drugs

If you're taking other prescription drugs, make sure you let your doctor know. Many prescription drugs can affect (raise or lower) blood sugar levels. Ask your pharmacist about all your prescription drugs, and ask whether any will affect other medications you're taking or your blood sugar levels.

One of the most important tools to self-care is understanding your medications. There's a lot to know, so the next chapter should be your next stop, whether you're taking oral hypoglycemic agents or oral anti-diabetic agents.

6

DIABETES MEDICATIONS

A great many people with Type 2 diabetes are unable to make the necessary lifestyle changes to keep their diabetes under control. The Canadian Diabetes Association recommends that if your blood sugar or glycemic targets are not achieved within two to three months after you've tried to alter your lifestyle management, anti-hyperglycemic medications should be initiated. This does not mean you've failed to control your diabetes. As we get older, it gets harder for us to change our eating habits, while many of us are not able to incorporate enough exercise or physical activity into our routines.

Today there are pills to help you manage your diabetes if the lifestyle changes you've made aren't doing the trick. Going on diabetes medication is in no way a cure-all; taking a pill will help you stay as healthy as possible in the event that you cannot or will not make the necessary lifestyle changes.

There are several kinds of medications that may be prescribed for you. It's crucial to note, however, that the medications discussed in this chapter can be prescribed only for people with Type 2 diabetes; this chapter does not address medication for anyone with Type 1 diabetes.

WHEN YOUR DOCTOR TELLS YOU TO TAKE A PILL

When diet and lifestyle changes make no impact on your blood sugar levels, you may be prescribed pills. Before you fill your prescription for oral diabetes medications, you should know that between

40 and 50 percent of all people with Type 2 diabetes require insulin therapy after 10 years. Continuing insulin resistance may cause you to stop responding to oral medications. Furthermore, these pills are meant to complement your meal plan, exercise routine, and glucose monitoring; they are not a substitute.

Bear in mind, too, that physicians who prescribe the medications discussed in this section without also working with you to modify your diet and lifestyle are not managing your diabetes properly. These medications should be prescribed only after you've been unsuccessful in managing your Type 2 diabetes through lifestyle modification and frequent blood sugar testing.

If you cannot get down to a healthy body weight, you are probably a good candidate for anti-diabetic medication. And anyone with Type 2 diabetes who cannot control his or her blood sugar levels *despite* lifestyle changes is also a good candidate.

Anti-hyperglycemic Agents

The term "anti-hyperglycemic agents" means "pills for high blood sugar." (These were formerly known as oral hypoglycemic agents, or OHAs.) There are several different types of anti-hyperglycemic agents. This section provides a general description of each class of oral anti-hyperglycemic agent used in Canada as of this writing; they are described in the order they are usually prescribed. *Note:* In some diabetes literature, the terms "anti-diabetic agents" or "anti-diabetic pills" are used; these terms refer to the list of medications provided in this section. The 2008 CDA Guidelines use the term "anti-hyperglycemic agents." There may be other terms used in the medical literature, but for the purposes of consistency in this book, this is what we will call the drugs used for lowering blood glucose levels.

Biguanides

Biguanides (metformin) are pills that help your insulin work better. This medication primarily stops your liver from producing glucose, and thus helps lower your blood sugar levels and increase glucose uptake by your muscle tissue. These pills also help your tissues respond better to your insulin. Metformin is generally well tolerated, is widely available, and is relatively inexpensive. The American Diabetes Association has recommended that metformin be initiated alongside lifestyle intervention at the time of diagnosis of Type 2 diabetes. This medication also seems to lower the "bad cholesterol" levels. These pills do not increase insulin levels and will not directly cause low blood sugar. A biguanide is appropriate for people who are obese and have milder levels of high blood sugar. That's because biguanides do not result in weight gain, which is typically associated with sulfonylureas (see below) and insulin therapy. The CDA's recommendation is to use metformin, despite potential gastrointestinal side effects, as the first medication, based on its effectiveness in lowering blood glucose, its relatively mild side effect profile, and its demonstrated benefit in overweight patients. Both the American and Canadian guidelines seem to be similar regarding the prescribing of metformin as a first-line therapy.

Biguanides should never be taken under the following conditions:

- alcoholism
- pregnancy
- kidney or liver failure

About one-third of all people taking this drug will experience gastrointestinal side effects (no appetite, nausea, abdominal discomfort, diarrhea). Adjusting dosages and taking your pills with your meals or afterward often clears up these symptoms. Biguanides are frequently prescribed in combination with any of the medications discussed further on, including insulin (see page 86).

Insulin Sensitizers

This class of drug is comprised of thiazoladinediones (TZDs), which are pills that make your cells more sensitive to insulin, thereby improving insulin resistance. When this happens, more glucose gets into your tissues, and less glucose stays in your blood. The result is that you'll have lower fasting blood glucose levels without the need to increase insulin levels. Both rosiglitazone (Avandia) and pioglitazone (Actos) work by stimulating muscle tissue to take in glucose. They also decrease glucose production from the liver and make fat tissue more receptive to glucose. The section further on (page 79) discusses some medical risks associated with Avandia, in particular.

The first generation of this drug, troglitazone (Rezulin), was released in 1997 and withdrawn from the market in March 2000 by its makers, Warner-Lambert Company, due to liver damage (hepatoxicity) in patients on the drug. Avandia and Actos, released in Canada in 2000, are very similar in chemical structure to troglitazone, but seem to have a much lower risk of liver damage than troglitazone. However, Avandia had other issues, noted on page 79. Nevertheless, it's very important to ask your doctor about the risks of either drug if they are prescribed. If you've ever had hepatitis (A, B, or C), you should not take this drug. A number of other factors in your history may prevent you from being on the drug, which you must discuss with your doctor. Trials with troglitazone showed that people with cardiovascular problems or who were immune-suppressed for any reason should not be on it. Therefore, please discuss the risks of Avandia or Actos if you have cardiovascular problems or are immune-suppressed, since the chemical structure of these drugs is similar to troglitazone. This drug may be prescribed with either biguanides as a combination therapy, or with biguanides and a sulfonylurea (see further) in a "triple therapy" cocktail.

Combination therapy with biguanides is so popular, in fact, that a new pill has been designed that mixes rosiglitazone and metformin, available in Canada by the brand name Avandamet. There is also Avandaryl, which is a mix of rosiglitazone and glimepiride. As with all of these medications, both on their own and in combined formulations, you should have a discussion with your doctor about which singular or combination therapy could work best for your diabetes.

The Latest Buzz on TZDs

The Canadian Diabetes Association strongly urges that all patients prescribed Actos or Avandia consult with their doctors about the safety of these medications. Here's what we know about TZDs as of this writing:

- They have a longer duration of glycemic control alone compared to metformin or glyburide (you need to be on this for six to 12 weeks to really see effects).
- They seem to help lower blood pressure.
- They don't lead to weight gain (waist-to-hip ratio not increased).

Now for the bad news:

- They may induce edema and/or heart failure.
- They should be avoided in anyone with heart failure.
- There are higher rates of heart failure when combined with insulin, but this is *not* an approved combination of drugs in Canada.
- They may lead to the rare occurrence of macular edema.
- They may lead to more fractures in women (see Chapter 13).

Special Problems with Avandia

Cardiovascular problems have been particularly observed with Avandia. The newest research available suggests that there are further complications to note about rosiglitazone (Avandia). In a November 2008 editorial in the journal *Lancet*, it was noted that Avandia was no longer recommended. For the first time, the American Diabetes Association (ADA) and the European Association for the Study of Diabetes (EASD) have issued guidelines that explicitly advise against the use of Avandia (rosiglitazone) for Type 2 diabetes. This is because further concerns about TZDs were raised this year when the ACCORD trial was terminated early after patients in the intensive-treatment arm (91 percent of whom received rosiglitazone) were at significantly increased risk of death, specifically from cardiovascular disease. As of October 2008, the consensus is to recommend Actos (pioglitazone) as a third-line treatment, but not Avandia. Since alternative effective options are available, the expert panel rightly felt that a drug with rosiglitazone's safety profile could no longer be advocated.

In a January 2009 issue of the *Canadian Medical Association Journal*, other problems were recognized with Avandia related to a 45 percent increase in fractures in women. Use of thiazolidinedione was also associated with significant bone loss. It's believed that for every 55 women at low risk of fracture who take TZDs for one year, one fracture would occur. Among women at high risk, one fracture would occur for every 21 women who take thiazolidinedione for one year. Essentially, TZDs may be associated with a higher risk of fracture in women with Type 2 diabetes. (See Chapter 13 for more information on osteoporosis and fracture prevention.)

Until further evidence of their net benefit is available, the appropriate role for these drugs is unclear.

Clinical drug trials are often underpowered to detect unanticipated and rare adverse effects, and a standardized post-marketing surveillance process is needed.

Who Should Take TZDs

If you have tried other therapies that have failed, there may be a role for TZDs, but the experts agree that the risks may outweigh the benefits. If you're considering a TZD, pioglitazone (Actos) has been shown to increase the risk of cardiovascular problems, and is the preferred option. Anyone considering these medications, however, needs to have an in-depth consultation with his or her doctor to discuss the latest risks and potential benefits.

Insulin Secretagogues

These are pills that help your pancreas release more insulin. The most commonly prescribed insulin secretagogues are sulfonylureas. The sulfonylureas available in Canada are gliclazide (Diamicron, Diamicron MR, generic), glimepiride (Amaryl), and glyburide (Diabeta, Euglucon, generic). Older generations of sulfonylureas that are still available but rarely used include chlorpropamide and tolbutamide. Short-acting insulin secretagogues, also called meglitinides in the 2008 CDA Guidelines, are available in Canada as repaglinide (GlucoNorm) and nateglinide (Starlix).

Here's what's currently known about insulin secretagogues:

- They lead to a relatively rapid lowering of your blood glucose level.
- Nateglinide is not as effective as other meglitinides.

- Post-prandial (post-meal) blood sugar is especially reduced by nateglinide and repaglinide.
- Hypoglycemia and weight gain are especially common with glyburide.
- People who are elderly or in renal/hepatic failure should not be on this class of drug, but if there isn't an alternative, glicazide is the most tolerated in this situation.
- Nateglinide and repaglinide are associated with less hypoglycemia in the context of missed meals.

Alpha-glucosidase Inhibitor (Acarbose)

Introduced in 1996, these pills delay the breakdown of sugar in your meal. Acarbose was the first oral diabetes medication to be introduced since the introduction of sulfonylureas and biguanides in the 1950s. Acarbose goes by the brand name Glucobay (the name used internationally), which was changed from Prandase, in Canada and is very similar in structure to the sugars found in foods. Acarbose reduces high blood sugar levels after you eat. Glucose, the main sugar in blood, is a simple sugar that is made from starch and sucrose (table sugar). Starch and sucrose are turned into glucose by enzymes in the lining of the small intestine called alpha-glucosidase. Acarbose stalls this process by forcing the starch and sugar you eat to "take a number" before they're converted into glucose. This slows down the absorption of glucose into the cells, preventing a rise in blood glucose after a meal, but in order to work, acarbose must be taken with the first bite of each main meal. You'll also need to test your blood sugar two hours after eating to see how well you're responding to the medication. Research is underway to determine if acarbose can be used worldwide as a preventive for people with impaired glucose tolerance (IGT).

Acarbose is prescribed for people who cannot seem to get their after-meal (that is, post-meal or post-prandial) blood sugar levels down to acceptable levels. A major benefit of acarbose is that it may reduce the risk of hypoglycemic episodes during the night, particularly in insulin users. Investigators are studying whether acarbose may be used one day as a substitute for that "morning insulin." The usual rules apply here: Acarbose should complement your meal plan and exercise routine; it is not a substitute or way out and does not, by itself, cause hypoglycemia.

Who Should Take Acarbose?

- Anyone who cannot control his or her blood sugar through diet and lifestyle modification alone
- Anyone who is on an insulin secretagogue, but is still experiencing high blood sugar levels after meals
- Anyone who cannot take any other type of anti-hyperglycemic agent, and for whom diet and lifestyle modifications have failed
- Anyone who is not doing well on his or her current anti-hyperglycemic medication, but who wants to avoid starting insulin treatment

Who Should Not Take Acarbose?

Anyone with the following conditions should not be taking this drug:

- inflammation or ulceration of the bowel (that is, inflammatory bowel disease, ulcerative colitis, or Crohn's disease)
- any kind of bowel obstruction
- any gastrointestinal disease
- kidney or liver disorders
- hernias
- pregnancy or lactation
- Type 1 diabetes

For best results, it's crucial that you take acarbose with the first bite of each main meal. In fact, if you swallow your pill even five to 10 minutes before a meal, acarbose will pass through your digestive system and have no effect. It's also important that you take acarbose with a carbohydrate; the medication doesn't work if there are no carbohydrates in your meal. You shouldn't take acarbose between meals either because it won't work. Also, acarbose should not be used as a weight-loss drug.

Side Effects

The good news is that acarbose doesn't cause hypoglycemia. However, since you may be taking this drug along with an insulin secretagogue, you may still experience hypoglycemia as acarbose doesn't prevent it either. (See the section "Recognizing the Symptoms" in Chapter 14 for warning signs and treatment for hypoglycemia.)

The only side effects that acarbose causes are gastrointestinal: gas, abdominal cramps, softer stools, or diarrhea. Acarbose, combined with metformin, can produce unacceptable gastrointestinal symptoms. You'll notice these side effects after you've consumed foods that contain lots of sugar. Avoid taking antacids; they won't be effective in this case. Adjusting the dosage and making sure you're taking acarbose correctly will usually take care of the side effects.

As of this writing, here's the latest on Acarbose:

- This is not recommended as an initial therapy in people with marked hyperglycemia (A1C ≥ 9.0 percent).
- This is ideal as a combination therapy with other anti-hyperglycemic agents.
- Acarbose doesn't cause weight gain or weight loss.
- There are gastrointestinal side effects to take into consideration.

COMING SOON TO CANADA: WHAT'S HOT IN THE US

There are new classes of drugs coming onto the scene that are being used in diabetes management outside of Canada. Currently, the following drugs are not yet recommended by the CDA, but probably will be soon. Here's what to watch out for:

Incretin-Based Injectable Therapies

In 2005, two new diabetes medications—exenatide (brand name Byetta) and pramlintide (Symlin)—became available. Both work differently from any previously approved diabetes drugs. Both are known as incretin-based therapies because they imitate natural hormones called incretins.

Exenatide

Exenatide (Byetta) is the first in a new class of drugs for the treatment of Type 2 diabetes known as incretin-based therapies, or GLP-1 analogue (aka GLP-1 receptor agonists). Glucagon-like peptide 1 (GLP-1) is an incretin hormone released by the gastrointestinal tract in response to eating, and is a potent insulin secretagogue. GLP-1 stimulates insulin secretion when the blood glucose level is high. A naturally occurring hormone known as exendin-4, isolated from the saliva of a lizard known as a Gila monster, has similar activity to GLP-1. Exenatide is the synthesized form of exendin-4, and is the first FDA-approved incretin-based therapy, although many more are in development.

Exenatide lowers blood glucose levels primarily by increasing insulin secretion the way GLP-1 naturally works. Because it has this effect only in the presence of elevated blood glucose levels, it does not tend to increase the risk of hypoglycemia on its own, although hypoglycemia can occur if exenatide is taken in conjunction with a sulfonylurea. The primary side effect of exenatide is nausea, which tends to improve over time. Exenatide is injected with meals and people using exenatide have generally experienced modest weight loss as well as improved glycemic control. Exenatide has been approved for use by people with Type 2 diabetes who have not achieved their target A1C levels using metformin (see above) or a combination of metformin and a sulfonylurea. Exenatide (Byetta) is an injectible diabetes drug, but it is not yet part of any international guidelines for diabetes treatment.

Pramlintide (brand name Symlin)

Pramlintide is a synthetic amylin analog, meaning it is chemically identical to a hormone produced by the pancreas called amylin, which is produced along with insulin by the beta cells in the pancreas. Amylin, insulin, and another hormone, glucagon, work in an interrelated fashion to maintain normal blood glucose levels. Pramlintide injections taken with meals have been shown to modestly improve A1C levels without causing increased hypoglycemia or weight gain and even promoting modest weight loss. The primary side effect is nausea, which tends to improve over time and as an individual patient determines his or her optimal dose. Pramlintide helps to reduce the rise in blood glucose after meals in the following ways:

- It slows the speed with which food leaves the stomach.
- It suppresses the secretion of glucagon after meals, which decreases the amount of glucose released from the liver.
- It decreases appetite, so that less food is eaten. This can also lead to a small weight loss in some people.

Pramlintide is approved for use in any adult who has either Type 1 or Type 2 diabetes who cannot achieve adequate blood glucose control when using intensive insulin therapy (see further on). Again, pramlintide is not yet recommended by the Canadian Diabetes Association.

QUESTIONS TO ASK ABOUT ANY DIABETES MEDICATION

Before you fill your prescription, it's important to ask your doctor or pharmacist the following:

1. *What does this drug contain?* If you are allergic to particular ingredients, such as dyes, it's important to find out the drug's ingredients before you take it.
2. *Are there any medications I shouldn't combine with this drug?* Be sure to ask about interactions with cholesterol or hypertension medications, as well as any anti-depressants or anti-psychotics.
3. *If this drug doesn't work well, would insulin ever be prescribed along with this pill?* In cases where blood sugar remains too high in spite of medication, insulin is used in combination with an anti-hyperglycemic agent. This has become standard care, but was once controversial.
4. *How will you measure the effectiveness of my drug?* You should be testing your blood sugar with a glucose monitor, particularly two hours after eating, to make sure that the lowest effective dose can be prescribed. Your doctor should also be doing a glycosylated hemoglobin or A1C test two or three times per year (see Chapter 4).

5. *How should I store my drugs?* All pills should be kept in a dry place at a temperature between 15°C and 25°C (59°F and 77°F). Keep these drugs away from children, don't give them out as "samples" to your sister-in-law (or anyone else!), and don't use tablets beyond their expiry date.

6. *What symptoms should I watch out for while on these drugs?* You'll definitely want to watch for signs of high or low blood sugar.

WHEN YOUR DOCTOR PRESCRIBES INSULIN

Let me dispel a common fear about insulin: Since insulin is not a blood product, you don't have to worry about being infected with a blood-borne virus such as HIV or hepatitis.

Many doctors often delay insulin therapy for as long as possible by giving you maximum doses of the pills discussed above. This isn't considered good diabetes management. If you need insulin, you should take insulin. The goal is to get your disease under control. Therefore, anyone with Type 2 diabetes with the following conditions is a candidate for insulin:

- high blood sugar levels, despite maximum doses of oral hypoglycemic agents
- fasting glucose levels consistently over 9 mmol/L
- illness or stress (insulin may be needed until you recover)
- major surgery
- complications of diabetes (see Part 3)
- pregnancy (insulin may be temporary)

If going on insulin will affect your job security, you should discuss this issue with your doctor so that appropriate notes or letters can be drafted to whomever it may concern. You should also keep in mind that if insulin therapy does not bring your diabetes under control within six months of treatment, it may be necessary to return to your oral drug therapy after all.

Most people think insulin needs to be prescribed by a doctor. Doctors will prescribe insulin, but you can walk into any pharmacy, identify yourself as a person with diabetes, and get at least one dosage of insulin over the counter anywhere in Canada. This policy is designed for emergencies, since people can damage or lose insulin while travelling, and so on. Insulin is not a patentable drug, which is one reason it remains an over-the-counter product. It is also not the sort of product that people would want unless they had diabetes. By supplying it over the counter, it remains a life-giving product that is not withheld from those in need; that doesn't mean it's given out free, but it is given out *hassle-free,* without the need to reach your doctor for permission. See Table 6.1 for the types of insulin approved for use in Canada.

Table 6.1: Types of Insulin (Approved for Use in Canada)

Insulin Type/Action (appearance)	Brand Names (generic name in brackets)	Dosing Schedule
Rapid-acting analogue (clear) Onset: 10–15 minutes Peak: 60–90 minutes Duration: 3–5 hours	Apidra (insulin glulisine) Humalog (insulin lispro) NovoRapid (insulin aspart)	Usually taken right before eating, or to lower high blood glucose *Author's Note: This is the "roadrunner." It gets there fast, but disappears quickly.*
Short-acting (clear) Onset: 30 minutes Peak: 2–3 hours Duration: 6.5 hours	Humulin®-R Novolin®ge Toronto	Taken about 30 minutes before eating, or to lower high blood glucose *Author's Note: This is the "hare." It gets there fast, but tires easily.*
Intermediate-acting (cloudy) Onset: 1–3 hours Peak: 5–8 hours Duration: Up to 18 hours	Humulin®-N Novolin®ge NPH	Often taken at bedtime, or twice a day (morning and bedtime) *Author's Note: This is the "tortoise." It gets there at a slower pace, but it lasts longer.*
Long-acting analogue (clear and colourless) Onset: 90 minutes Peak: none Duration: Up to 24 hours (Lantus 24 hours, Levemir 16–24 hours)	Lantus (insulin glargine) Levemir (insulin detemir)	Usually taken once or twice a day *Author's Note: This is the "two-legged turtle." It's really slow, and it hangs around for a long time.*

(continued)

Table 6.1: (continued)

Insulin Type/Action (appearance)	Brand Names (generic name in brackets)	Dosing Schedule
Premixed (cloudy) A single vial or cartridge contains a fixed ratio of insulin (the numbers refer to the percent of rapid- or fast-acting insulin to the percent of intermediate-acting insulin)	PREMIXED REGULAR INSULIN - NPH Humulin (30/70) Novolin®ge (30/70, 40/60, 50/50) PREMIXED INSULIN ANALOGUES Humalog Mix25 and Mix50 NovoMix 30	Depends on the combination

Sources: 1. Adapted from the Canadian Diabetes Association 2008 Clinical Practice Guidelines for the Prevention and Management of Diabetes in Canada.
2. Adapted from The Canadian Type 2 Diabetes Sourcebook, 2nd Edition, 2004.

The Right Insulin

The goal of a good insulin program is to try to mimic what your pancreas would do if it were working properly. Blood sugar rises in a wave pattern. The big waves come in after a big meal; the small waves come in after a small meal or snack. The insulin program needs to be matched to your own particular wave pattern, so what you eat—and when—has a lot to do with the right insulin program. Therefore, the right insulin for someone who eats three square meals a day may not be appropriate for someone who tends to graze all day. And the right insulin for an active 47-year-old man in a stressful job may not be the right insulin for a 67-year-old woman who does not work and whose heart condition prevents her from exercising regularly.

You and your health care team will also need to decide how much control you need over your blood sugar. Insulin "recipes" depend on whether you need tight control (4–6 mmol/L), medium control (6–10 mmol/L), or even loose control (11–13 mmol/L). Loose control is certainly not encouraged, but on rare occasions, when a person is perhaps quite elderly and suffering from a number of other health problems, it is still a goal that is discussed. To determine the appropriate insulin recipe for you, your health care team should look at who you are as a person—what you eat, where you work (do you work shifts?), your willingness to change your eating habits, and other lifestyle factors.

There are many kinds of insulins available. Every manufacturer has a different brand name of insulin and a separate letter code for the insulin action. Refer to Table 6.1 on page 87. Once you and your diabetes health care team choose the right insulin for you, you will need to have a mini-course on how to use and inject insulin. This is usually done by a certified diabetes educator (CDE).

Insulin Brands

As you can see, insulin is highly individualized. It's simply not possible for me to tell you in this book which insulin you need to be on any more than I can tell you what, exactly, you need to eat each day. This is why a diabetes health care team, discussed in Chapter 4, is so crucial. Your meal plans, medications, and insulin (when needed) are tailored to suit *you*, and that has everything to do with who you are, not which brand of insulin is popular. The following is a description of what's available as of this writing.

Human Insulin

All human insulin is biosynthetic, which means that the biochemically created product normally made by the human pancreas has been recreated in a test tube through DNA technology.

Today, most manufacturers produce only these insulins, which are considered the purest form of insulin available. Human insulins come in four different actions: immediate-acting, short-acting (clear fluid), intermediate-acting (cloudy fluid), and long-acting (cloudy fluid). Short-acting means that it stays in your body for the shortest duration of time; long-acting means that it stays in your body for the longest duration of time. See Table 6.1: Types of Insulin, for details.

Insulin Analogues

These are synthetic insulins that do not have an animal or human source. With traditional human insulins, you need to be extremely good at calculating when you're going to eat, how much you're going to eat, and how much insulin to inject. Basically, you need to be in excellent control of your diabetes. The problem with traditional, longer-acting insulin is that you can wind up with too much of it in your system, which can cause insulin shock or hypoglycemia (low blood sugar; see Chapter 14). Insulin lispro (Humalog) and insulin aspart (NovoRapid in Canada and Novolog in the US) are immediate-acting insulins, which means that you inject them about 15 minutes before you eat (while you're cooking dinner or when ordering food in a restaurant). Therefore, some experts consider these easier insulins to work with. A "slowest-acting" insulin analog, called glargine (Lantus), is available in the US. The benefit of glargine over human long-acting insulin is that it starts working in two hours, it has no peak, and it has a duration of 18–24 hours. That means you can eat at any time after injecting it.

Premixed Insulin

Premixed insulin means that both the short-acting insulin and the intermediate-acting insulin are mixed together. These are extremely popular insulins for people with Type 2 diabetes. They work well for people who have a very set routine and don't want to take more than one or two insulin injections daily.

Premixed insulins are labelled as 10/90 (10 percent short-acting; 90 percent intermediate-acting), 20/80, 30/70, 40/60, and 50/50. Premixed insulin is always cloudy. It's also possible to mix together short-acting with long-acting, or long-acting with intermediate-acting.

A Word about Beef/Pork Insulin

As new diabetes-related drugs are developed and marketed, manufacturers are correspondingly discontinuing old product lines. (For example, with the introduction of human/genetic insulin, the production of most animal insulin was discontinued.) Beef-pork insulins are no longer marketed worldwide. However, Hypurin Beef insulin is available to Canadians from Wockhardt UK Ltd. via Health Canada's Special

Access Program (SAP). Wockhardt UK will now have a licensed importer/distributor in Canada to distribute the pork insulins and that may facilitate access of beef insulin to patients who use the Special Access Program. For more information on the Special Access Program, please visit their website
(http://www.hc-sc.gc.ca/dhp-mps/acces/drugs-drogues/index-eng.php).

Learning to Use Insulin

Insulin must be injected. It cannot be taken orally because your own stomach acids digest the insulin before it has a chance to work. Your doctor or a registered nurse (frequently a CDE is a registered nurse, too) will teach you how to inject yourself painlessly. Don't inject insulin by yourself without a training session. One convenient way to use insulin is with an insulin pen, but not all insulin can be used with the pen. If you use the pen, your insulin (if human or biosynthetic) will come in a cartridge. If you are not using a pen, your insulin will come in a bottle and you will need a needle and syringe. Always know the answers to these questions before you inject your insulin:

1. How long does it take before the insulin starts to work? (Known as the *onset of action.*)
2. When is this insulin working the hardest? (Known as *the peak.*)
3. How long will my insulin continue to work? (Known as the *duration of action.*)

How Many Injections Will I Need?

This really depends on what kind of insulin you're taking and why you're taking it. A sample routine may be to take an injection in the morning, a second injection before supper, and a third before bed. What you want to prevent is low blood sugar while you're sleeping. You may need to adjust your insulin if there is a change in your food or exercise routine, which could happen if you're sick. Your insulin schedule is usually carefully matched to your mealtimes and exercise periods.

Where to Inject It

The good news is that you do not have to inject insulin into a vein. As long as it makes it under your skin (but *not* in your muscle), you're fine. This is called a subcutaneous injection. Thighs and tummies are popular injection sites. These areas are also large enough that you can vary your injection site. (You should space your injections 2–3 cm apart.) Usually you establish a rotating pattern. Other injection sites are the upper outer area of the arms, the upper outer surfaces of the buttocks, and the lower back area. Insulin injected in the abdomen is absorbed more quickly than insulin injected in the thigh. In addition, strenuous exercise will speed up the rate of absorption of insulin if the insulin is injected into the limb you've just worked out. Other factors that can affect insulin's action are the depth of injection, your dose, the temperature (it should be room temperature or body temperature), and what animal your insulin came from (human or pig). A hardening of skin due to overuse will affect the rate of absorption. Your doctor or CDE will show you how to inject your insulin (angles, pinching folds of skin, and so on). There are lots of tricks of the trade to optimize comfort. With the fine needle points available today, injection doesn't have to be an uncomfortable ordeal. The needle length also affects the absorption rate; the longer the needle, the deeper it goes, and the faster it's absorbed. With shorter needle lengths, patient advocates with diabetes recommend leaving the needle in for about five seconds to increase the rate of absorption.

Side Effects

The main side effect of insulin therapy is low blood sugar, which means that you must eat or drink glucose to combat symptoms. This side effect is also known as insulin shock. Low blood sugar or hypoglycemia is discussed in Chapter 14. Additionally, when you use insulin to lower your blood sugar, the sugar in your bloodstream enters cells in your body instead of being excreted in your urine. Your body converts the sugar your cells don't use for energy into fat, which can lead to weight gain. To limit weight gain, closely follow your exercise and diet regimen. (See chapters 7, 8, 9, and 11.)

Questions to Ask about Insulin

The answers to the following questions will depend on your insulin brand. Pharmacists and doctors should know the answers to all these questions, but if they don't, call the customer care 1-800 number provided by your insulin manufacturer.

- How do I store this insulin?
- What are the characteristics of this insulin (that is, onset of action, peak, and duration of action)?
- When should I eat after injecting this insulin?
- When should I exercise after injecting this insulin?
- How long are opened insulin bottles or cartridges safe at room temperature?
- What about the effect of sunlight or extreme temperatures on this insulin?
- Should this insulin be shaken or rolled?
- What should I do if the insulin sticks to the inside of the vial or cartridge?
- Should this insulin be clear or cloudy? And what should I do if the appearance looks "off" or has changed?
- What happens if I accidentally inject out-of-date insulin?
- What other medications can interfere with this particular brand?
- Who should I see about switching insulin brands?
- If I've switched from animal to human insulin, what dose should I be on?

Your Insulin Gear

If you've graduated to insulin therapy, here's what you'll need to buy:

- a really good glucose monitor that is made for people who test frequently
- lancets and a lancing device for testing your blood sugar
- insulin pens and cartridges (this is far easier) or traditional needles and syringes (a diabetes educator will need to walk you through the types of products available)
- the right insulin brand for you

Air Travel with Insulin

Travelling by air gets worse every year. If you are planning to travel by air, review the latest Transport Canada and Canadian Air Transport Security Authority information about packing your supplies and what is permitted (and not permitted) in carry-on and checked baggage. First, make sure you pack identification in the form of a doctor's note, plus a MedicAlert bracelet that clearly states you have diabetes. In fact, many experts suggest that for a trip, you switch to an insulin pen, if you can. (Not all insulins work with the pen.) Transport Canada recommends that you should clearly state to all security personnel that you have diabetes and are carrying your supplies on board. Have your letter and MedicAlert bracelet or card ready for security to inspect.

Next, organize your supplies in your carry-on luggage so that they are easy to get at for security scanning. You must ensure that you have needle guards in place, and your needles must be accompanied by the insulin in order for you to pass through security. Your insulin and other diabetes medications must be in a container with professionally printed label from your pharmacy, clearly identifying what it is. If the pharmacy places its label on the outside of the box containing the insulin, the insulin must be carried in the original packaging. All lancets must be capped and must be accompanied by a glucose meter that has the manufacturer's name imprinted on the meter. Prior to travelling outside of the country, contact the airlines and find out what precautions they require in order for you to pass through security with your supplies.

Advice from the Transportation Safety Association

The Transportation Safety Association (TSA) makes the following recommendations to airline passengers with diabetes.

- Before you go through security, notify the screener that you have diabetes and are carrying your supplies with you.
- Insulin and insulin-loaded dispensing products (vials or box of individual vials, jet injectors, pens, infusers, and preloaded

syringes) must be clearly identified with a prescription label containing a name that matches the passenger's name on his or her ticket.

- Other liquid prescription medicines must be clearly identified with a prescription label containing a name that matches the passenger's name on his or her ticket.
- Essential non-prescription liquid medicines (such as regular insulin) should be clearly labelled.
- Multiple containers of liquids and gels to treat hypoglycemia can be taken on board. If containers are more than 80 mL (3 oz), then passengers need to declare these items to security checkpoint personnel.
- You can take unlimited number of unused syringes when accompanied by insulin or other injectable medication.
- Blood glucose meters, blood glucose meter test strips, continuous blood glucose monitors, lancets, alcohol swabs, meter-testing solutions, and monitor supplies can all be taken on board.
- Insulin pump and insulin pump supplies (cleaning agents, batteries, plastic tubing, infusion kit, catheter, and needle) can all be taken on board.
- Urine ketone test strips can be taken on board.
- Unlimited number of used syringes when transported in Sharps disposal container or other similar hard-surface container can be taken on board.

Other Things to Keep in Mind

Security scanners used at check-in will not normally damage your insulin or blood glucose meter. If baggage remains in the path of the X-ray for longer than normal, or if the baggage is repeatedly X-rayed, the insulin may lose potency. Insulin is affected by extreme temperatures and should never be stored in the unpressurized baggage area of the aircraft. As always, it is important to inspect your insulin before injecting each dose. If you notice anything unusual about the appearance of your insulin, or notice that your insulin needs are changing, contact your doctor.

If you use an insulin pump, notify the screening officer in advance, as the walk-through metal detector and the hand-held metal detector may affect the functioning of an insulin pump, so you can ask the screening officer to perform a physical search in a private location.

Try to do some form of activity during your journey: walk around in the terminal before boarding, consider doing simple stretching exercises in your seat, or move your ankles in circles and raise your legs occasionally.

The American Diabetes Association (ADA) (www.diabetes.org) offers the following interesting tips:

- Learn to say "I have diabetes" and "Sugar or orange juice, please" in the language or languages of the countries you'll visit.
- Note that the prescription laws may be very different in other countries. If you're going out of the country, write for a list of International Diabetes Federation groups by visiting their website (www.idf.org).
- Before you leave, get a list of English-speaking foreign doctors from the International Association for Medical Assistance to Travelers (IAMAT) (www.iamat.org).

Food and Meals while Travelling by Air

Airlines usually offer special meals for people with diabetes, but most often the regular airline meals are not on flights shorter than four hours, while the snacks offered on many flights are highly variable and not appropriate for people with diabetes. You will need to bring all your food with you. Even if you're planning a short trip, always have appropriate snacks with you in case your flight or in-flight meal is delayed, or the meal provided does not have enough carbohydrates. Be aware of time zone changes, and schedule your meals and medication accordingly. If you choose to sleep while travelling by air, use a travel alarm clock or ask the flight attendant to wake you at meal or medication time.

The Traveller's Checklist

Before you leave, remember to get:
- a medical checkup
- travel health insurance from the Canadian Diabetes Association
- an identification card and MedicAlert bracelet or necklace
- information on the local foods and drinking water
- a list of your medications
- a letter from your doctor
- any needed vaccinations
- information on local medical facilities or organizations

Ask your doctor or health care team about:
- illness management
- hypoglycemia management (glucagon for insulin users)
- adjustments for meals, insulin, and medications in different time zones
- avoiding illness caused by contaminated food and water
- tips for adjusting your medication if required

Packing list:
- extra supply of insulin or oral agent for diabetes
- extra supply of syringes, needles, and an extra insulin pen if used*
- blood glucose testing kit and logbook
- fast-acting insulin for high blood glucose and ketones*
- fast-acting sugar to treat low blood glucose
- extra food to cover delayed meals such as a box of cookies or crackers and fruit juice
- urine ketone-testing strips*
- anti-nausea and anti-diarrhea pills
- pain medication
- sunblock
- insect repellent
- large amounts of bottled water, if necessary
- comfortable walking shoes
- glucagon*
- telephone numbers of your doctor and diabetes educator
- supplies for the trip home in case you run into any problems

* Supplies for insulin users
Source: The Canadian Diabetes Association, 2008.

7

CARBOHYDRATES AND LOW GLYCEMIC INDEX EATING

When you're diagnosed with Type 2 diabetes, there are three things to remember with respect to your diet: First, you need to reconsider the kind of carbohydrates you're eating. Only carbohydrates directly influence blood sugar levels, but excess carbohydrates are stored as fat. Second, you need to reconsider the types of fats you're eating as these foods influence your weight, cholesterol, and triglyceride levels. It is the types of fats in foods that can cause you to have high cholesterol levels. Finally, you should consider the sodium content of foods as sodium can increase your blood pressure. If sodium is a major concern, the DASH diet, discussed in Chapter 2, can be reviewed.

There is only one diet you need to follow that will keep all three of these things in check: a healthy diet that is based on the principles of a low glycemic index (GI) diet and a "good fats" diet, which is based on the principles of a low-fat diet and a Mediterranean diet. This chapter focuses on the carbohydrates in your diet and low glycemic eating. Chapter 8 addresses the "good fats" diet. Diets that provide more than 60 percent of total daily energy from low glycemic index and high-fibre carbohydrates are considered the optimal diet for people with diabetes.

THE CARBOHYDRATE-DIABETES CONNECTION

Before the discovery of insulin in 1921, people with diabetes went on the Allen diet, a very low-calorie diet that required low quantities of carbohydrates, followed by exercise. Dr. Frederick Madison Allen, a leading diabetologist who spent four years working with diabetic patients at the Rockefeller Institute in New York City, published a 600-plus-page paper in 1919 called "Total Dietary Regulation in the Treatment of Diabetes." Allen's work showed that diabetes was largely a problem of carbohydrate metabolism. Allen and his predecessors understood something central to diabetes meal planning: *Carbohydrates were key*, and they are. Allen recognized the ability of carbohydrates to convert into glucose. The timing of this glucose conversion will affect how quickly and how high the blood glucose level rises after eating.

What Food Does

To live, you need three basic types of foods: carbohydrates, protein, and fat. Carbohydrates are the main source of fuel for muscles. Protein is the cell food that helps cells grow and repair themselves. Fat is a crucial nutrient that can be burned as an alternative fuel in times of hunger or famine. Simple sugars that do not contain any fat will convert quickly into energy or be stored as fat. Your body will change carbohydrates into glucose for energy. If you eat more carbohydrates than you can burn, your body will turn the extra into fat. The protein your body makes comes from the protein you eat. As for fats, they are not broken down into glucose and are usually stored as fat. The problem with fatty foods is that they have double the calories per gram compared with carbohydrates and protein, so you wind up gaining weight. Too much saturated fat can increase your risk of developing cardiovascular problems. What we also know is that the rate at which glucose is absorbed by your body from starch and sugars is affected by other parts of your meal, such as the protein, fibre, and fat. If you're eating only carbohydrates and no protein or fat, for example, your blood sugar will go up faster.

Low Fat versus Low Carb

A diet is considered low fat when it restricts calories from fat to less than 30 percent of daily totals. There are dozens of established low-fat diets on the market, but they vary from extremely low-fat diets, which restrict calories from fat to about 10 percent, to more moderate low-fat diets, which restrict calories from fat to 15–30 percent. Very low-fat diets (restricting calories from fat to 7–10 percent) are modelled after the originators of the very low–fat diet as we know it today—Nathan Pritikin, who popularized low-fat eating in the 1950s, and Dean Ornish, who reframed the original Pritikin diet in the late 1970s. Ornish- and Pritikin-styled diets remain the most well-known and most effective diets for people who are extremely obese and at high risk of dying from an obesity-related health problem, *but they are generally too restrictive for people with Type 2 diabetes*. The Center for Science in the Public Interest rated a number of diets for the masses in 2000. Very low-fat diets such as Pritikin's and Ornish's were actually found to be acceptable, but were found to restrict some healthy foods, such as seafood, low-fat poultry, and calcium. For people with high triglycerides, it was suggested that they cut out some carbohydrates and replace them with unsaturated fats.

The main problem with *very* low-fat diets (7–10 percent calories from fat) is that they are too restrictive for the general public because they are extremely difficult to stick to unless you are very knowledgeable about low-fat cuisine and are a creative chef. Also, new information about the benefits of monounsaturated fats and omega-3 fatty acids (the "good fats") has caused nutritionists to rethink the rules governing fat in the diet. In the 1970s and 1980s, the limitations of the very low-fat diet (which was never intended for the masses, but as heart disease therapy) led people to gorge on "bad carbs" (meaning carbs that are high on the glycemic index) because they were led to believe that so long as a food was "fat-free," it was healthy. Also, too few calories from fat left people hungry and craving food. Unfortunately, the huge consumption of carbs, which peaked in the 1980s and early 1990s, led to a sharp increase in insulin resistance from carbohydrate overload in the diet.

Then came the diet backlash: the low-carb diet, or the Atkins diet. Low-carbohydrate diets are the opposite of low-fat diets; they restrict carbohydrates (which a healthy diet ought to be based on) to about 5 percent, and encourage mostly high-fat foods—the more saturated fat, the better. These diets are also known as high-protein diets, and in clinical circles *ketogenic diets* because they trigger ketosis, discussed on page

70, which, in the non-diabetic population, occurs when the insulin hormone is shut down, forcing the liver to produce ketone bodies. People without diabetes certainly lose weight while in ketosis, but living in a state of ketosis is not exactly what nature intended for a healthy human body. *But when you do have Type 2 diabetes, living in a state of ketosis is dangerous and life-threatening, particularly since it puts tremendous strain on your kidneys.*

In addition to the dangers of ketosis, the Atkins diet can cause terrible constipation in the first phase. Also, consuming high levels of saturated fat spells disaster for people with Type 2 diabetes, especially for those with high levels of LDL. In addition, many people have a genetic condition that causes high triglycerides, which cannot be controlled through diet alone; in these people, the Atkins diet can be life-threatening (while a very low-fat diet has been shown, since the 1950s, to be life-saving) even in those without Type 2 diabetes. Other groups who are warned against following the Atkins diet are those who suffer from any disease that puts a strain on the kidneys: hypertension, cardiovascular disease, bladder infections, or bladder conditions. Of course, anyone who is pregnant should definitely stay away from this diet.

The Center for Science in the Public Interest rates the low-carbohydrate diets, such as Atkins, unacceptable in the non-diabetic population because of the high quantities of saturated fat and low quantities of fibre and essential nutrients. People become constipated; they may burn fat due to ketosis, but at the same time, they are depriving their bodies of essential nutrients, many of which are known to decrease incidences of diseases such as certain cancers. People who are loading their bodies with saturated fats known to be associated with higher rates of cancers are obviously putting themselves at risk for certain cancers.

Carbohydrates 2.0

In the past, diabetes associations were encouraging people with diabetes to count carbs in order to follow meal plans or specific types of diets in the 40/30/30 range (40 percent carbs, 30 percent protein, 30 percent fat). The CDA used to encourage people with diabetes to follow their "Food Choice Values and Symbols" (in previous editions of this book), which was used as a carb-counting tool. Dieticians provided their patients with a carb goal per meal and snack. This has become antiquated advice, and none of this is encouraged anymore. Today, it's been shown that simply following a low glycemic index diet (low GI diet) is much simpler and less confusing. Selecting from types of foods is much easier than counting carbs.

THE GLYCEMIC INDEX AND LOW GI EATING

This glycemic index, developed at the University of Toronto, measures the rate at which various foods convert to glucose, which is assigned a value of 100. Higher numbers indicate a more rapid absorption of glucose. This is not an index of food energy values or calories; some low GI foods are high in fat, while some high GI foods are low in fat.

Low GI eating emphasizes foods containing carbohydrates that break down slowly, and thus release sugar into the bloodstream slowly, keeping the blood sugar more stable. These foods are called *low GI* foods. The glycemic index (see page 116) ranks foods with a value of 0–100 according to their effect on blood sugar levels. Changes in blood sugar produced by a given food are measured against the rise in blood sugar produced by a load of sugar, or sucrose, which is 100 percent. To qualify as low GI, foods should have an index of 60 percent or less; those above 60 percent are considered high GI.

One of the important influences of a low GI diet is its effect on the body's capacity to secrete insulin. A high GI diet results in large peaks of insulin secretion by the pancreas, whereas low GI eating results in a steady secretion of insulin. This means that on a high GI diet you might experience sugar crashes where you find that after a meal, you get tired or sleepy, and then a few hours later become very hungry, resulting in the need to eat more to keep your blood sugar stable.

The obesity epidemic over the last three decades has coincided with an overall increased intake of carbohydrate-containing foods, many of which are high GI. What's made matters worse is our tendency to eat one or two large meals a day. This results in tsunami-size insulin peaks, which predispose us to weight gain, as well as a host of symptoms and side effects that are a result of excess insulin in the blood. To address these symptoms and side effects, low GI eating also calls for frequent healthy, low GI snacks to maintain steady low levels of insulin in the blood. Low GI eating will also decrease insulin levels, making it easier for your body to burn fat.

Low GI Packaged Foods

The glycemic index runs from 0–100 and usually uses pure glucose, which has a GI value of 100, as the reference. The effect other foods have on blood sugar levels are then compared with this. In simple terms, the GI index tells us whether a food raises blood sugar levels dramatically, moderately, or just a little bit. Foods that have only a slow, small effect on blood sugar have a *low GI value*, while those causing a rapid and massive rise in blood sugar have a *high GI value*. There are many books and websites that list the GI index for different foods, and I provide some tables of commonly used foods. The GI covers only carbohydrates, such as fruits and juices, potatoes, rice, pasta, breads, cereals, etc., which contain sugars, starches, and different types of fibre.

Food values may vary slightly depending on the source, but in general they should be roughly the same. Many lists divide the foods into categories of low, medium/moderate, and high. Foods in the low category usually have a GI value of 55 or less; in the medium/moderate category, a GI value of 56–69 (see page 118); and in the high category, a GI of 70 or more (see page 118).

You might be surprised by some of the foods included in the low and high categories. Rice cakes and bran flakes actually have a high GI value, even though you may have learned that these foods are great weight-loss choices. Meanwhile, salted peanuts and milk chocolate have a low GI value, but they're still very high in calories. Many of the foods that have a low GI value but are high in fat should be limited as well. *Remember: foods appear on the GI index only if they contain carbohydrates.* This explains why you won't find foods like fresh meat, chicken, fish, eggs, and cheese in GI lists, even though they have dense calories, but they *are* low GI! To further complicate matters, you may find certain processed foods, like sausages or chicken nuggets, on some GI lists because they contain flour! Some foods cause glucose levels to rise quickly after you eat them. The result is a virtual gush of glucose into the bloodstream, which in turn results in a rating of these foods as high GI. Other carbohydrate foods cause glucose levels to rise more slowly—more like a small wave—which results in a rating of these foods as low GI.

How can you tell what the GI value of a packaged food item, which contains many different ingredients, will be? First, the overall nutrient content of a food will affect its GI. For example, fat and protein affect the absorption of carbohydrate. This helps to explain why chocolate, which is high in fat, has a low GI value.

How you cook a food and the degree of processing it has undergone also affect its GI. So does, for example, the ripeness and variety of a fruit. Even the structure of the carbohydrate itself influences the GI. For example, processed instant oatmeal has a higher GI than traditional rolled oats. This is because, as a result of the processing, the starch in instant oats is more easily exposed to digestive enzymes, causing it to break down and enter the bloodstream more rapidly. Meanwhile, some foods have low GI values because they're packed with fibre. Fibre acts as a physical barrier, slowing down the absorption of carbohydrate into the blood.

Eyeballing Glucose

There are several kinds of sugars in the foods we eat; some are natural, and some processed. Natural sugars include fructose (fruit sugar), lactose (milk sugar), and maltose (grain sugar). These natural sugars have lower GI values, and will not cause a spike in blood sugar levels to the extent that sucrose (or ordinary table sugar) will. So, in packaged food items, what you especially need to watch for are foods *high in sucrose* or foods that come with the phrase "added sugar" on their packaging; these are sugars that manufacturers add to foods during processing.

Foods containing fruit juice concentrates, invert sugar, regular corn syrup, honey or molasses, hydrolyzed lactose syrup or high-fructose corn syrup (made out of highly concentrated fructose through the hydrolysis of starch) all have added sugars. And many people don't realize that pure, *unsweetened* fruit juice is still a potent source of sugar, even when it contains no added sugar. Extra lactose, dextrose, and maltose are also contained in many of our foods. In other words, these products may have naturally occurring sugars anyway, and then *more* sugar is thrown in to enhance consistency, taste, and so on. The best way to know how much sugar is in a product is to look at the nutritional label. If sugars aren't mentioned on the label, look at "total carbohydrates."

However, *how fast* that sugar ultimately breaks down and enters your bloodstream greatly depends on the amount of fibre in your food, how much protein you've eaten, and how much fat accompanies the sugar in your meal. This is what helps determine the overall *GI rating* of a meal.

Why Are Sugars Added?

Sugars are added to foods because they can change their consistency and, in some instances, act as a preservative, as in jams and jellies. Sugars can increase the boiling point or reduce the freezing point in foods; sugars can add bulk and density, and make baked goods do wonderful things, including help yeast to ferment. Sugars can also add moisture to dry foods, making them crisp, or balance acidic tastes in foods like tomato sauce or salad dressing. Invert sugar is used to prevent sucrose from crystallizing in candy; corn syrup is used for this purpose as well.

Since the 1950s, a popular natural sugar in North America has been fructose, which has replaced the sucrose in many food products in the form of high-fructose syrup (HFS), made from corn. HFS was developed in response to high sucrose prices and is very cheap to make. In other parts of the world, the equivalent of high-fructose syrup is made from whatever starches are local, such as rice, tapioca, wheat, or cassava. According to the International Food Information Council in Washington, DC, the average North American consumes about 37 g of fructose daily.

"Sugar-Free"

Sugar-free in the language of labels simply means "sucrose-free." However, this doesn't mean the product is carbohydrate-free, as in dextrose-free, lactose-free, glucose-free, or fructose-free. Check the labels for all ingredients ending in *-ose* to find out the sugar content; you're not looking just for sucrose. Watch out for "no added sugar," "without added sugar," or "no sugar added." This simply means: "We didn't put the sugar in, God did." Again, reading the number of carbohydrates on the nutrition information label is the most accurate way to find out the amount of sugar in the product. Fruits and vegetables are discussed at the end of this chapter.

Sweeteners

Products with certain sweeteners are an option, but only if they are in liquid or tablet form. Sweeteners in granulated forms (e.g., Splenda) should not be used at all since these substitutes contain maltodextrin as a bulking agent. According to dieticians who specialize in low GI meal planning, maltodextrin is a very high GI product, and should be avoided. In fact, from a GI rating standpoint, a small amount of sugar may even be a better choice.

Most artificial sweeteners will be classified as low GI because they don't affect your blood sugar levels since they don't contain sugar, but they may contain a few calories. It depends on whether a given sweetener is classified as nutritive or non-nutritive.

Nutritive sweeteners have calories or contain natural sugar. Sorbitol, mannitol, xylitol, lactitol, isomalt, and maltitol are all sugar alcohols. Like ordinary sugar, sugar alcohols contain only 4 calories per gram, and will affect your blood sugar levels like ordinary sugar. How *much* sugar alcohols affect your blood sugar levels depends on how much is consumed, and the degree of absorption from your digestive tract.

Non-nutritive sweeteners are sugar substitutes or artificial sweeteners; they don't have any calories and will not affect your blood sugar levels. Examples of non-nutritive sweeteners are saccharin, cyclamate, aspartame, sucralose, and acesulflame potassium.

Table 7.1: Non-nutritive Sweeteners

Sweetener	Intake Based on mg/kg Body Weight
Aspartame	40
Acesulfame potassium	15
Cyclamate	11
Saccharin	5
Sucralose	9

Source: Canadian Diabetes Association, 2008 Clinical Practice Guidelines:S41.

Foods in Jars and Tins

There are many canned and jarred foods available to the low GI dieter. Here are things to have on hand and pick up when strolling the aisles:

- Tuna (preferably in water)
- Salmon (preferably in water)
- Sardines (preferably in water)
- Tomatoes and tomato paste
- Corn
- Fruits (not packed in syrup)
- New white potatoes
- Vegetables (asparagus, carrots, green beans mushrooms, etc.). Marinated vegetables packed in jars are great as snacks and side dishes. An added benefit is the vinegar they contain, which helps lower the GI of the foods you eat with them. Examples include sun-dried tomatoes, artichoke hearts, and olives.
- Dried fruits and nuts, especially walnuts and nut bars
- Capers
- Marinated vegetables
- Roasted peppers
- Pickles

The Outside Aisles

What you need to eat on the low GI diet is usually found in the outside aisles of any supermarket or grocery store. Outside aisles stock the foods you can buy at outdoor markets: fruits, vegetables, meat, eggs, fish, breads, and dairy products. Natural fibre is also found in the outside aisles. But remember: Foods you buy in the outside aisles can be high in fat unless you select wisely. Fat content may also affect the GI values. Whole milk, for example, has a low GI value because it's packed with protein and fat.

How Ingredients Affect the GI Value of a Meal

The outside aisles will help you select low GI ingredients wisely. But how you cook a food, the degree of processing, and the ripeness and variety of a fruit, for example, can also affect its GI value. Yellowish green bananas are a good example. They have a lower GI value than the darker yellow, spotty bananas. Processed instant oatmeal has a higher GI value than traditional rolled oats because the starch in instant oats is more easily exposed.

Meanwhile, some foods have low GI values because they're packed with fibre (discussed further on), which acts as a physical barrier, slowing down the absorption of carbohydrate into the blood. It's important to remember that GI charts identify the effect different foods have on bloods sugar levels only when they're eaten *on their own*. Once you put them together in a meal, the mixture of foods will completely change the GI value of what you're eating. As a guideline, the more low GI foods you include in a meal, the lower the overall GI value of that meal.

Food Acidity

The more acidity there is in food, the more slowly it's emptied from the stomach—and the more slowly it's digested and turned into blood sugar. Foods that are acidic, such as oranges and sourdough breads, have low GI values. Adding acid to a meal in the form of vinegar (found in many salad dressings) or lemon juice, can therefore help lower the GI value of that meal. Adding roughly 20 mL (4 tsps) of vinegar in the form of vinaigrette dressing at an average meal can actually lower blood sugar by 30 percent. Recipes with acidic foods can also balance higher GI ingredients. So just to recap, adding pickles and other acidic vegetables to meals can lower the GI values of those meals. Adding lemon juice or vinegar to recipes has the same effect—the GI values of those meals are lowered.

Baking Ingredients

If you're planning to bake, and the recipe uses whole-wheat flour or plain white flour, be aware that these both have high GI values. (The insoluble fibre added to whole-wheat flour does not lower the GI.) *The flour needs to be 100 percent stone ground.* It *is* acceptable to have plain flour if there's a soluble fibre component to the recipe. Recipes using flour labelled as all-purpose flour, flour, bread flour, whole-wheat flour, etc., are all high GI flours. However, if enough soluble fibre is in the recipe to counteract the high GI effect of the flour used, the recipe is acceptable. Examples would be ingredients such as rolled oats, a number of apples, applesauce, wheat germ, raw carrots, protein foods such as yogourt or buttermilk, and other acidic ingredients.

Many baking recipes contain cornstarch, which is a high GI thickening agent. Yet when there are relatively small amounts of cornstarch in a recipe that contains a lot of protein, the GI will still be kept relatively low. But as a general rule, be aware that low GI thickening agents are flour or oat bran.

Again, as far as baking is concerned, powdered sugar substitutes or sweeteners should not be used as they contain substantial amounts of maltodextrin, a high GI bulking agent. These sweeteners have a higher GI than sugar itself. However, liquid sweeteners usually do not contain maltodextrin, nor do tablet sweeteners. Tablet sweeteners need only be dissolved in a very small quantity of water and added to the recipe. If bulk is required for the recipe, it's preferable to use sugar or fructose rather than powdered sugar substitutes or sweeteners.

Pastas and Rice

Whole-wheat pastas are lower in carbs, and brown rice is lower in carbs than white pasta or white rice. There are now a variety of low GI pastas and rice to choose from. As long as pasta is made of durum wheat and is cooked *al dente* (firm) it's low GI. A good medium GI choice of rice is basmati, brown, or long-grain rice. As a general rule, avoid any quick-cooking or instant starches.

For even lower carb options, spaghetti squash, steamed spinach, broccoli, or other cooked vegetables can substitute for pastas, rice, or other carbs normally required for sauces. As a general rule, cooked foods have higher GIs than uncooked foods. One of the reasons is because cooking causes starches to swell, which makes them easier to digest and they therefore convert into glucose more quickly. The amount of cooking time can affect the GI, too. When pasta is cooked only until it's *al dente*, it has a low GI; when pasta is overcooked and becomes soft and mushy, it has a higher GI.

Beverages

The general advice is to drink 2–5 L (.5–1.3 gal.) of water per day. Caffeine is to be kept to a minimum (no more than two cups per day). Sodas, including diet sodas, are not recommended as they contain phosphates that leach calcium from the bones. In addition, recent studies have shown that even diet sodas appear to contribute to obesity, although it is not clear why. Some experts I've consulted theorize that the sweetness of even a 0 calorie sweetener may prompt an insulin response, but this has yet to be studied. Alcohol is discussed further on.

Bulk Food Items

Bulk food items are generally more affordable than the processed or packaged variety you may be used to eating. They're also high-fibre items, and when properly stored, they last forever! When preparing for a low GI diet, here are some suggestions:

- Dried beans and peas (great for soups and stews)
- Rolled oat flakes over packaged or instant cereal
- Barley (for use in soups as well as on its own); it's also high in fibre
- Basmati rice, brown or wild rice, and whole-grain pastas; in general, it's always a good idea to opt for those grains that have undergone the least amount of processing
- Whole grains, such as bulgar and couscous, as another alternative to breads or a common white starch; both of these grains, when added to vegetables, can transform a healthy starch into a hearty meal
- Natural peanut butter, as long as it comes without any added sugars

Fruits and Vegetables

The lowest GI fruits to choose from include all varieties of citrus fruits (e.g., grapefruits and oranges) as well as apples, apricots, cherries, mulberries, peaches, pears, plums, strawberries, and kiwi. Dried fruits such as apple slivers, apricots, and sultanas are low GI, but raisins are not.

And as for vegetables, most leafy green and cruciferous vegetables are low GI, including beans (with the exception of haricot beans or refried beans), lentils, and chickpeas. It's best not to opt for sweet corn and peas as both have a higher GI value. There are certain root vegetables, such as parsnips and beets, which are also high GI.

THE IMPORTANCE OF FIBRE

A key component in lower GI foods is fibre. Complex carbohydrates are foods that are high in fibre. Fibre is the part of a plant your body can't digest. It comes in the form of both water-soluble fibre (which dissolves in water) and water-insoluble fibre (which doesn't dissolve in water but instead absorbs water). Soluble fibres, such as those found in apples, rolled oats, and beans and other legumes, tend to slow digestion, resulting in a low GI. Including kidney beans or chickpeas in a salad or adding an apple as the dessert to a meal will lower that meal's overall GI, thus producing a slower and more subtle rise in after-meal blood sugar levels.

Soluble fibre also lowers the "bad cholesterol," or LDL, in your body. Experts aren't entirely sure how soluble fibre works its magic, but one popular theory is that it gets mixed into the bile the liver secretes, and forms a type of gel that traps the building blocks of cholesterol, thus lowering your LDL levels. It's akin to a spider web trapping smaller insects. Sources of soluble fibre include oats or oat bran, legumes (dried beans and peas), some seeds, carrots, oranges, bananas, and other fruits. Soybeans are also high sources of soluble fibre. Soluble fibre helps delay the absorption of glucose into your bloodstream, which not only improves blood sugar control, but helps to control post-meal peaks in blood sugar. This stimulates the pancreas to produce more insulin.

Insoluble fibre doesn't affect your cholesterol levels at all, but it does regulate your bowel movements. As insoluble fibre moves through your digestive tract, it absorbs water like a sponge and helps form your waste into a solid matter faster, making the stools larger, softer, and easier to pass. Without insoluble fibre, your solid waste just gets pushed down to the colon or lower intestine as usual, where it's stored and dried out until you're ready to have a bowel movement. High-starch foods are associated with drier stools. Ignoring "the urge" only makes the situation worse, as the colon will continue to dehydrate the waste. This makes it harder and more difficult to pass, a condition known as constipation. Insoluble fibre will help to regulate your bowel movements by speeding things along. It's also linked to lower rates of colorectal cancer. Good sources of insoluble fibre are wheat bran and whole grains, skins from various fruits and vegetables, seeds, leafy greens, and cruciferous vegetables (cauliflower, broccoli, or Brussels sprouts).

Finding High-Fibre, Low GI Grains and Breads

Rethinking bread is critical for people on a low GI diet. Even breads made with whole-grain flour can still be high GI. Flour has to be 100 percent stone-ground whole wheat, or another soluble-fibre product (such as oats, oat bran, wheat germ, or All-Bran) needs to be used in order for a bread to be low GI. For a bread to be low GI, it needs to be labelled as whole grain, multigrain, or 100 percent stone ground. Rye bread can also be low GI, but must be labelled as whole meal or sourdough rye. Other types of acceptable breads include those made with soya, sunflower seeds, or linseeds.

Although whole-grain breads are good sources of insoluble fibre (flax bread is particularly good because flaxseeds are a source of soluble fibre, too), they may not be low GI unless they're 100 percent whole grain. The problem lies in understanding what is actually "whole grain." For example, there's an assumption that because bread is dark or brown, it's more nutritious; this isn't so. In fact, many brown breads are simply enriched white breads dyed with molasses. ("Enriched" means that nutrients lost during processing have been replaced.) Whole-wheat pita breads are considered classic low GI breads. A good rule is to simply look for the phrase "whole wheat," which means that the wheat is, indeed, whole.

AT THE LIQUOR STORE

Many people with diabetes think they have to avoid alcohol completely because it converts into glucose. This is not so. Alcohol *alone* doesn't increase blood sugar since alcohol cannot be turned into glucose. It's the sugar in that alcoholic beverage that can affect your blood sugar level.

Red wine, in particular, has been proven to raise your "good cholesterol" (HDL). Red wine is believed to have a heart-healthy effect in three ways: it is antioxidant (fights free-radicals), vasodilating (widens blood vessels), and anti-thrombotic (blood thinning). The two most studied compounds in wine are resveratrol and quercitin. Resveratrol apparently increases HDL cholesterol by preventing LDL cholesterol from oxidating. The tannins in red wine, which are not present in white wine or other liquor, seem to help blood flow and de-clog arteries. Grape juice and de-alcoholized red wine apparently confer some of the same benefits as the alcoholic version. In general, a maximum of two glasses of red wine per day is fine for people with Type 2 diabetes.

It's crucial to note that alcohol can cause hypoglycemia (low blood sugar) if you're on medication or insulin. Please discuss the effects of alcohol and hypoglycemia with your health care team.

Fine Wine

Dry wines can be considered low GI if they are listed as 0, meaning no added sugar (in Ontario and British Columbia) or if they are "dry," and are fine to ingest if you are diabetic. Wine is the result of natural sugar in fruits or fruit juices fermenting. Fermentation is a process in which natural sugar is converted into alcohol. A glass of dry red or white wine has calories (discussed below), but no sugar. And unless extra sugar is added to the wine, there's no way that alcohol will change back into sugar, even in your digestive tract. The same thing goes for cognac, brandy, and dry sherry that contain no sugar.

On the other hand, a sweet wine listed as 3 in Ontario or British Columbia means that it contains 3 g of sugar per 100 mL (3.5 oz) portion. Dessert wines or ice wines are really sweet; they contain about 15 percent sugar or 10 g of sugar for a 60 mL (2 oz) serving. Sweet liqueurs are 35 percent sugar. All of these would be considered high GI drinks.

A glass of dry wine with your meal adds about 100 calories, or the equivalent calories of fat or oil. Half soda water and half wine (a spritzer) contains half the calories. When you cook with wine, the alcohol evaporates, leaving only the flavour.

At the Pub

If you're a beer drinker, you're basically having some corn, barley, and a couple of teaspoons of malt sugar (maltose) when you have a bottle of beer. The corn and barley ferment into mostly alcohol and some maltose. Calorie-wise, that's about 150 calories per bottle plus 15 mL (3 tsp) of malt sugar. A light beer has fewer calories, but contains at least 100 calories per bottle. De-alcoholized beer still has sugar.

The Hard Stuff

The stiffer the drink, the more fattening it gets. Hard liquors, such as scotch, rye, gin, and rum, are made out of cereal grains—the grains ferment into alcohol; vodka, the Russian staple, is made out of potatoes. Hard liquor averages about 40 percent alcohol, but has no sugar. Nevertheless, you're looking at about 100 calories per small shot glass, so long as you don't add fruit juice, tomato or Clamato juice, or sugary soft drinks.

The Glycogen Factor

If you recall from Chapter 1, glycogen is the stored sugar your liver keeps handy for emergencies. If your blood sugar needs a boost, the liver will tap into its glycogen stores and convert it into glucose. Alcohol in the liver *blocks* this conversion process. So, if you've been exercising and then go out with friends for a few drinks, unless you've eaten something after your exercise, you may need that glycogen. If you drink to the point of feeling tipsy, that glycogen can be cut off by the alcohol, causing hypoglycemia. What complicates matters even more is that your hypoglycemia symptoms can mimic drunkenness. This glycogen problem can affect people with either Type 1 or Type 2 diabetes because it can result when either insulin or oral hypoglycemic agents are used. (See Chapter 227 for details on hypoglycemia, and below for the alcohol and diabetes rules.)

CHAPTER SEVEN

Don't Drink and Starve

If you're going to drink, *eat!* Always have food with your alcohol. Food delays absorption of alcohol into the bloodstream, providing you with carbohydrates and therefore preventing hypoglycemia.

Diabetes experts also recommend the following:
- Avoid alcohol when your blood sugar is high.
- Remember that two drinks a day is fine for someone with a healthy liver, but less is recommended for liver health.
- Choose dry wines or alcoholic beverages with no sugar.
- Remember that juice has sugar, even tomato and Clamato juice.
- Never substitute alcohol for food if you're taking insulin or pills.
- Talk to your doctor about how to safely balance alcohol and insulin, and alcohol and any medication you're taking.

SAMPLE GLYCEMIC INDEX TABLES

The following is a sample of glycemic index tables, which abound on the Internet. Simply use "GI Table" or "Glycemic Index Table" as a search term and several will pop up.

Low Glycemic Index Foods (55 or Less)

Note: The following foods are listed alphabetically. Their corresponding GI values are based on a standard single serving.

All-Bran: 42
Apple: 38
Apple juice, unsweetened: 40
Baked beans in tomato sauce: 48
Banana: 55
Butter beans: 31

Carrots, boiled: 49

Cherries: 22

Chickpeas, canned: 42

Dried apricots: 31

Fettucine pasta, cooked *al dente*: 32

Grapefruit: 25

Green grapes: 46

Kiwi fruit: 52

Lentil soup: 44

Low-fat fruit yogourt: 33

Low-fat yogourt with low GI sweetener: 14

Macaroni: 45

Milk chocolate: 49

Noodles: 40

Oatmeal made with water: 42

Orange: 44

Orange juice: 46

Peach: 42

Pear: 38

Pearl barley: 25

Peas: 48

Potato chips: 54

Raw oat bran: 55

Red lentils: 26

Roasted and salted peanuts: 14

Skimmed milk: 32

Special K: 54

Stone-ground whole-grain bread: 53

Sweet corn: 55

Tomato soup, canned: 38

White spaghetti, cooked *al dente*: 41

Whole-grain spaghetti, cooked *al dente*: 37

Whole milk: 27

Medium/Moderate Glycemic Index Foods (56–69)

Note: The following foods are listed alphabetically. Their corresponding GI values are based on a standard single serving.

Apricots, canned in syrup: 64

Basmati rice: 58

Boiled potatoes: 56

Cantaloupe melon: 67

Cheese and tomato pizza: 60

Coca-Cola: 63

Couscous: 65

Croissant: 67

Crumpet, toasted: 69

Digestive biscuit: 59

Honey: 58

Ice cream: 61

Mars bar: 68

Muesli, untoasted: 56

New potatoes: 62

Pineapple, fresh: 66

Pita bread: 57

Raisins: 64

Rye bread: 65

Shortbread biscuit: 64

Shredded Wheat: 67

Sultanas: 56

Whole-grain bread: 69

High Glycemic Index Foods (70 or More)

Note: The following foods are listed alphabetically. Their corresponding GI values are based on a standard single serving.

Bagel: 72

Baguette: 95

Bran flakes: 74

Cheerios: 74

Cornflakes: 84

French fries: 75

Jacket potato: 85

Jelly beans: 80

Mashed potato: 70

Parsnips, boiled: 97

Puffed wheat: 89

Rice cakes: 82

Rice Krispies: 82

Watermelon: 72

White bread: 70

White rice, steamed: 98

Source: Reprinted with permission from Farid, N. and Norene Gilletz, *The PCOS Diet Cookbook,* Your Health Press/Trafford, Victoria pp. 291–294, 2008.

8

IN DEFENCE OF FAT: RIGHT
FATS AND WRONG FATS

The previous chapter looked at low glycemic eating, which focuses on rethinking carbohydrates. Instead of counting carbs, the focus is now on selecting low glycemic index carbohydrates instead of high glycemic index carbs. The second part of the food puzzle is reassessing the fat in your diet. Reducing your intake of certain fats, and increasing your intake of others, can dramatically reduce the risk of cardiovascular disease, one of the chief complications of Type 2 diabetes. This chapter looks at the right fats rather than low-fat foods. When you put this together with the information in the previous chapter, you're on your way to adopting a healthy diet for life.

UNDERSTANDING FATS

Fat is technically known as *fatty acids,* which are crucial nutrients for our cells. We cannot live without fatty acids. Fat is therefore a good thing—in moderation, but like all good things, most of us want too much of it. Excess dietary fat is by far the most damaging element in the Western diet. A gram of fat contains twice the calories as the same amount of protein or carbohydrate. Fat in the diet comes from meats, dairy products, and vegetable oils. Other sources of fat include coconuts (60 percent fat), peanuts (78 percent fat), and avocados (82 percent fat). There are different kinds of fatty acids in these sources of fats: saturated, unsaturated, and trans-fatty acids (or trans fat).

The trans-fatty acids are like a saturated fat in disguise. Some fats are harmful, while others are considered beneficial to your health. The terms "good fats" and "bad fats" began to be used when research into diets higher in monounsaturated fats were closely observed. These monounsaturated fats were found, in spite of being "fats," to raise good cholesterol, or HDL, which protects against heart disease.

Understanding fat is a complicated business. This section explains everything you need to know about fats, and a few things you probably don't want to know but should.

Saturated Fats

Saturated fat is solid at room temperature and stimulates cholesterol production in your body. Foods high in saturated fat include processed meats, fatty meats, lard, butter, margarine, solid vegetable shortening, chocolate, and tropical oils (coconut oil is more than 90 percent saturated). Saturated fat should be consumed only in very small amounts. The CDA recommends that saturated fat be restricted to less than 7 percent of total daily intake.

Meats

All fresh meats are fine. Lean meats are preferable; choose from:

- Chicken, Cornish hen, and turkey (all without skin). You can also substitute ground turkey for ground beef in burgers.
- Lean beef (round, sirloin, chuck, loin). Look for "choice" or "select" grades instead of "prime," and lean or extra-lean ground beef (with no more than 10 percent fat).
- Lean veal, ham, pork (tenderloin, loin chop), and lean lamb (leg, arm, loin).
- Red meats, but only once or twice per week; pork and lamb are particularly fattening.
- Chicken breast or drumstick instead of chicken wing or thigh.
- Exotic meats, such as emu, buffalo, rabbit, pheasant, and venison. These have less total fat than animals commonly raised for market.

Unsaturated Fats

Unsaturated fat is partially solid or liquid at room temperature. This group of fats includes monounsaturated fats, polyunsaturated fats, and omega-3 oils (fish oil), all of which protect you against heart disease (see below). Sources of unsaturated fats include vegetable oils (canola, safflower, sunflower, corn) and seeds and nuts. To make it easy to remember, unsaturated fats, with the exception of tropical oils, such as coconut, come from plants. The more liquid the fat, the more polyunsaturated it is, and the more it *lowers* your cholesterol levels. However, if you have familial hyperlipidemia (high cholesterol), which often occurs alongside diabetes, unsaturated fats may not make a difference in your cholesterol levels.

In Mediterranean diets, for example, which are considered among the healthiest diets, olive oil, herbs, and spices are routinely used in place of butter as spreads or dips for breads. Properties of olive oil were found to contain a host of protective factors and "catalyst" ingredients, which allowed phytochemicals from plant-based foods to work their magic in the body. The virtues of a Mediterranean diet, with its good fats became the basis for a revolution in dietary fat guidelines, which now recognize that healthy diets should have some monounsaturated fats, the best of which is olive oil. Other monounsaturated oils are canola, peanut, sesame, soybean, corn, cottonseed, and safflower, but olive oil is 74 percent monounsaturated, while the next best oil, canola, is only 59 percent monounsaturated. The CDA stresses that polyunsaturated fats should be restricted to less than 10 percent of your daily diet, and that most fats in your daily intake should be monounsaturated fats, such as fatty fish, or plant oils, both rich in omega-3 fatty acids. Basically, your total fat intake is not as important as the types of fat you take in daily.

Fish Fat (Omega-3 Oils)

Fish that swim in cold waters have a layer of fat to keep them warm. These fats are known as omega-3 fatty acids (crucial for brain tissue) or fish oils, which are all polyunsaturated. They lower your cholesterol levels and protect against heart disease. Mackerel, albacore tuna, salmon, sardines, and lake trout are all rich in omega-3 fatty acids. In fact, whale meat and seal meat are enormous sources of omega-3 fatty acids and were once the staples of the Inuit diet. Overhunting and federal moratoriums on whale and seal hunting have dried up this once-vital source of Inuit food, which clearly offered real protection against heart disease.

Artificial Fats

An assortment of artificial fats have been introduced into our diet, courtesy of food producers who are trying to give us the taste of fat without all the calories or harmful effects of saturated fats. Unfortunately, artificial fats offer their own horrors.

Trans-fatty Acids (Hydrogenated Oils)

These are harmful fats that not only raise the level of "bad cholesterol" (LDL) in your bloodstream, but lower the amount of "good cholesterol" (HDL) that's already there. Trans-fatty acids are what you get when a liquid oil, such as corn oil, is changed into a more solid or spreadable substance, such as margarine. Trans-fatty acids, you might say, are the "road to hell paved with good intentions." Someone, way back when, thought that you could take the good fat—unsaturated fat—and solidify it so it could double as butter or lard. That sounds like a great idea. Unfortunately, to make an unsaturated liquid fat more solid, you have to add hydrogen to its molecules. This is known as *hydrogenation,* the process that converts liquid fat to semi-solid fat. That ever-popular chocolate bar ingredient, hydrogenated palm oil, is a classic example of a trans-fatty acid. Hydrogenation also prolongs the shelf life of a fat. Polyunsaturated fats can oxidize when exposed to air, causing rancid odours or flavours. Deep-frying oils used in restaurants are generally hydrogenated.

Trans-fatty acid is sold as a polyunsaturated or monounsaturated fat with a descriptor such as "Made from polyunsaturated vegetable oil." Your body treats trans-fatty acids as a saturated fat. This is why trans-fatty acids are a saturated fat in disguise. The advertiser may, in fact, say that the product contains "no saturated fat" or is "healthier" than the comparable animal or tropical oil product with saturated fat, so be careful: *Read your labels.* The magic word you're looking for is "hydrogenated." If the product lists a variety of unsaturated fats (mono-unsaturated X oil, polyunsaturated Y oil, and so on), keep reading. If the word "hydrogenated" appears, count that product as a saturated fat; your body will!

Several companies are now banning the use of trans fats in their manufacturing, and labels are more likely to scream these days: "No trans fats." Since the news of trans-fatty acids broke in the late 1980s, margarine manufacturers began to offer some healthier margarines; some contain no hydrogenated oils, while others have much smaller amounts of them. More recently, many margarines are now using good fats with omega-3 oils. In general, select a margarine that does not have trans fats, and is made with omega-3 oils or monounsaturated oils.

Fake Fats

We have artificial sweeteners; why not artificial fat? This question has led to the creation of an emerging yet highly suspicious ingredient: *fat substitutes,* designed to replace real fat and hence reduce the calories from real fat without compromising the taste. This is done by creating a fake fat that the body cannot absorb.

Many foods have been created using fat replacers, which simulate many of the properties of fat in food, for example, they make it creamy or smooth.

Carbohydrate-based gums and starches, like guar gum and modified food starch, are common. These gums and starches include sugar-like compounds, fibres, and even fruit purées and applesauce. Carbohydrates can be used as thickeners, bulking agents, moisturizers, and stabilizers. For example, a new carbohydrate-based fat replacer, oatrim (marketed by Golden Jersey Products under the brand name Replace), is an oat-flour ingredient added to some brands of skim milk in the US. Oatrim contains a type of fibre called beta-glucan, which may help lower blood cholesterol. Oatrim provides fat-like creaminess. Unless they are new to the food supply, most carbohydrate-based fat replacers do not require government approval because they are already in use and are safe. In the US this is called Generally Recognized as Safe (GRAS). A few fat replacers, including carageenan (a seaweed derivative) and polydextrose, were submitted to the FDA for food additive approval because they were new to the food supply.

Protein-based fat replacers are made from milk, whey, egg, soy, and other types of protein that have been manipulated to create texture, appearance, and mouth feel (their texture and consistency in your mouth).

Then there are fat-based fat replacers. Salatrim and caprenin are fat replacers; they contain fatty acids that are partially but not completely digested, supplying 5 versus 9 calories per gram. These fat replacers cannot be used to fry or sauté foods, but are used in products such as reduced-fat chocolate chips.

OLESTRA

The calorie-free fat substitute, olestra, is a fat-based fat replacer. It was developed by Procter & Gamble and approved for use in the US by the FDA, but olestra is a potentially dangerous ingredient that most experts feel can do more harm than good. Canada has not yet approved it.

Olestra is made from a combination of vegetable oils and sugar. It is known as a sucrose polyester. It tastes just like the real thing, but the biochemical structure is a molecule too big for your liver to break down, so olestra just gets passed into the large intestine and is excreted. Olestra is more than an empty molecule, however. It can cause diarrhea and cramps and may deplete your body of vital nutrients, including vitamins A, D, E, and K; the last is necessary for blood to clot. Some nutrition experts fear a greater danger with olestra: Instead of encouraging people to choose nutritious foods (such as fruits, grains, and vegetables) over high-fat foods, products like olestra encourage a high *fake-fat* diet that's still too low in fibre and other essential nutrients. And the no-fat icing on the cake is that these people could wind up with a vitamin deficiency to boot. Olestra is the only fat replacer that entirely replicates fat; it can be used for frying, which is why it can be used in salty snacks. Olestra required FDA approval because it is a new food ingredient, not a combination of ingredients that already were in the food supply. A 30 g (1 oz) portion of potato chips has no fat when made with olestra and 10 g when made with oil.

Health Canada is taking the same stance as many nutrition experts, who find that the long-term consequences of olestra in the food supply haven't been addressed. Many experts feel that approving olestra would be tantamount to springing an untested chemical onto the public. Currently, olestra is still not available in Canada.

The position of the American Dietetic Association (ADA) is that fat-reduced or fat-replaced foods can only be part of a diet that includes plenty of fruits, vegetables, and grains (see Chapter 7). Fat replacers enable you to eat lower-fat versions of familiar foods without making major changes in the way you eat, but these lower-fat versions should not be eaten in excess.

Critics of olestra argue that people will make the mistake of thinking that "no fat" is healthy; they'll choose olestra-containing Twinkies over fruits and think they're eating well. Olestra is currently being used only in snack foods, but potential uses for olestra could include restaurant foods touted as "fat-free" fries, fried chicken, fish and chips, and onion rings. At home, olestra could be used as cooking oil for sautés, as a butter substitute for baking, or as a fat-free cheese. Potentially, we could be facing a future of eating "polyester foods." In fact, Procter & Gamble filed for olestra to be approved as a fat substitute for up to 35 percent of the natural fats used in home cooking and up to 75 percent of the fats used in commercial foods. The company did not ask for approval to use olestra in table spreads or ice creams, however. The FDA did not approve olestra for use in the products Procter & Gamble requested. A new request—to use olestra only in salty snack foods—was submitted. In 1996, the FDA approved olestra for use in savoury snacks; Procter & Gamble proceeded to market olestra under the trade name Olean. By 1998, Frito-Lay and Procter & Gamble announced the release of Olean products in dozens of snack foods, and the FDA approved this under the proviso that a warning label about olestra's health consequences should be on each Olean product. (Current warnings that the products, when eaten in large amounts, cause fecal leakage, are affixed to all Olean products.) When the 1999 sales of Olean were disappointing, Proctor & Gamble sought to have the warning removed; the FDA agreed to revise, but not remove the label. The Center for Science in the Public Interest has been opposed to the approval of olestra because of safety concerns. Studies have not found that olestra substantially reduces fat intake for the same reasons many low- or no-fat products have failed: People just eat more. Although olestra-made snacks taste identical to their originals, they still have plenty of calories from carbohydrates. People treat olestra-based snacks the same way they treat other low-fat snacks.

Types of Fat Replacers Available

Carbohydrate-Based Fat Replacers

Maltodextrins: Baked goods

Starches: Baked goods, margarines, salad dressing, frozen desserts

Cellulose: Frozen desserts, sauces, salad dressings

Guar, xanthan, or other gums: Salad dressings

Polydextrose: Baked goods, cake mixes, puddings, frostings

Oatrim: Milk

Protein-Based Fat Replacers

Protein concentrate (whey, egg white, soy): Frozen desserts, reduced-fat dairy products, salad dressings

Fat-Based Fat Replacers

Caprenin: Chocolate

Salatrim: Chocolate

Olestra (not in Canada): Snack chips, crackers

Table 8.1: Recommendations for Fat

Type of Fat	How Much to Eat
Saturated	No more than 7 percent daily
Polyunsaturated fat	No more than 10 percent daily
Monounsaturated fat	As much as possible
Omega-3 fatty acids	As much as possible
Trans-fatty acids	Limit as much as possible

Source: Canadian Diabetes Association, 2008 Clinical Practice Guidelines:S41.

THE MEDITERRANEAN DIET: GOOD FOR DIABETES AND HEART DISEASE

The Mediterranean diet has been dubbed "the healthiest diet in the world." Many controlled studies that placed one group of people on a Mediterranean diet for two years or more and another group on a regular North American diet for that time frame found that the heart disease rates dramatically dropped in the Mediterranean group. Olive oil, rich in linolenic and oleic acids; vitamin E and antioxidants; garlic, fresh fruits and vegetables, and relatively lower meat consumption all add up to a low GI diet rich in the good fats. In a Mediterranean diet, saturated fat consumption is low, and monounsaturated consumption is high, which elevates "good cholesterol" and thus protects against heart disease.

The Mediterranean diet was so dubbed because it refers to diets within olive-growing regions of the Mediterranean, which explains the diet's heavy reliance on olive oil. But if you look at the components of a healthy diet (see Chapter 8), the Mediterranean diet has them all: a large consumption of salads and legumes, whole grains (wheat), olives (whole), grapes, and other fruits. The total fat consumption in a Mediterranean diet is higher than our fat guidelines in North America: around 40 percent in some regions, such as Greece, but right on target—about 30 percent in Italy. In Spain, where fish is eaten more, fat consumption is also closer to 40 percent.

A Brief History of the Mediterranean Diet

Physician Ancel Keys, who, in 1959, developed heart-healthy dietary guidelines that mirror today's, pioneered international heart study research as early as 1947, when he noticed a sharp rise in heart disease in the US. When he travelled to Italy in 1952, he observed the Mediterranean diet and concluded that it was the healthiest diet in the world, calling it the "good Mediterranean diet." His heart-healthy dietary guidelines, based on the findings of his Italy trip, were published in his book, *How to Eat and Stay Well the Mediterranean Way*. In the late 1950s, Keys and his colleagues undertook a 15-year project in which they collected data on more than 12,000 men from seven countries—Finland, Greece,

Italy, Japan, Yugoslavia, the Netherlands, and the US. Known as the Seven Country Study, published in 1984, Keys noted that the lowest rates of heart disease in the world were in Mediterranean countries, notably Greece, and the second-lowest were in Japan, yet Japan's heart disease rate was twice that of Greece. In 1986, a follow-up analysis on the Seven Country Study found that intakes of monounsaturated fat, such as olive oil, were the reason for such low heart disease rates.

Keys took note of Greece's high olive oil consumption and low saturated fat consumption. Keys noted olive oil consumption as high as 20 kg per person per year, compared to France's consumption, which was far lower. In Greece, the olive tree is associated with peace because it takes olive trees 30 years to mature and bear olives; thus, they were planted in Greece only when society was stable, or so legend has it.

The major fatty acid in olives is oleic acid, a monounsaturated fatty acid comprising 56–83 percent of olive oil. The polyunsaturated fatty acids in olive oil are represented by the omega-6 fatty acid, linoleic (3.5–20 percent), and the omega-3 fatty acid, alpha-linolenic (0–1.5 percent). Fatty fish are also high in omega-3 fatty acids, but olive oil provides all the good fats you need without going fishing! Studies confirm that when you replace saturated fats with monounsaturated fats, you lower your total cholesterol and LDL, the "bad cholesterol" (see Chapter 2). If you used only monounsaturated fats, such as olive oil, you can preserve HDL cholesterol levels better, and reduce both total and LDL cholesterol.

Other monounsaturated oils are canola, peanut, sesame, soybean, corn, cottonseed, and safflower, but olive oil is 74 percent monounsaturated, while the next best oil, canola, is only 59 percent monounsaturated. Olive oil also makes the carotenes in vegetables come alive, while nonfat dressings or the absence of monounsaturated oils on salad actually make the salad's nutrients inferior. In fact, dressing your salads with olive oil is one of the best ways to protect your heart.

Oily fish high in polyunsaturated omega-3 fatty acids are also part of the Mediterranean diet, as are nuts, garlic, and snails. In short, if we're well-oiled, we'll apparently run better and resist "rust." Olive oil literally helps to offset oxidation, which is a natural process in the body that leads to breakdown. That's why antioxidants are considered so valuable.

The only hole you can poke in the Mediterranean diet studies, which all conclude that olive oil is great for our health, is that other factors such as lifestyle (more activity, less depression due to a more community-oriented society, or plain genetics) could be operating. But studies on North Americans who have adopted the Mediterranean diet confirm the same health benefits.

Foods on the Mediterranean Diet

People interested in trying out the Mediterranean diet will find that it's not that different than what you already eat and are exposed to, and meets all the requirements of a low GI diet. A typical daily menu plan from such a diet looks something like this. Breakfast would be pretty close to what you might already have: a high-fibre cereal, granola, or hot cereal with fruit and skim milk. Or a couple of soft-boiled eggs on whole-wheat toast (they can be poached or hard-boiled, or fried in a non-stick pan). You can have plain yogourt with fruit, or toast with jam. Lunch could be a big salad with olive oil and vinegar dressing (60 mL [1/4 cup] vinegar to 175 mL [3/4 cup] olive oil with herbs and spices as you wish). Lunch might consist of a lentil soup with bread dipped in olive oil or one of the following with a fruit: roast pepper and cheese sandwich, pasta salads (cooked pasta with vegetables and the olive oil dressing), potato salad (same as pasta salad, only with potatoes); tuna salad (substitute the olive oil dressing for the mayo); baked potato (substitute olive oil and salt for the butter and sour cream). Dinner might consist of any grilled or broiled fish, shrimp or seafood, or chicken, seasoned with olive oil and spices; baked potato with olive oil and salt instead of butter and sour cream; and a salad with olive oil dressing and some feta cheese. Or you can grill or broil any vegetable (fresh or frozen), lightly brushed with olive oil, which makes them delicious. Instead of meat or fish, you can make any type of pasta with a marinara sauce, olive oil, and garlic and herbs sauce, etc. Add some meat to the pasta for garnish and/or vegetables. Bread dipped in olive oil can be an accompaniment. You can have fruit for dessert, and a glass of red wine with dinner. There are hundreds of things you can easily make. When shopping for a Mediterranean meal plan, the best items to stock up on include: frozen vegetables, beans and legumes (for soups especially), some cheeses such as feta, Parmesan, Romano, or Provolone (you can buy these all as non-fat cheeses); seafood such as canned clams for marinara sauces; fruits; garlic; red wine or grape juice; poultry, game, and fish of your choice; lemons; salad fixings; mushrooms, olives and olive oil (of course); balsamic vinegar; rice; peppers (for roasting); spinach; tomatoes; tuna; and yogourt. Get yourself a Mediterranean cookbook with plenty of Italian and Greek recipes, and you should be able to eat interesting foods without getting bored. Most women do well on about 1,500 calories per day, while men should be on about 2,000 calories per day.

Walking Mediterranean Style

Activity within the Mediterranean lifestyle is routine in the form of a walk around the community before dinner or after dinner. In Italy, the *passeggiata* is the daily stroll around a neighbourhood or shopping area. It lasts for about an hour and is usually with a friend or family member, window shopping, buying certain foods for dinner, and so forth. We North Americans can do this easily in most cities. If you live in a suburban area of strip malls, plan a walk around the neighbourhood, walk your dog, etc. For your daily activity, you can substitute something else, such as a bike ride, dancing lessons, etc., instead of a walk. The point is that the Mediterranean diet incorporates about an hour of moderate activity per day, which used to be just part of everyone's life.

DIETARY SUPPLEMENTS

Countries where high-fibre and plant-rich diets are the norm have far lower rates of cancer, heart disease, and diabetes. This fact has led to research into specific foods or food ingredients that you can now buy in pill or capsule form: Garlic capsules, broccoli pills, and hundreds of other food supplements have sprung onto the health food market. Should you be taking supplements or simply eating a healthy diet? It depends on you. Ideally, if you adopt a low glycemic index diet (see

Chapter 6), and combine it with a right fats diet, most food supplements are unnecessary. Fibre supplements, however, are considered beneficial for most people with Type 2 diabetes. There are a variety of fibre supplements now on the market.

Phytochemicals

Phytochemicals, or "plant chemicals" (*phyto* is Greek for "plant"), are the natural ingredients found in plant foods such as tomatoes, oats, soya, oranges, and broccoli. Researchers are finding all kinds of disease-fighting chemicals in common fruits and vegetables; this sometimes leads to misleading claims on food labels, such as an ad a few years earlier by a ketchup company, claiming it prevented prostate cancer because it contained lycopene. While phytochemicals, such as *isoflavones* (found in soybeans), *allylic sulphides* (found in garlic, onions, and chives), *isothiocyanates* (found in cruciferous vegetables like Brussels sprouts, cabbage, and cauliflower), *saponins* (spinach, potatoes, tomatoes, and oats), *lignin* and *alpha-linolenic acid* (flaxseeds), sound exotic, you can easily get them by simply eating a variety of fruits, grains, and vegetables.

Another hot phytochemical right now is *beta-glucan* (found in legumes, oats, and other grains). Beta-glucan is believed to help prevent diabetes by delaying gastric emptying and by slowing down glucose absorption in the small intestine, so if you have diabetes, it can help to regulate your blood sugar.

In fact, biologically engineered foods, which alter the natural genetic codes in vegetables, may interfere with these natural phytochemicals.

PUTTING IT ALL TOGETHER

When you look at all the government food guidelines, and at the sound diet programs, they all say the same thing: Eat largely plant-based foods because they're low in calories but high in vitamins, minerals, fibre, and phytochemicals. Cut down on saturated fat (or foods of animal origin); use unsaturated or fish fats instead, and cut down on refined sugars. That still means eating low GI foods and the right fats. The most important component to any diet, however, is activity: Using more energy (calories) than you ingest will maintain your body weight or lead to weight loss. This is what dieticians of the 1950s and 1960s called a "sensible" or "balanced" diet. By 1990, it was called a low-fat diet, *but it's the same diet.*

Original food guidelines and serving suggestions were designed in the early twentieth century to prevent malnutrition from vitamin deficiencies. By 1950, the problem of overnutrition, meaning too much of every type of food available leading to overeating, began to be evident. Overnutrition led to a rise in obesity-related diseases such as Type 2 diabetes. In his 1959 book on heart disease, *Eat Well and Stay Well,* Ancel Keys and his wife, Margaret Keys, authored the guidelines for a "healthy heart," which were almost identical to today's dietary guidelines: maintaining normal body weight; restricting saturated fats and red meat; using polyunsaturated fats instead to a maximum of about 30 percent of daily calories; eating plenty of fresh fruits and vegetables and non-fat milk products; and avoiding overly salted foods and refined sugar. The Keys' guidelines even stressed doing exercise, stopping smoking, and reducing stress.

Saturated fats are the building blocks of clogged arteries and cardiovascular problems; unsaturated fats are heart-protective. We can therefore choose the right type of fat over the wrong type of fat, but overall weight loss *by simply eating less* will have more of an impact on reducing obesity and obesity-related health problems. I discuss this more in Chapter 11.

9

THE ROLE OF ACTIVE LIVING

The purpose of this chapter is to explain how exercise affects your body when you have diabetes. It is not intended as a workout program, however. Anybody reading this chapter needs to design a doable exercise program that is appealing and convenient; for most people, that will mean combining some kind of simple stretching routine with some aerobic activity. As one expert aptly put it on her video, the program you can do is the one you will do.

Most people who have been sedentary most of their lives are intimidated by health-and-fitness clubs. Walking into a room with complex machines, filled with young, fit, supple bodies, is not exactly an inviting atmosphere for somebody who doesn't understand how to program a StairMaster. And the language of exercise is intimidating, too. Not only do you need an anatomy lesson to understand which movements stretch which group of muscles, but you need to take a crash course in cardiology to understand exactly how long you have to hyperventilate and have your pulse at X beats per minute, with the sweat pouring off you, before you burn any fat. The concept of gaining muscle over existing fat is also a hard one to grasp. (My stupid question is always: "How come, if I've been doing my program for six months, I weigh *more* than when I started?")

You're wearing all the equipment you will ever need to exercise. If you can breathe, stretch, and walk, you can become a lean, mean exercise machine without paying a membership fee.

WHAT DOES EXERCISE *REALLY* MEAN?

The *Oxford English Dictionary* defines exercise as "the exertion of muscles, limbs, etc., especially for health's sake; bodily, mental, or spiritual training." In the Western world, we have placed an emphasis on "bodily training" when we talk about exercise, while completely ignoring mental and spiritual training. Only recently have Western studies begun to focus on the mental benefits of exercise. (It's been shown, for example, that exercise creates endorphins, hormones that make us feel good.) But we in the West do not encourage meditation or other calming forms of mental and spiritual exercise, which have also been shown to improve well-being and health.

In the East, for thousands of years, exercise has focused on achieving mental and spiritual health *through* the body, using breathing and postures, for example. Fitness practitioners maintain that posture is extremely important for organ alignment. Standing correctly—with the ears aligned over the shoulders, and the shoulders over the hips, with the knees slightly bent and the head straight up—naturally allows you to pull in your abdomen. Nor should we ignore the Aboriginal and Northern traditions known to improve mental health and well-being, such as traditional dances, active prayers that incorporate physical activity, circles that involve community and communication, and even sweat lodges, which are believed to help rid the body of toxic by-products through sweating. These are all forms of wellness activities that you should investigate.

The Meaning of Aerobic

If you look up the word "aerobic" in the dictionary, what you'll find is the chemistry definition: "living in free oxygen." This is certainly correct; we are all aerobes—beings that require oxygen to live. Some bacteria, for example, are anaerobic; they can exist in an environment without oxygen. All that jumping around and fast movement in aerobic exercise is done to create faster breathing, so we can take more oxygen into our bodies.

Why are we doing this? Because the blood contains *oxygen!* The faster your blood flows, the more oxygen can flow to your organs.

But when your health care practitioner tells you to exercise or to take up aerobic exercise, he or she is not referring solely to increasing oxygen but to exercising the heart muscle. The faster it beats, the better a workout it gets, although you don't want to overwork your heart either.

Why We Want More Oxygen

When more oxygen is in our bodies, we burn fat (see below), our breathing improves, our blood pressure improves, and our hearts work better. Oxygen also lowers triglycerides and cholesterol, increasing our high-density lipoproteins (HDL) or the "good cholesterol," while decreasing our low-density lipoproteins (LDL) or the "bad cholesterol." This means that your arteries will unclog and you may significantly decrease your risk of heart disease and stroke. More oxygen makes our brains work better, so we feel better. Studies show that depression is decreased when we increase oxygen flow into our bodies. Ancient techniques such as yoga, which specifically improve mental and spiritual well-being, achieve this by combining deep breathing and stretching, which improves oxygen and blood flow to specific parts of the body.

With Type 2 diabetes, more oxygen in the body increases your cells' sensitivity to insulin, causing your blood glucose levels to drop. More oxygen can also improve the action of insulin-producing cells in the pancreas. As you continue aerobic exercise, your blood sugar levels will become much easier to manage. You can also use exercise to decrease blood sugar levels in the short term, over a 24-hour period. People who are taking oral hypoglycemic pills may find that their dosages need to be lowered or that they no longer need the medication.

Exercise has been shown to dramatically decrease the incidence of many other diseases, including cancer. This is demonstrated widely in the medical literature. In the latest 2007 *Food, Nutrition, Physical Activity, and the Prevention of Cancer Report,* published by the American Institute for Cancer Research and The World Cancer Research Fund, physical activity (including occupational, household, transport, and recreational) modifies the risk of colon cancer and breast cancer, in particular. In fact, about 25 percent of cancer cases globally are due to excess weight and a sedentary lifestyle—the very same causes of Type 2 diabetes, so the fringe benefit of exercise is that you'll reduce your risk of cancer, too.

Exercise is found to reduce the risk of the following cancers and other diseases: 75 percent for breast cancer, 49 percent for cardiovascular and heart diseases, 35 percent for diabetes, and 22 percent for colorectal cancer. Increased physical activity also prevented weight gain associated with aging by at least two times more in individuals who were more active compared with those who were inactive. Physical activity also reduces fall-related injuries, depression, and emotional distress.

In fact, there is "irrefutable evidence" that regular exercise prevents several chronic diseases. The current Health Canada physical activity guidelines are ideal guidelines to follow.

Burning Fat

The only kind of exercise that will burn fat is aerobic exercise because *oxygen burns fat*. If you were to go to your fridge and pull out some animal fat (chicken skin, red-meat fat, or butter), throw it in the sink, and light it with a match, it would burn. What makes the flame yellow is oxygen; what fuels the fire is the fat. That same process goes on in your body. The oxygen will burn your fat however you increase the oxygen flow in your body (through jumping around, increasing your heart rate, or employing an established deep-breathing technique).

Of course, when you burn fat, you lose weight, which can also cause your body to use insulin more efficiently and lower your blood sugar levels.

The Western Definition of Aerobic

In the West, an exercise is considered aerobic if it makes your heart beat faster than it normally does. When your heart is beating fast, you'll be breathing hard and sweating and will officially be in your target zone or ideal range.

If you are on heart medications of any kind, be sure to discuss what target to aim for with your health professional.

Finding Your Pulse

You have pulse points all over your body. The easiest ones to find are those on your neck, at the base of your thumb, just below your earlobe, or on your wrist. To check your heart rate, look at a watch or clock and begin to count your beats for 15 seconds. Then multiply by 4 to get your pulse.

Other Ways to Increase Oxygen Flow

This will come as welcome news to people who have limited movement due to joint problems, arthritis, or other diabetes-related complications ranging from stroke to kidney disease. You can increase the flow of oxygen into your bloodstream without exercising your heart muscle by learning how to breathe deeply through your diaphragm. Many yoga-like programs and videos can teach you this technique, which does not require you to jump around. You would be increasing the oxygen flow into your bloodstream, which is better than doing nothing at all to improve your health, and gain many health benefits, according to myriad wellness practitioners. Core-strengthening exercises that are emphasized in Pilates are also important.

An Aerobic Activity versus Active Living

The term "aerobic activity" means that the *activity* causes your heart to pump harder and faster and causes you to breathe faster, which increases oxygen flow. Activities such as cross-country skiing, walking, hiking, and biking are all aerobic.

Health promoters are trying to get people away from terms such as "aerobic" and just stress "active living" because that's what becoming un-sedentary is all about. There are many ways you can adopt an active lifestyle. Here are some suggestions:

- Limit the time that you and your family spend watching TV, being online, texting, etc.
- Investigate working with a trainer at your local YMCA or YWCA and see if a program can be designed for you. You may need to meet with the trainer only a couple of times per year.

- If you drive everywhere, pick a parking space farther away from your destination so you can work some daily walking into your life.
- If you take public transit everywhere, get off one or two stops early so you can walk the rest of the way to your destination.
- Choose stairs more often over escalators or elevators.
- Park at one side of the mall and walk to the other.
- Take a stroll after dinner around your neighbourhood.
- Volunteer to walk the dog.
- On weekends, go to the zoo or get out to flea markets, garage sales, farmers' markets, and community events.

For activities in the workplace that you may be able to fit into your day, try:

- Using part of your lunch break to be active: either go for a quick, brisk walk, or simply climb a set of stairs in your office.
- Take the stairs in the office instead of the elevator whenever possible.
- Start a walking club with a group of work friends, and choose different routes outside around your workplace.
- Get up and do some stretching and bending every few minutes every hour at your desk.

If you are an employer, here are some tips on promoting an active living lifestyle for your employees:

- If you've already got a company-sponsored plan in place, put together a kit that could include an inspirational letter from management encouraging all employees to participate.
- Arrange for fitness assessments either on site or at a local community facility.
- Buy one or two bikes and helmets for employees to use at work for a little exercise, or perhaps to run some errands.
- Subsidize employee enrolment in walking or running programs in the community.

- Offer a weight-management program that would focus on keeping active and that would also give nutrition advice.
- Link to activity and nutrition sites on your company intranet.

The Canadian Health Network outlines exactly how we can go about encouraging and cultivating an active living community. Some of the examples that they cite on their website—like bike racks at shops, schools, and workplaces; parks with maintained and accessible trails; workplaces that provide active spaces (e.g., a fitness facility with showers and lockers, picnic tables, a basketball hoop, and walking paths); preservation of green spaces; and the encouragement of active transportation to, from, and at work—are precisely the kinds of practices put into play in cities across North America. Communities are taking more initiative and have progressively displayed interest in creating healthier towns and cities, more green spaces, and placing more focus on the outdoors and exercise.

Get a Pedometer

Pedometers have been gaining in popularity since the mid-1990s, and across Canada, there are many programs in place to encourage their usage for both kids and adults. There is a great deal of information to be found on the Internet, from places like The Alberta Centre for Active Living (www.centre4activeliving.ca), for example. The site offers excellent information in general on physical activity, and it also has an in-depth "Pedometer Information Sheet" with great tips and information on:

- what a pedometer is
- how it works
- creative ways to wear your pedometer
- how to test it
- the health benefits of walking
- how to get started on a program and progress safely
- how to care for your pedometer
- the 10,000-step goal!

And although achieving the recommended goal of 10,000 steps per day may seem insurmountable, people generally cover about half of that in their typical day, so you only have to come up with about 4,000–6,000 extra steps! As the Alberta Centre notes on their website, among the many physical health benefits that walking can bring, it can also boost your mood!

The Toronto Public Health's "Walk into Health" program offers valuable information on their website as well. They offer a pedometer-lending program through a number of branches of the Toronto Public Library throughout the city. You can borrow a pedometer for a three-week period, and anyone can download a fantastic and comprehensive brochure put together in 2007 at this link: http://www.toronto.ca/health/walkintohealth/pdf/walkintohealth_booklet.pdf, which outlines the benefits of walking, how to use a pedometer to track your steps throughout the day, safety tips while out walking in the daytime and nighttime, and how to set walking goals.

What about Muscles?

Forty percent of your body weight is made from muscle, where sugar is stored. The muscles use this sugar when they are being worked. When the sugar is used up, the muscles, in a healthy body, will take in sugar from your blood. After exercising, the muscles will continue to take in glucose to replenish the glucose that was there before exercise.

But when you have insulin resistance, glucose from your blood has difficulty getting inside your muscles; the muscles act like a brick wall. As you begin to use and tone your muscles, they will become more receptive to the glucose in your blood, allowing the glucose in. Studies show that the muscles specifically worked out in a given exercise take up glucose far more easily than another muscle in the same body that has not been worked out.

Doing weight-bearing activities is also encouraged because it builds bone mass and uses up calories. Building bone mass is particularly important; as trainers have told me, "If you want a strong house, you need a strong frame!" Women who are vulnerable to osteoporosis (loss of bone mass) as a result of estrogen loss after menopause (unless they are on hormone-replacement therapy) will benefit from these activities. The denser your bones, the harder they are to break or sprain. As we age, we are all at risk for osteoporosis unless we've either been building up our bone mass for years or are maintaining current bone mass. For information on osteoporosis, visit www.osteoporosis.ca.

By increasing muscular strength, we increase flexibility and endurance. For example, you'll find that your legs may feel sore the first time you ride your bike from home to downtown. Do that same ride 10 times, and your legs will no longer be sore. That's what's meant by building endurance. Of course, you won't be as out of breath either, which is another way of building endurance.

Hand weights or resistance exercises (using rubber-band products or pushing certain body parts together) help increase lean body mass, body tissue that is not fat. That is why many people find their weight does not drop when they begin to exercise. As your muscles become bigger, your body fat decreases.

Sugar and Muscle

When you think "muscle," think "sugar." Every time you work any muscle in your body, either independent of an aerobic activity or during an aerobic activity, your muscles use up glucose from your bloodstream as fuel. People with high blood sugar prior to muscle toning will find that their blood sugar levels are lower after the muscle has been worked.

On the downside, if you have normal blood sugar levels prior to working a muscle, you may find that your blood sugar goes too low after you exercise *unless* you eat something; this should be carbohydrates. In fact, your muscles prefer to use carbohydrates rather than fat as fuel. When your muscles use up all the sugar in your blood, your liver will convert glycogen (excess glucose it stores up for these kinds of emergencies) back into glucose and release it into your bloodstream for your muscles to use.

To avoid this scenario, eat before and after exercising if your blood sugar level is normal. How much you eat prior to exercising largely depends on what you're doing and how long you do it. The general rule is to follow your meal plan, eating smaller, more frequent meals through-out the day to keep your blood sugar levels consistent.

Athletes without diabetes will generally consume large quantities of carbohydrates before an intense workout. In fact, it's a known strategy in the athletic world to eat 40–65 g (1.5–2 oz) of carbohydrate per hour to maintain blood glucose levels to the point where performance is improved. It's also been shown that consuming glucose, sucrose, maltodextrins, or high-fructose corn syrup during exercise can increase endurance. After a training session, athletes will typically consume more carbohydrates to replenish their energy and carry on throughout the day.

Athletes who have Type 1 diabetes do exactly the same thing, ex-cept they must be more careful about timing their food intake with insulin to avoid either too low or high blood sugar.

If your blood sugar is low, don't exercise at all as it may be life-threatening. Do not resume exercise until you get your blood sugar levels under control.

Exercises That Can Be Hazardous

These are activities, such as wrestling or weightlifting, which can wors-en diabetes eye disease. In addition, they are short but very intense. As a result, unless you fuel up ahead of time, they will force your body to use glycogen (see Chapter 1), which is the stored glucose your liver keeps handy. When you have diabetes, it's not a great idea to force your liver to give up that glycogen. This can actually increase your blood pressure and put you at risk for other health problems, including hypoglycemia. To avoid this, you'll need to eat some carbohydrates prior to these exer-cises, which will provide enough fuel for the muscles.

Getting a Trainer

Consulting a personal trainer could very well help get you started on a concrete exercise regimen. Here are some tips on working with a trainer:

- Ask your friends, colleagues, or people that you may already work out with at a gym or community centre for references.

Word-of-mouth really helps to find out if someone has had a positive or negative experience with a particular trainer.

- Try it out first. A trainer either working on his or her own, or as part of a gym or community centre, should let you try out his or her services first. If you like the atmosphere, then continue.
- Definitely check the trainer's credentials. Many trainers don't renew their certification on a regular basis or don't even have any in the first place.

The following organization has certification programs in Canada: The Canadian Society for Exercise Physiology (www.csep.ca). Another place you could check to find out about certification and personal trainers is the Certified Professional Trainers Network (www.cptn.com). There is a very detailed personal trainer search form on the website that will allow you to locate someone in your area, based on the type of training regime you'd like to pursue.

LET'S GET PHYSICAL

Clearly the benefits of exercise and an active living lifestyle in general are hugely beneficial. The new CDA Guidelines are very clear in their recommendations for exercise, but modifications can be made according to decisions you make with your health care provider. The Guidelines recommend that people with diabetes should do a minimum of 150 minutes of moderate- to vigorous-intensity aerobic exercise each week, spread over at least three days of the week, with no more than two consecutive days without exercise. The examples, also noted at the end of this chapter, are for moderate intensity: biking, brisk walking, raking leaves, dancing, water aerobics, and, for vigorous intensity, jogging, hockey, basketball, fast swimming, and fast dancing.

But, as mentioned earlier, the fitness industry has done an excellent job of intimidating inactive people. Some people are so put off by the health club scene that they become even more sedentary. This is similar to diet failure when you become so demoralized that you cheat and binge even more.

If you've been sedentary most of your life, there's nothing wrong with starting off with simple, even leisurely activities such as gardening, feeding the birds in a park, or a few simple stretches. Any step you take to be more active is a crucial and important one.

Experts also recommend that you find a friend, neighbour, or relative to get physical with you. When your exercise plans include someone else, you'll be less apt to cancel plans or make excuses for not getting out there. Whoever you choose, teach this person how to recognize hypoglycemia just in case. (See Chapter 14.)

Things to Do before "Moving Day"

1. *Choose an activity that's right for you:* Whether it's walking, chopping wood, jumping rope, or folk dancing, pick something you enjoy. You don't have to do the same thing each time either. Vary your routine to avoid monotony. Just make sure that whatever activity you choose is continuous for the duration. Walking for two minutes and then stopping for three isn't continuous. It's also important to choose an activity that doesn't aggravate a pre-existing problem, such as eye problems. Lowering your head in a certain way (as in touching your toes) or straining your upper body can increase blood pressure and/or aggravate eye problems. If foot problems are a concern, perhaps an activity that doesn't involve walking, such as canoeing, is better. And so on.

2. *Choose the frequency:* Decide how often you're going to do this activity. (Twice, three, or four times a week? Or once a day?) Try not to let two days pass without doing something. And pick a duration. If you're elderly or ill, even a few minutes are a good start. If you're sedentary but otherwise healthy, aim for 20–30 minutes.

3. *Choose the intensity level that's right for you:* This is easy to do if you're using an exercise machine of some kind by just setting the dial. If you're walking, the intensity would mean how fast you are planning to walk, or how many hills you will incorporate into your walk. In other words, how fast do you want your heart to beat?

4. *Work your activity into your diet and nutrition regimen:* Once you decide what kind of exercise you'll be doing and for how long, see your dietitian about incorporating your exercise needs into your nutritional regimen. Snack prior to and after exercise if you're planning to be active for longer than 30 minutes. If you are overweight, you do not need to consume extra calories before exercising unless your blood sugar level is low.

5. *Tell your doctor what you're doing:* Your doctor may want to monitor your blood sugar more closely (or want you to do so) or adjust your medication. Don't do anything without consulting your doctor first. Before beginning a program of physical activity more vigorous than walking, people with diabetes should be assessed for conditions that might be contraindications to certain types of exercise, predispose them to injury, or be associated with increased likelihood of cardiovascular disease (CVD). An exercise electrocardiogram (ECG) stress test should be considered for previously sedentary individuals with diabetes at high risk for CVD who wish to undertake exercise more vigorous than brisk walking. Several large studies have demonstrated that in people with Type 2 diabetes, regular physical activity and/or moderate to high cardiorespiratory fitness are associated with reductions in cardiovascular and overall mortality of 39–70 percent over 15–20 years of follow-up.

When Not to Exercise

Everyone can and should exercise, but your diabetes may get in the way at times, especially if you're taking insulin, so here are some alarm bells to listen for. If they go off, skip your exercise and do what you have to do to get back on track:

- Keep track of where you're injecting insulin. Insulin injected into an arm or leg that is being worked out will be used up. Any signs of low blood sugar mean *stop exercising!*
- Check your blood sugar after 30 minutes to make sure it's still normal. If it's low, eat something before you resume exercising. (Blood

sugar below 4 mmol/L is low; anything that's 3 mmol/L or less means you should stop exercising or not start exercising at all.)

- If your blood sugar level is high, exercise will bring it down, but if it's greater than 14 mmol/L, check your urine for ketones and don't exercise. When your body is stressed, the blood sugar level can go even higher.

Table 9.1: Aerobic Exercise

Definition and Frequency	Intensity	Examples
Rhythmic, repeated, and continuous movements of the same muscle group for at least 10 minutes	Moderate (50–70 percent of a person's maximum heart rate)	Biking Brisk walking Swimming Dancing Raking leaves Water aerobics
Recommended for 150 minutes/week	Vigorous: >70 percent of heart rate	Brisk walking up an incline Jogging Aerobics Hockey Basketball Fast swimming Fast dancing

Table 9.2: Resistance Exercise

Definition	Frequency	Examples
Activities that use muscular strength to move a weight or work against a resistant load	Three times/week Start with 1 set of 10–15 repetitions at moderate weight Progress to 2 sets Progress to 3 sets of 8 reps at heavier weight	Weight machines Weightlifting

Source: Canadian Diabetes Association, 2008 Clinical Practice Guidelines: S38.

PART II

PEOPLE IN SPECIAL CIRCUMSTANCES

10

TYPE 2 DIABETES IN ABORIGINAL CANADA

It's not possible to write a book about Type 2 diabetes without address-ing the impact of this disease on Canada's Aboriginal population. Since I originally began writing about diabetes in Aboriginal Canada in 1997, things have only worsened. There are even higher numbers of cases of Type 2 diabetes and an epidemic of Type 2 diabetes in Aboriginal chil-dren (see Chapter 3). As stated earlier, among Aboriginal peoples in Canada, the rate of diabetes is three to five times that of non-Aboriginal Canadians, which is one of the highest rates of diabetes worldwide, and as high as 26 percent in individual communities.

A POPULATION AT RISK

Canadian Aboriginal peoples are comprised of individuals of First Nations, Inuit, and Métis heritage living in a range of environments from large cities to small, isolated communities. The Métis, Aboriginal people of both French and Aboriginal ancestry, are represented by the Métis National Council. The Inuit people in Canada who live in the Northwest Territories and northern Quebec are represented by the Inuit Tapirisat of Canada, while the Inuit in what is now Nunavut are represented by the Kivalliq Inuit Association.

This chapter may read more like a history textbook than a health book, but it's not possible to understand the explosion of Type 2 diabe-tes in Canada's Aboriginal population without some history.

According to extremely conservative estimates, overall, Type 2 diabetes prevalence in this population is three to five times higher than in the general Canadian population. But on many reserves, such as Akwesasne, Quebec, near Cornwall, Ontario, *more than 75 percent of residents older than 35 have diabetes*, up from 50 percent in 1989. In the First Nations community of Kahnawa:ke, in Quebec, the prevalence of diabetes in men aged 45–64 years is 14 percent, twice the corresponding rate for non-Aboriginal Canadian men, although since aggressive diabetes education programs have been initiated, incidence rates have decreased in this particular community from 1986–2003.

Overall, Aboriginal women are twice as likely to develop gestational diabetes, while exposure to diabetes in utero can predispose children to developing Type 2 diabetes. Because the symptoms of diabetes can be vague and develop slowly, many Aboriginal peoples have the disease, but do not realize it. For every known case of diabetes among Aboriginal peoples, at least one goes undiagnosed. And when you consider that Type 2 diabetes was not a recognized health problem in this community until the 1940s, this is a staggering increase. In Manitoba, it's estimated that between 1996 and 2016, there will have been a 10-fold increase in heart disease and amputations, and a five-fold increase in blindness.

Aboriginal Canadians also suffer more end-stage renal disease (ESRD), a common complication of diabetes, discussed in Chapter 19, than non-Native Canadians. Chronic renal failure among Aboriginal peoples is 2.5–4.0 times higher than in the general Canadian population, mostly due to Type 2 diabetes. The United States reports similar statistics among its indigenous populations, such as Pacific Islanders or Pima Indians.

The Aboriginal population is most at risk for this disease because of thrifty genes, which is also discussed in chapters 2 and 11. Centuries of living off the land, eating seasonally and indigenously, bred metabolisms that weren't able to adapt to nutrient excess and a sedentary lifestyle. Yet prior to contact with Europeans, Canada's Aboriginal peoples were leading the kind of healthy lifestyle that may ultimately prevent diabetes from developing in the first place.

A BRIEF HISTORY OF CANADIAN ABORIGINAL HEALTH

Aboriginal history in Canada is broken down into two periods: the pre-European or pre-contact period, and the post-contact period. We refer to the meeting of European and Aboriginal societies as "first contact." Europeans failed miserably in their first contact mission because they interfered, took over, and ruined a culture, with both health and environmental consequences for *all* peoples.

At the time of their first contact with Europeans, Aboriginal peoples enjoyed good health. Infections were rare; fevers were unheard of; while mental, emotional, and physical vigour was status quo. For any ailment, a common remedy was to enter a smokehouse and sweat it out. Sweat lodges are still a traditional form of healing.

Before being exposed to European foods, Aboriginal peoples lived on the ideal diet of seasonal foods native to Canada. Eating foods seasonably indigenous to the land is a concept widely written about in several disease-prevention health books. In pre-European Canada, there was no cholera, typhus, smallpox, measles, cancer, or skin problems, while fractures were also rare. Mental illness among Aboriginal peoples during this time was also unheard of. Interestingly, more than 500 drugs used in pharmaceuticals today were originally used by Aboriginal peoples.

The Diseases

As European ships arrived in Canada, they brought with them a smorgasbord of strange and new bacteria and viruses, causing terrible epidemics among Aboriginal peoples. (This is not unlike what happens to Europeans when they go into Africa and Asia and are exposed to micro-organisms to which they have no immunity.) Many European explorers and settlers were weak and sick when they first met Aboriginal peoples because they'd survived a long voyage in crowded, unsanitary ships with contaminated drinking water and food that had gone bad. Nevertheless, thousands of Aboriginal peoples got sick and died from infections they caught from Europeans. Influenza, measles, polio, diphtheria, smallpox, and other diseases were brought to Canada from the public health disaster areas of European slums. In a sense, the result was genocide as Aboriginal peoples died by the thousands during the eighteenth and nineteenth centuries. And thus began an incredible transformation: Healthy people became steadily unhealthy as more Europeans came to Canada. Sources of food and clothing from the land diminished, while centuries of a traditional economy dissolved. And, worst of all, once-mobile, active people were confined to small plots of land with limited natural resources and poor sanitation. *Fit people became unfit.* Amid this physical deterioration, centuries of spiritual practices and beliefs were actually outlawed as Christianity took over. With ceremonial and spiritual activity banned (elders and healers were prosecuted by Christians for engaging in unlawful spiritual ceremonies), self-respect and cultural pride began to disappear.

The early twentieth century was one of the worst periods in Canadian Aboriginal history. Epidemics and disease were rampant, and the Canadian government responded with feeble attempts to improve Aboriginal peoples' health. From the end of the nineteenth century to the middle of the twentieth, semi-trained RCMP agents, missionaries, and officers tried to administer health care. The 1918 influenza epidemic was particularly harsh, and thousands of Aboriginal peoples succumbed to influenza.

By 1930, the first nursing station was opened on a Manitoba reserve. Fearing the spread of tuberculosis from Aboriginal communities into the general population, by 1950 the Canadian government was operating 33 nursing stations, 65 health centres, and 18 small regional hospitals for what were then known as "registered Indians" and Inuit. Virtually all providers of health and social services for Aboriginal peoples were White Europeans, people who had no knowledge of Aboriginal healing skills, herbal medicines, or other traditional treatments.

From Disease to Diseased Environment

As waters became polluted and environmental raping of resources continued, the diseases changed from infectious to chronic. "Country food," traditional food indigenous to Canada, such as wild game, fish, root vegetables, fruit, whale meat, and blubber (now known to contain omega-3 oils, which are linked to low levels of heart disease and cholesterol and hence are heart-protective foods), became increasingly unavailable, forcing Aboriginal peoples to eat the processed, refined foods of Europeans. Cut off from their habitat, fishing, hunting, ceremonies, and indigenous food supply, and exposed to infections, alcohol, and overprocessed foods high in fat and sugar, Aboriginal peoples developed poor eating habits, and became obese and inactive. The main risk factors for Type 2 diabetes are obesity, poor eating habits, and physical inactivity.

On the Akwesasne reserve, for example, diabetes exploded in the population as Mohawks turned to fast foods after their traditional diet of perch became contaminated with PCBs. Yellow perch was the staple of the Mohawk diet for centuries until the 1950s, when the St. Lawrence Seaway was constructed and became polluted by industry. In 1980, scientists deemed the perch unsafe for human consumption. What happened on Akwesasne has happened all over North America. Today, there's a project in place to raise healthy perch in tanks to replenish the once-healthy and traditional diet. Similar projects are springing up all over the country and are crucial in helping to contain the Type 2 diabetes epidemic among Native peoples.

The Issue of Cash Crops

Cash crops have further deteriorated indigenous food supplies. By the early twentieth century, chemical agriculture and factory farming revolutionized food production, a practice that has had a detrimental effect on the traditional Aboriginal diet. Canada's corn production over the last 40 years is a good example of the nutritional perils of overfarming.

Corn used to be the grain staple of Canada's Aboriginal peoples in the Gananoque region, and was an industry controlled by them until the introduction of hybrid corn during the 1930s and early 1940s. Hybrid corn replaced the open-pollinated varieties that naturally flourished in Ontario. Before 1960, corn was a fairly minor crop in Canada, mostly limited to Ontario. But because of new technology and the development of better-yielding and earlier-maturing hybrids, corn boomed throughout the 1960s and 1970s, transforming itself from a regional crop into a cash crop as it became the most popular feed grain for livestock (beef, pork, and poultry). By 1980, more than 30 percent of cultivated farmland was seeded annually to corn. But corn is also used to make paper and cardboard, automobiles, clothing, absorbents (in diapers and sanitary napkins), non-petroleum-based plastics, and now ethyl alcohol as an alternative fuel. The problem with this type of farming is that corn soon became the *only* crop on several farms, causing a number of environmental problems. The soils in which corn was planted each year became overworked and nutrient-poor, leading to crop failures and unstable farm income. Corn rootworm, a pest common to one type of corn, became rampant in the 1970s and early 1980s, necessitating the use of pesticides. But the more pesticides were used, the more resistant the pests became, and the more exotic the pesticide concoctions became. Soon, these pesticides were detected in rivers and streams, getting into fish and groundwater, destroying important sources of food in that region and beyond.

The Impact of Poverty and Isolation

Because poverty is also rampant among Aboriginal peoples, the food supply is further diminished. Another problem is the cost involved in transporting fresh vegetables and fruits to remote locations, where many Aboriginal peoples reside. Shipping costs and poor supplier selection aggravate matters. There is a real problem in understanding how to shop for Western food, too. Reading labels and interpreting ingredients create so much confusion that grocery shopping tours are now being conducted by volunteers. In the Sandy Lake Project, for example, people were shown how to walk down grocery aisles, select food, and read labels. Projects regarding health food choices labelling are also being initiated.

Planting vegetable gardens that can provide natural foods for communities sounds like a good idea, but in many communities, gardening is associated with a time when gardening was done out of necessity, when White culture killed off Native hunting, so it is not a desirable activity.

Meanwhile, a lack of familiarity with European food preparation aggravates matters, too. In the same way that most Europeans would be unfamiliar with whale blubber recipes, many Aboriginal peoples are not up on their vegetarian lasagna recipes. Cooking methods for imported foods are also unfamiliar to many Aboriginal peoples. Therefore, high-protein, low-fat foods and quality game meats (which are much lower in fat than livestock-raised meats, and high in iron and vitamin C) have been replaced with starches, fats, sugar, and alcohol. As mentioned above, the traditional diet of Aboriginal peoples was far superior to the Western diet that made everyone fat (see Chapter 11). Today's diet, coupled with a sedentary lifestyle, is shown not only to increase the incidence of obesity—and hence diabetes—but to increase blood pressure and dental problems. Aboriginal peoples are also burdened with an alarming list of heart diseases, cancer, infant morbidity, and mortality in higher frequencies than non-Aboriginal Canadians.

Genetics

To our genes, 200 years is an exceedingly short amount of time to ask our immune systems and metabolisms to adjust. Aboriginal peoples have not built up an immunity to an overabundance of food—particular nutrient-poor foods, such as junk food, known as "overnutrition," which encourages overeating. Europeans, for the most part, haven't lived nomadically for thousands of years and have therefore developed metabolisms to adjust to more sedentary lifestyles in response to urbanized living.

This is why it is said that Aboriginal peoples have an inherited tendency toward diabetes, known as thrifty genes. Because Aboriginal peoples lived seasonably on indigenous diets for so many centuries, their bodies are still behaving as though they were living in seventeenth-century Canada. To date, two distinct genetic mutations linked to Type 2 diabetes were found among the Oji-Cree in northern Ontario.

HEALING ABORIGINAL COMMUNITIES

As I have stressed throughout this book, diet is one of the most crucial aspects in managing Type 2 diabetes, yet Aboriginal peoples with Type 2 diabetes often do not understand the concept of low GI eating, for example, or meal planning. That's because the role of food is different in Aboriginal culture. For one thing, there are strong cultural beliefs that equate health and prosperity with being overweight. The more central problem is that many Aboriginal peoples do not have information about the cost and availability of many of the foods recommended in these meal plans.

The traditional Aboriginal diet consisted mostly of high-protein game meat with very few vegetables. In fact, fruits and vegetables are not usually available in the small stores on most reserves, and if they are, they are so expensive that nobody buys them.

As a result, projects such as the Northern Food, Tradition, and Health Kit, which encourages traditional foods for health and well-being, were developed for the Northwest Territories. This kit is far more relevant for people with diabetes in this culture and was developed by the Nutrition Section, Department of Health, Government of the Northwest Territories, after elders and Northern educators requested it. The kit incorporates traditional regional foods, cooking, and preserving practices. Food items include small land mammals, sea mammals, three kinds of fish, sea urchins, fish eggs, birds, wild greens, berries, and bannock. Pictures of the foods are in an accompanying booklet to increase comprehension, while a resource booklet provides a lot of background information, worksheets, posters, and various other components to promote cultural pride in Northern foods and food preparation.

In Zuni First Nation children, an educational component targeting sugary soft drinks, awareness of risk factors, and a youth-oriented fitness centre helped to significantly decrease insulin resistance. These programs are designed to reduce childhood obesity. Other programs look at reducing obesity in women prior to their first pregnancies and help to promote breastfeeding in the first year of life.

In Australia, one study initiated a temporary return to a traditional hunter-gatherer lifestyle among Australian Aboriginal males, and was shown to significantly improve glucose levels and overall health. A number of American studies have looked at introducing a more carbohydrate-restrictive diet that mirrors the hunting diet that was more indigenous to this population; the results are similar with respect to improved glucose readings. As a result, the traditional Aboriginal diet that is carbohydrate-restrictive is being considered as one way to manage diabetes in this population. Returning the body to the diet it once knew and thrived on is the general idea.

Overall, diabetes education programs in Aboriginal communities need to incorporate local traditional activities and foods, and be taught in the languages of the individual communities.

Traditional Healers

Treating diabetes in the Aboriginal population is not possible within the current Western framework. Many Aboriginal peoples with Type 2 diabetes usually do not follow a doctor's orders regarding medication, diet, and exercise, but it's not because there's a problem with the patient; there is a problem with the way Western medicine is *communicating* with that patient.

Aboriginal peoples approach their health from a cultural perspective; the health of the culture and community is reflected in the individuals of that community. Therefore, telling an Aboriginal person to "work out" every day is not as effective as planning, say, a community walk. Health and wellness programs must be connected to the health and wellness of the community and environment. Western-trained health care providers are beginning to recognize that they are woefully unequipped to deliver health care to the Aboriginal community. In fact, Aboriginal doctors and nurses have clearly identified that the diabetes educational and prevention materials available to their patients are not culturally relevant. Individual self-care can take place only if there is *community* self-care.

Nor does the West provide health care services in accordance with the Circle of Life or the Medicine Wheel, which have guided the health and wellness of Aboriginal Canadians for generations. In fact, the Circle of Life is a far more progressive and sophisticated approach to health than Western medicine. It incorporates physical, emotional, social, and spiritual aspects of health. The premise of the Circle of Life is that good health occurs when there is balance and harmony within the self, the society, and the natural environment. When there is no harmony, there is ill health.

The role of spirituality is central to Aboriginal health, while traditional healing methods and therapies can make an enormous contribution to managing diabetes in the Aboriginal population.

The majority of traditional healers went underground when they were persecuted by Canadian governments and the Christian Church for using ceremonies, herbal treatments, and other Native therapies. By the 1960s, healers were almost wiped out. In the 1980s, some members of the Peguis First Nation community in Manitoba began exploring their cultural roots, and a new movement began to bring back the practices of traditional medicine. Today, with explosive interest in complementary and alternative medicine, traditional healing is encouraged by Western health care providers. Now, traditional healers come under the Non-insured Health Benefits Program for Aboriginal peoples. There is a movement for traditional healers to be recognized by the College of Physicians and Surgeons in each province. It is hoped that healing centres and lodges will be accessible in urban, rural, and reserve settings to all Aboriginal peoples, and that they will deliver integrated health and social services.

Aboriginal/Community Diabetes Programs

The most recent trend in treating Aboriginal peoples with Type 2 diabetes is to combine Western medicine with Northern traditions. Right now, professional organizations such as the Native Physicians Association in Canada (NPAC), the Native Psychologists in Canada (NPC), and the Aboriginal Nurses Association of Canada (ANAC) play a crucial role in marrying the West and North. The NPAC includes over 100 physicians of Aboriginal ancestry; most members are women working in primary care, who are actively involved in Aboriginal health.

Several programs, such as the Northern Diabetes Health Network, utilize Aboriginal Canadians as diabetes educators who tailor education for the community. That means that culturally appropriate questions such as "Did you have any bannock [a traditional bread] today?" will be asked of patients.

The Diabetic Education Program for Native People is based on the Standards and Guidelines of the Canadian Diabetes Association and includes a cultural component throughout.

The Sioux Lookout Diabetes Program (SLDP) was one of the first model programs, which served Ojibway and Cree First Nations people from 30 remote communities in northwestern Ontario, many of which can be reached only by plane. This program established a registry of people with diabetes within the community and was one of the first to have a multidisciplinary approach, with full-time dieticians and staff who travelled to the communities to provide education; in the past, the communities were expected to come to one out-of-the-way hospital for education. This community-based diabetes program involved the community's input with respect to educational materials. Instead of pictures of people in aerobics classes, materials showed people doing familiar activities such as chopping wood. The materials were also translated into the community's first language—Cree rather than English or French.

Today, a number of Aboriginal communities provide similar comprehensive diabetes training for local lay people, who can then combine their knowledge of diabetes with their knowledge of their own culture.

Healing Circles are also used to explain blood sugar monitoring in a bloodletting ceremony. Walking groups have also been started in a few communities; during these events the whole community, not just one individual, becomes more active. Other culture-specific programs involve elders in diabetes education, who remind their community about traditions of food patterns and fitness. Traditional feasts are also used to teach diabetes education, using only traditional, and not Western, foods.

These programs have proven beyond a doubt that when education gaps created through cultural and language barriers are closed; when diet and activity are better suited to the cultural environment of Aboriginal communities; and when the intimidating Western health practitioner is removed, diabetes education and management can work.

11

"DIABESITY": THE OBESITY-DIABETES CONNECTION

Eighty to 90 percent of those with Type 2 diabetes are overweight or obese. The connection between Type 2 diabetes and obesity is so profound that the term "diabesity" emerged a few years ago, which refers to a linked problem rather than obesity in isolation. It's been shown that as soon as people with diabetes begin to lose weight, Type 2 diabetes can often be reversed. In fact, studies that have looked at people with diabetes who have undergone bariatric surgery have found that Type 2 diabetes can virtually disappear within two weeks after surgery. This chapter looks at the causes of obesity and the best methods for weight loss, including bariatric surgery, for those who are morbidly obese.

WHY WE ARE GETTING FATTER?

Today, there is no question that the North American lifestyle is considered the single largest contributing factor to obesity. Although social, behavioural, metabolic, cellular, and molecular factors all contribute to obesity, obesity genes were turned on only when they were exposed to an environment conducive to weight gain, such as the North American environment.

North Americans have the highest obesity rates in the world. More than half of North American adults and about 25 percent of North American children are now obese (see Chapter 3). These figures reflect a doubling of adult obesity rates since the 1960s, and a doubling of the childhood obesity rate since the late 1970s, a staggering increase when you think about it in raw numbers. Obese children will most likely grow up to become obese adults, according to the most recent research.

For many years, people have been hearing that obesity is caused by sedentary living and eating too much of the wrong things. In other words, obesity is caused by an energy imbalance: consuming more calories than can be burned off through regular activity. That's still true, but now researchers who look at nutrition through a socio-political and ethical lens are beginning to hold the food industry more accountable for the obesity increase through their advertising, spending, and lobbying practices, as well as their questionable influence on schools and nutritional researchers. All of this is corrupting the way our children live and eat, and the way nutrition labelling and guidelines are developed. As adult consumers, we have become confused by what we see on food labels and in printed guidelines. Even when we consciously try to select what we think are more nutritious foods, we frequently wind up consuming hidden calories.

Other changes in our society have contributed to obesity, too. We are more sedentary due to long commutes, bigger and better televisions, strip mall living, which makes it harder to do errands on foot (endemic in the suburbs), as well as more time spent on the computer. Our children are no longer encouraged to walk to school or play outside in many neighbourhoods because of safety concerns. Many parents are opting for indoor, safer activities, fearing their children will vanish along with thousands of others. In many communities, budget cuts have led schools to cut their physical education programs and facilities. In urban communities, there is less green space and parks, replaced by malls (always with food courts) and parking lots. People are working harder to make the same wages, and two-income families are more stretched and stressed each year. Alongside these changes, the fast-food industry has experienced enormous growth, making more high-fat, inexpensive meals widely available to all. Thus, convenience foods, as they are also called, have become the standard North American diet. The socio-economic causes of obesity are more complex than you might think.

Defining Obesity

Obesity refers to a body size that is too fat for good health. Obese people have greater incidences of heart attacks, strokes, peripheral vascular disease (circulation problems, leading to many other health problems), Type 2 diabetes, and certain types of cancers.

At one time, being defined as "obese" applied to people who weighed 20 percent more than their ideal weight for their age and height, but this is not as accurate an indicator as the body mass index (BMI), which is now the best measurement of obesity The BMI is calculated by dividing your weight (in kilograms) by your height (in metres) squared. (The formula used is: BMI = kg/m^2 if you're doing this on your calculator.) BMI charts abound on the Internet, the backs of cereal boxes, and in numerous health magazines. Most people can now easily find BMI converters on the Internet, where you simply type in your weight in pounds, as most of the online BMI calculators are generated in the United States, which does not use the metric system, and your height to arrive at your BMI.

Currently, a BMI of 18.5 or less indicates that you are underweight. A BMI between 18.5 and 24.9 is normal weight. The most recent clinical guidelines define people with a BMI between 25 and 29.9 as overweight; those with a BMI between 30 and 34.9 as Class I obese; 35–39.9 as Class II obese; and 40 or greater as Class III obese.

Morbid Obesity

People with BMIs in the high thirties or over 40 are classified as morbidly obese. Another method to calculate morbid obesity is using ideal body weight: When people exceed their ideal weight by over 45 kg (100 lbs), they are considered morbidly obese. People who are morbidly obese are at the highest risk of health complications. For example, morbidly obese men aged between 25 and 35 have 12 times the risk of dying prematurely than their peers of normal weights. Morbid obesity also causes a range of medical problems, such as breathing difficulties, gastrointestinal ailments, endocrine problems (especially diabetes), musculoskeletal problems, hygiene problems, sexual problems, and so on. For these reasons, bariatric surgery may be an option. (See page 179.)

OVERNOURISHMENT

Nutrition experts call North Americans malnourished through *nutrient excess*. In the early twentieth century, public health initiatives sought to lower rates of infectious diseases such as TB and diphtheria by improving nutrition. In 1900, life expectancy was under 50; nutritionists encouraged people to eat a greater variety of foods so that infectious diseases would not be made worse by malnutrition. Improvements in sanitation also led to fewer outbreaks of infectious diseases. By the 1970s, life expectancy rose to about 70, which was considered a huge improvement. Foods became fortified with vitamins, and minerals such as iron, and school lunch programs were introduced, which helped to virtually eliminate North American children dying from starvation and undernourishment. Once the food supply became more abundant, fortified, and accessible, sedentary living and a "diet of leisure" became the norm.

The seeds of sedentary life were already planted in the 1920s as consumer comforts, mainly the automobile and radio, led to more driving, less walking, and more sedentary recreation. The Depression interrupted what was supposed to be prosperous times for everyone. It also intercepted obesity and all diseases related to obesity as most industrialized nations barely ate enough to survive.

The Depression years, which ended in Canada when Britain declared war on Germany in 1939, combined with six long years of war, led to an unprecedented yearning for consumer goods such as cars, refrigerators, stoves, radios, and washing machines. As the boys marched home, they were welcomed with open arms into civilian bliss. By 1948, university enrolment had doubled in a decade, leading to an explosion in desk jobs and the commuter economy that exists today. The return of the veterans led to an unprecedented baby boom, driving the candy, sweets, and junk-food markets for decades to come. Moreover, a sudden influx of money from Victory Bond investments and veterans' re-establishment grants coincided with the first payments of government pensions and family allowances. Never before had North Americans had so much money.

Manufacturers and packaged-goods companies were looking for better ways to compete and sell their products. The answer to their prayers arrived in the late 1940s with the cathode ray tube: television.

In the end, television would become the appliance most responsible for dietary decline and sedentary lifestyle as it turned into a babysitter that could mesmerize the baby boom generation for hours.

The Diet of Leisure

Naturally, after the war, people wanted to celebrate. They gave parties, they drank wine, they smoked, they went to restaurants. More than ever before, our diets began to include more high-fat items, refined carbohydrates, sugar, alcohol, and chemical additives. And as people began to manage large families, easy-fix meals in boxes and cans were being manufactured in abundance and advertised on television to millions.

The demand for the diet of leisure radically changed agriculture, too. Today, 80 percent of our grain harvest goes to feed livestock. The rest of our arable land is used for other cash crops such as tomatoes, sugar, coffee, and bananas. Ultimately, cash crops have helped to create the modern Western diet: an obscene amount of meat, eggs, dairy products, sugar, and refined flour.

Since 1940, chemical additives and preservatives in food have risen by 995 percent. In 1959, the Flavor and Extract Manufacturers Association of the United States (FEMA) established a panel of experts to determine the safety status of food flavourings to deal with the overwhelming number of chemicals that companies wanted to add to our foods.

One of the most popular food additives is monosodium glutamate (MSG), the sodium salt of glutamic acid, an amino acid that occurs naturally in protein-containing foods such as meat, fish, milk, and many vegetables. MSG is a flavour enhancer that researchers believe contributes a "fifth taste" to savoury foods such as meats, stews, tomatoes, and cheese. It was originally extracted from seaweed and other plant sources to function in foods the same way as other spices or extracts. Today, MSG is made from starch, corn, sugar, or molasses from sugar cane or sugar beets. MSG is produced by a fermentation process similar to that used for making products such as beer, vinegar, and yogourt. While MSG is labelled "Generally recommended as safe" (GRAS) by the United States Food and Drug Administration (FDA), questions about the safety of ingesting MSG have been raised because food sensitivities to the substance have been reported. This fact notwithstanding, the main problem with MSG is that it arouses our appetites even more. Widespread in our food supply, MSG makes food taste better. And the better food tastes, the more we eat.

Hydrolyzed proteins are also used as flavour enhancers. These are made by using enzymes to chemically digest proteins from soy meal, wheat gluten, corn gluten, edible strains of yeast, or other food sources. This process, known as hydrolysis, breaks down proteins into their component amino acids. Today, there are several hundred additive substances like these used in our food, including sugar, baking soda, and vitamins.

Of course, one of the key functions of food additives is to preserve foods for transport. The problem is that once we begin to eat foods that are not indigenous to our country, the food loses many of its nutrient properties. Refrigerators make it possible for us to eat tropical foods in Canada and Texas-raised beef in Japan. As a result, few industrialized countries eat indigenously anymore.

Eating More

Today, concerns over overnourishment have become a public health crusade. In 1997, North American children got 50 percent of their calories from added fat and sugar; only 1 percent of children surveyed had a diet that resembled "variety" based on government nutritional guidelines, such as Canada's Food Guide or the US Food Pyramid. Both Canada and the US have almost parallel recommendations stressing a diet that relies mostly on plant-based foods (grains, fruits, and vegetables), some dairy, and less meat. Snack foods and sweets are not in these guidelines.

Another public health puzzle is that in spite of the overabundance of food, many poor children in North American still do not have enough nutritious foods to eat; however, diets of poverty are relying on cheaper, high-fat, overprocessed foods, which contribute to childhood obesity. Overall, roughly 3 million Canadians live in poverty, and the majority are women; two-thirds of food bank users are single mothers, while close to half a million children in this country, mostly all in households headed by single mothers, are considered "food insecure" by Statistics Canada. According to The National Population Health Survey, half a million Canadians did not have enough money for food.

The diet-related medical costs for the six main obesity-related conditions total over 70 billion. As a population, if we reduced our saturated fat intake by just 1 percent, we could shave more than $1 billion off health care costs. The North American food supply is so abundant that we could feed everyone in the world twice over. Add to that an affluent society that can afford to buy "nice-to-have" foods versus "must-have" foods, and you have a competitive food marketplace, which, by the way, was the industry that first labelled its end-user the "consumer" based (of course) on how much of their product we literally consumed.

The food industry would not make money if it told us to eat less food. Therefore, it must tell us to eat more food in order to profit. Marion Nestle, nutritionist and author of *Food Politics*, calls this the politics of "eat more," which dominates the food industry. To get us to eat more, food companies sometimes have to get us to eat more of one product instead of another. Distorted facts from various health studies may be combined with labelling to achieve this. Tomato sauce and ketchup producers tell us that lycopene in the tomatoes will protect us from prostate cancer, so we are instructed to *eat more* of that and less of something else. Manufacturers of cereals with oats (no matter how much sugar and calories are mixed in with those oats) tell us that if we *eat more* of that product, we'll prevent heart disease (also a distortion). Studies looking at whether certain foods are of benefit to our health are frequently sponsored by food companies.

We will also eat more to get more value for our dollar. "Dollar meals" or getting an obscene size of a particular product for "just a dollar/quarter/dime more" pushes us to eat more. Adding side products to the meal and selling it as a package also gets us to eat more. Fast-food chains purchase commodities in bulk, so they are able to offer value portions, which offer much bigger portions for just a few cents more per person, translating into profit for the food companies. In the late 1950s, for example, adult-sized soft drinks were 250 mL (8 oz);

today child-sized drinks at McDonald's are 360 mL (12 oz), and a large soft drink is 960 mL (32 oz). A large portion of fries at McDonald's in 1972 was three times smaller than the supersize fries most people purchase today, which contains 610 calories and 29 g of fat per serving. If you ordered a regular hamburger, fries, and a 360 mL (12 oz) Coke, you would ingest 600 calories. Now, most orders are rarely for regular hamburgers; most people order a Quarter Pounder with Cheese (440 calories), a Big Mac (580 calories), and so on. Add the supersize fries and supersize drink, and you're eating more.

In sit-down restaurants (particularly in the United States), the portions are enormous, often enough to feed four people. People feel obliged to finish the portions in order to get value for their dollar, or so they won't feel as though they're wasting money. Many restaurants now have "no sharing" signs posted on menus, thus discouraging people from eating less. I visited one restaurant that offered a huge breakfast for just $2.99, allowing the customer to order between one and six eggs for the same price, with strict admonitions that one couldn't share. (Hopefully this might ensure fewer people would take advantage of the six-egg deal.) All-you-can-eat buffets are popping up faster than you can say "all you can eat." I have referred to these types of restaurants in the past as "obesity delivery systems." The value of the buffet is more economical than ordering from the menu, so everyone winds up at the buffet—at least twice—no matter how disciplined they try to be.

Companies have also found ways to market their "sub products." For example, Timbits, one of the most popular fast-food items sold in Canada, are marketed as "doughnut holes." Timbits were introduced in Canada in 1976. (Dunkin' Donuts, the largest doughnut chain in North America, which is US-based, has a similar product called a "munchkin.") Today, people are encouraged to buy them in bulk in a snack pack of 20 or a family pack of 45.

Pizza companies now routinely offer dipping sauces for the pizza crusts, a common throwaway item for many. The dipping sauces thereby encourage people who would normally toss their crust or not finish it to *eat more*. Pizza companies now routinely offer an oxymoron: "dessert pizza," which, incredibly, has taken off. Consumers actually will order a pizza for dinner, which packs more than enough calories into it for the whole family. And then they complete their meal with a dessert pizza, which takes the form of large danishes or pies. There is an entire generation of children who think that "dessert pizza" is a natural second course to regular pizza.

Currently North Americans order roughly 3 billion pizzas a year from more than 60,000 pizzerias that are either chains (such as McDonald's-owned Donatos) or individually owned. One out of every six restaurants is a pizzeria; annual sales reach $30 billion, and are topped only by hamburger sales. Although some nutritionists argue that pizza represents all food groups, many feel it is simply a high-calorie food that no one needs. At Pizza Hut, three pieces of pizza have 12 g of saturated fat.

The Impact of "Low-Fat" Products

Since the late 1970s, North Americans have been deluged with low-fat products. In 1990, the United States government launched Healthy People 2000, a campaign to urge manufacturers to double their output of low-fat products by the year 2000. Since 1990, more than 1,000 new fat-free or low-fat products have been introduced into North American supermarkets annually. Data show that with regard to absolute fat, the intake has increased from 81 g per day in 1980 to 83 g per day in the 1990s. Total calorie intake has also increased, from 1,989 calories per day in 1980 to 2,153 calories per day in the 1990s. In fact, the data show a drop in the percentage of calories from fat only because of the huge increase in calories per day. The result is that as a population, we weigh more today than in 1980, even though roughly 10,000 more low-fat foods are available to us now than in 1980.

Most of these low-fat products, however, actually encourage people to eat more. For example, if a bag of regular chips has 9 g of fat per serving (one serving usually equals five or six chips or one handful), we will more likely stick to that one handful. However, if we find a low-fat brand of chips that boasts "50 percent less fat" per serving, we're more likely to eat the whole bag because they are low-fat chips, which can easily triple your fat intake.

Low-fat or fat-free foods trick our bodies with ingredients that mimic the functions of fat in foods. This is often achieved by using modified fats that are only partially metabolized, if at all. While some foods have the fat reduced by removing the fat (as in skim milk and lean cuts of meat), most low-fat foods require a variety of "fat copycats" to preserve the taste and texture of the food. These fat replacers are discussed in Chapter 8.

There's no question that low-fat foods are designed to give you more freedom of choice with your diet, supposedly allowing you to cut your fat intake without compromising your taste buds. Studies show that taste ranks higher than nutrition in your brain. Many experts believe that in the long-term, low-fat products create more of a barrier to weight loss.

Researchers at the University of Toronto suggest that these products essentially allow us to increase our calories even though we are reducing our overall fat intake. For example, in one study, women who consumed a low-fat breakfast food ate more during the day than women who consumed a higher-fat food at breakfast.

LIFE IN THE FAST LANE

In Eric Schlosser's *Fast Food Nation*, he tells us how we became a society ruled by fast-food chains, which have infiltrated every aspect of our culture to the detriment of our health or what he refers to as "the McDonaldization of America" (a term coined by farm activist Jim Hightower). Indeed, the obesity epidemic hit North America when we began eating meals outside the home.

Today, half our meals are prepared outside the home and 25 percent are fast foods. We depend on prepackaged sandwiches, salads, entrées, and desserts. Supermarkets now have salad bars, hot food bars, takeout chicken, and prepared "home meal replacements." And then there are takeout foods.

If you look at the prices of grocery-bought convenience foods, such as frozen foods or supermarket-prepared "home meals," they're often not as cheap and predictable as fast foods. That is why they proliferate. But even when we try to choose more nutritious offerings, the hidden fat in fast foods has made us fatter.

In surveys on dietary patterns conducted between 1970 and the late 1990s, people report eating less fat, but, in fact, dietary fat has increased during that time frame by 25 percent. USDA nutritionists account for these discrepancies by concluding that the fat is hidden. Although people think they are eating less fat because they are choosing products they believe have less fat, they are actually eating more hidden fat within the products they choose.

With the exception of salads, fast foods are prepared elsewhere, and arrive at the chain in a frozen or freeze-dried state. We are not actually eating what we think we are. If you're a vegetarian, for example, you might be upset to learn that McDonald's fries are cooked in beef extract, which is what gives its fries a characteristic taste. Wendy's Grilled Chicken Sandwich also contains beef extract. Chicken McNuggets, introduced in 1983, are reconstituted chicken held together with stabilizers. They're breaded, fried, frozen, and then reheated. People select McNuggets thinking that they're chicken, and ergo, lower in fat, but a Harvard study that analyzed the contents of McNuggets revealed that they were cooked in beef tallow, and were more beef than fowl in the final analysis. Now McNuggets are cooked in vegetable oil, but beef extract is still used to make them. Chicken McNuggets, a favourite menu item for children, actually have twice as much fat as a regular hamburger.

Hamburgers have problems, too. About 25 percent of the ground beef used for hamburgers sold in fast-food chains comes from "dried-up" dairy cows, who are not as healthy as free-range cattle raised specifically for beef. Dairy cows frequently have antibiotic residue in their meat because of the antibiotics used in the dairy industry to prevent or treat infections involving the cows' nipples or breasts. Meat from dozens of different cows is all ground up together, so one hamburger could come from several different animals, which accounts for a rise in the notorious *E. coli* bacteria.

Obesity rates go up wherever fast foods are available. Between 1984 and 1993, the number of fast-food chains in the United Kingdom doubled, and so have its obesity rates. Britain, notorious for expensive, bad food and small portions (by our standards), is now eating more fast foods than any other country outside of North America. Asian diets are considered ideal, and Asian populations have also enjoyed the lowest obesity rates in the world among First World countries. But in China, obesity rates among its teenagers have tripled since the 1990s, along with the fast-food restaurants. Similarly, in Japan, obesity rates have doubled since the arrival of Ronald McDonald in 1971. Now, Japan is witnessing the first generation of men who are obese.

Schlosser notes that in 1960, the typical North American ate only 2 kg (4 lbs) of frozen french fries per year; today the typical North American consumes roughly 22 kg (49 lbs) of frozen fries per year, 90 percent of which are purchased at fast-food restaurants. North Americans spent $6 billion on fast foods in 1970; that number climbed to $110 billion by 2000, more than North Americans spent on education, high-tech equipment, cars, or other items.

In Canada, the first McDonald's opened in 1967. By 2000 there were 1,100 outlets. At least 25 percent of the North American adult population go to a fast-food restaurant once a day. Unfortunately, most people don't go to fast-food chains to get the lighter fare items; they are there to satisfy a craving for brand-name items they hate to love.

BIOLOGICAL CAUSES OF OBESITY

The physiological cause of obesity is eating more calories than you burn. People gain weight for two reasons: they may eat excessively (often excessive amounts of nutritious foods), which results in daily consumption of just too many calories; or they may eat moderately, but are too inactive for the amount of calories they ingest. Genetic makeup can predispose some body types to obesity earlier in life because of "thrifty genes" (see below). But in general, experts in nutrition agree that genetics plays only a *small* role in the sharp increase in obesity. Since genetic changes take place over centuries, and our obesity rate has at least doubled since the 1960s, it's fairly obvious that lifestyle factors are the chief culprit. Furthermore, as we age, our metabolisms slow down, which means that unless we decrease our calories or increase activity levels to compensate, we will probably gain weight. Hormonal problems can also contribute to obesity, such as an underactive thyroid gland (called hypothyroidism), which is very common in women particularly.

Thrifty Genes

Thrifty genes were first introduced in Chapter 2, pp. 31–32. Again, genetics plays a role in obesity when it comes to Aboriginal and other minority groups, due to what some researchers call the "thrifty gene." This is the gene thought to be responsible for the higher rates of obesity and obesity-related conditions in the Aboriginal and non-European populations. For more on this, please refer back to chapter 2.

Asian populations generally have the lowest rates of obesity, but that is also because they are frequently able to maintain their dietary habits when they emigrate to North America. In fact, European North Americans tend to benefit when they adopt the same Asian diets. That said, when Asian and South East Asian populations begin eating the North American way—pizzas, hamburgers, fries, sweet drinks, and snack foods—their obesity rates begin to soar, too, and they are more prone to Type 2 diabetes.

Thrifty genes are evident when you look at the obesity patterns in the United States. There, obesity is more prevalent in African Americans, Latinos, Native Americans, Native Hawaiians, and American Samoans; these groups have higher incidences of diabetes and cardiovascular disease, as well. For example, almost 63 percent of Native Hawaiian women are obese, and between 61 and 75 percent of Yaqui Indians are overweight. Among Hispanics, Mexicans have the highest rates of obesity (48.2 percent), followed by Puerto Ricans (40.2 percent).

Diets of poverty may also be a factor, particularly on reserves in northern Canada, where food availability in northern stores is a problem. Diets of poverty typically rely on calories from high-fat, low-nutrient foods instead of fresher foods, fruits, and vegetables. Aboriginal, African, and Hispanic populations tend to have much lower incomes, and are therefore eating lower-quality foods, which, when combined with the thrifty gene, can lead to obesity and obesity-related health problems. When epidemiologists look at these same thrifty gene groups in higher income levels, the obesity rates are lower.

Leptin and Other Hormones

The most promising anti-obesity treatment once involved the "anti-fat hormone," leptin. Its discovery led to a surge of obesity-drug research. Leptin, discovered in 1994, seemed promising because it was the first anti-fat hormone that surfaced. The leptin hormone receptor was developed in 1997. Leptin was discovered when a mutant strain of extremely obese mice, who lacked the gene to make leptin, were able to shed their weight when given leptin. When on leptin, the mice's appetite decreased while their metabolic rates increased. Researchers wondered whether all obese people would lose weight on leptin, but not everyone did. It turns out that like the mutant obese mice, there are only a few rare cases of human obesity caused by leptin deficiency. Everyone else becomes obese by eating too much and being too sedentary. Some rare cases of human obesity are caused by defects in leptin production. The leptin discovery led to a successful treatment for rare, terribly sad cases of obesity in leptin-deficient individuals who, in the past, had not been able to lose weight.

Most people who are obese actually have higher than normal blood levels of leptin, a hormone that is produced by fat cells, and are resistant to its actions. In leptin trials, the hormone was given to overweight people, and it was found that they were leptin-resistant because they had too much of it already. In fact, obesity researchers now believe that leptin has more to do with protecting against weight loss in times of famine than with protecting against weight gain in times of plenty. When fat stores increase, so does leptin; when fat stores shrink, so does leptin. Appetite will increase and metabolism will decrease when leptin levels shrink, but the opposite does not occur; appetite is not suppressed when leptin increases, nor is metabolism increased. Leptin, it seems, is one of those evolutionary hormones designed to keep our species alive by protecting us from starvation. Discovering leptin has led obesity researchers into finding out more about how appetite, fat stores, and famine-protection mechanisms work in the body.

Crash Dieting: Altering Your Fat Metabolism

The road to obesity is also paved with crash dieting, which typically begins in the teens and twenties by individuals who are at healthy body weights, but who want to be model thin. Because of society's unrealistic beauty standards and the societal pressures on women to meet them, women are particularly vulnerable to crash dieting.

The crash-and-burn approach to diet is what we do when we want to lose a specific amount of weight for a particular occasion, for example, so we can wear a particular outfit. The pattern is to starve for a few days and then eat what we normally do. Or we eat only certain foods (such as celery and grapefruit) for a number of days and then eat normally after we've lost the weight. Most of these diets do not incorporate exercise, which means that we burn up some of our muscle as well as fat. Then, when we eat normally, we gain only fat. And over the years, the fat cells simply grow fatter. The bottom line is that when there is more fat than muscle on your body, you cannot burn calories as efficiently. It is the muscle that makes it possible to burn calories. Diet your muscle away, and you diet away your ability to burn fat.

If we starve ourselves to lose weight, our bodies become more efficient at getting fat (similar to what happens in thrifty genes). Starvation triggers an intelligence in the metabolism; our bodies suddenly think we're living in a war zone and go into super-efficient nomadic mode. When we return to our normal caloric intake, or even a lower than normal caloric intake after we've starved ourselves, *we gain more weight.* Our bodies say, "Oh look—food! Better store that as fat for the next famine." Some researchers believe that starvation diets slow down our metabolic rates far below normal so that weight gain becomes more rapid after each starvation episode.

This cycle of crash dieting or starvation dieting is known as the yo-yo diet syndrome and has been the subject of thousands of articles in women's magazines in the past 30 years. Breaking the pattern sounds easy: Combine exercise with a sensible diet, but it's not that easy if you've been sedentary for most of your adult years. Ninety-five percent of the people who go on such a diet gain back the weight they lost, as well as extra weight, within two years. Experts say that unless we are significantly overweight to begin with or have a medical condition, *we should not diet.* Just eat well. Again, the principles of eating discussed in chapters 7 and 8 are the healthy lifestyle diet to follow.

Psychological Causes of Obesity: Binge-Eating Disorder

When we hear the term "eating disorder," we usually think about anorexia or bulimia. Many people, however, binge without purging. This practice is also known as binge-eating disorder or compulsive overeating. The bingeing is still an announcement to the world that "I'm out of control." Someone who purges after bingeing is hiding his or her lack of control. Someone who binges and never purges is *advertising* his or her lack of control. The purger is passively asking for help; the binger who doesn't purge is aggressively asking for help. It's the same disease with a different result, but there is one more facet to compulsive overeating. This facet is controversial and often rejected by the overeater: The desire to get fat is often behind the compulsion. Many people who overeat insist that fat is a *consequence* of eating food, not a *goal*. Many therapists who deal with overeating behaviour disagree and believe that if a person admits to having an emotional interest in actually being large, he or she may be much closer to stopping the compulsion to eat.

Many who eat compulsively do not recognize that they are doing so. There are reams of materials for those with binge-eating disorder. For more information, a good place to start is Overeaters Anonymous at www.oa.org.

TREATMENT FOR OBESITY

There are a variety of approaches for treating obesity; the approach that is right for you depends on the degree of your obesity (moderate to severe), and the severity of your diabetes. For most people whose BMIs are in the 25–34 range, the first approach is simply diet modification, following the principles discussed in chapters 7 and 8, combined with exercise and activity, and perhaps a weight-loss program, such as Weight Watchers. The second approach may involve certain medications. However, drug treatment for obesity has not been shown to be that successful (discussed further on page 180). The most dramatic research in treating obesity while virtually eliminating diabetes has been in bariatric surgery, which is typically reserved for people with a BMI of 35 or higher, but the guidelines are changing in light of spectacular success with curing diabetes.

Bariatric Surgery: Curing Obesity and Type 2 Diabetes

Bariatric surgery involves two types of procedures: (1) the laparoscopic Roux-en-Y (RNY) gastric bypass and (2) the laparoscopic vertical banded gastroplasty (LAGB or lap band). In RNY, the stomach's upper part is transected, creating a small gastric pouch about a tenth of the size of the original stomach, bypassing the remaining stomach, duodenum, and a small portion of the jejunum. In LAGB, a smaller stomach is created by inserting a silicone band around it. In 2007, research revealed that RNY resulted in complete remission of Type 2 diabetes long before weight loss occurred. In fact, five to seven days was the time frame for remission in many. This is believed to be due to hormonal changes related to alterations in nutrient flow through the intestine. According to one of the first researchers to observe this at the University of Washington, roughly 80–85 percent of Type 2 diabetes is resolved or at least in long-term remission 10 years following RNY. This is in addition to patients losing 50–60 percent of their weight and keeping it off 10 years after their surgeries. Other benefits are also seen, such as reduction in hypertension in 78 percent of patients and improved cholesterol levels in more than 70 percent of patients, according to reports in *JAMA*.

Since the introduction of bariatric surgery, it's been perfected over the last decade, and several studies are tracking astounding benefits. In one seven-year follow-up study, diabetes was reduced by 92 percent, cancer by 60 percent, and heart disease by 56 percent. These benefits represent the results of cruder techniques in bariatric surgeries before laparoscopic techniques were developed. Therefore, the long-term benefits are predicted to exceed even what has been reported.

A Miracle Cure for Type 2 Diabetes?

Within days or weeks, people who have undergone RNY start to see normal blood glucose levels very quickly, and most can stop all diabetes medications (see Chapter 6). In fact, resolution of diabetes with this procedure is as certain as the weight loss that patients expect. This has led to more research into specific gastric bypass procedures that do not restrict the stomach size, with the goal of resolving diabetes.

Within the next decade, surgical resolution of Type 2 diabetes may be a common therapy.

Who Should Have this Surgery?

The guidelines for bariatric surgery candidates haven't been changed since 1991. In the past, the guidelines recommended that only those with a BMI over 40, or those with many health problems with a BMI 35 or over, should be candidates. Now, many experts are recommending that the surgery should be offered to anyone who may benefit, including those with lower BMIs who are interested in having their Type 2 diabetes go into remission. However, the surgery requires lifelong lifestyle changes. Those with binge-eating disorders, other mental health issues, or addiction problems are not considered suitable candidates. For these reasons, a team approach to assessing candidates for bariatric surgery is the norm, which includes a primary care doctor, a bariatric surgery team, and a psychologist and psychiatrist or other specialists, as necessary. Support groups for patients who have had this surgery are also recommended as the lifestyle changes required can be difficult for many patients to implement.

Potential Pitfalls of Bariatric Surgery

This is not risk-free surgery. In 5–10 percent of patients, hemorrhage, obstruction, leaks, infection, and pulmonary emboli are among some of the complications. Long-term risks can include serious vitamin deficiencies, calcium depletion, bone loss, hypoglycemia, and nerve damage, as well as hyperparathyroidism. Some people do regain their weight, and in some people, diabetes may return after 20 years, for reasons still unclear.

Drug Treatment for Obesity

Drug treatment for obesity has an awfully shady history. Women have been especially abused by the medical system's attempts to deal with weight gain. Throughout the 1950s, 1960s, and into the 1970s, women were prescribed thyroxine, which is thyroid hormone, to speed up their metabolisms. Unless a person has an underactive thyroid gland or no thyroid gland (it may have been surgically removed), this is a very dangerous medication that can cause heart failure. Request a thyroid function test before you accept this medication.

Doctors also pedalled amphetamines ("speed") to women. These drugs, too, are dangerous, and can put your health at risk.

One of the most controversial anti-obesity therapies was the use of fenfluramine and phentermine (Fen/Phen). Both drugs were approved for use individually more than 20 years ago, but since 1992, doctors have tended to prescribe them together for long-term management of obesity. In 1996, US doctors wrote a total of 18 million monthly prescriptions for Fen/Phen, and many of the prescriptions were issued to people who were not obese. This practice is known as "off-label" prescribing. In July 1997, the United States Food and Drug Administration and researchers at the Mayo Clinic and the Mayo Foundation made a joint announcement warning doctors that Fen/Phen can cause heart disease. On September 15, 1997, fenfluramine was taken off the market.

Approved Anti-obesity Pills

In 2000, Canada approved an anti-obesity pill that blocks the absorption of almost one-third of the fat people eat. One of the side effects of this new prescription drug, called orlistat (Xenical), is diarrhea when the fat content in a meal exceeds 20 percent. To avoid the drug's side effects, simply avoid fat! The pill can also decrease absorption of vitamin D and other important nutrients, however.

Orlistat is the first drug to fight obesity through the intestine instead of the brain. Taken with each meal, it binds to certain pancreatic enzymes to block the digestion of 30 percent of ingested fat. When people on orlistat combined it with a sensible diet, they lost more weight than those not on orlistat. This drug is not intended for people who need to lose a few pounds; it is designed for medically obese people. The safety of orlistat for people with diabetes is under debate. Although in studies orlistat was found to lower cholesterol, blood pressure, and blood sugar levels (as a result of weight loss), taking the drug can lead to pancreatitis (inflammation of the pancreas, discussed in Chapter 1) and inflammation of the gallbladder.

Another anti-obesity drug, sibutramine (Meridia), was approved for use in Canada in 2001. Sibutramine is meant for people whose BMI is 27 or higher.

Sibutramine's safety for people with Type 2 diabetes is debatable. Anyone with high blood pressure (Chapter 2) is cautioned against taking sibutramine because it can significantly raise blood pressure.

If you're taking medications for depression, thyroid problems, seizures, glaucoma, osteoporosis, gallbladder disease, liver disease, heart disease or stroke prevention, kidney disease, migraines, or Parkinson's disease, you are also cautioned against taking sibutramine and should discuss with your doctor whether the drug is safe.

WEIGHT-LOSS PROGRAMS FOR TYPE 2 DIABETES

There are some diets based on calorie restriction; this is not the right diet for you as you can consume 1,500 calories a day and select only high glycemic index foods, for example. Generally, this is not the type of diet that is encouraged for people with diabetes, although arguably, if weight loss is achieved, the body will still use insulin more effectively. Generally, the right diet for those with Type 2 diabetes is a balanced one. Anyone following Diabetes Association guidelines from any country will be eating low GI, good-fats meals. The very low-fat and low-carb diets discussed in Chapter 7, however, are not recommended for the masses or for people with Type 2 diabetes.

Programs such as Weight Watchers, Jenny Craig, or similar programs by brand-name weight-loss centres emphasize calorie reduction through different techniques, but it's important to make sure you're eating a balanced diet and not simply restricting calories.

The most popular program by its success rate, based on long-term sustainability and maintenance, is Weight Watchers, which used to be pure calorie counting before the introduction of its Core Plan, which is essentially a low GI eating program based on food selection and not calorie counting. The disadvantage to calorie counting is that a chocolate bar may contain the same calories/points as a large sandwich, but it's not as healthy or nutritious, although dark chocolate (with a cocoa content of 70 percent or more) has now been found to have some heart-health benefits. Nonetheless, by being aware of the calories, most people ultimately use their points more judiciously and the point system allows people some leeway for indulging without feeling that they blew their diets. Discouragement from dieting is what the Weight Watchers system helps to offset.

Programs like Jenny Craig are similar, but make most of their money from selling you their brand of low-calorie packaged foods or meals. All of their meal plans are based on their foods, but in principle, the foods are generally low glycemic index foods or good-fat foods.

But these weight-loss organizations have some added support group/motivational seminars or classes, weigh-ins to keep you focused and goal-oriented, and, most important, education about how to shop in today's confusing world of labels and overabundance of fast foods and restaurants, and behavioural counselling about eating habits. The support, in addition to the diet, can be beneficial, particularly to women, who generally like to share experiences. People who dislike discussion groups will probably not like Weight Watcher-like programs, but there are also online versions of many of these programs.

Ultimately, most people, regardless of the weight-loss program chosen, will probably wind up with a balanced, low GI, good-fats diet.

Some diets are advertised as "low carb" or "high protein," but are, in fact, balanced low GI, good-fats diets, too. One such example is The Zone, which the Center for Science in the Public Interest found to be too low in whole grains and calcium, but is fairly balanced. Any diet that limits calories, not entire food groups, is just fine. For example, a vegetarian diet may eliminate meats but not fats, which is a food group. Pick one you like and fly with it. You can judge a good diet based on these four simple questions:

1. Are all food groups—vegetables and fruits, grains and low GI carbs, proteins (lean meats), and healthful fats—included? If not, avoid it.

2. Are you encouraged to have *the least* number of calories from fats, and discouraged from eating junk foods and refined sugars? If so, this is sensible.

3. Is the average weight loss promised about .5–1 kg (1–2 lbs) per week, or is it 4.5 kg (10 lbs) or more per week? Anything more than .5–1 kg (1–2 lbs) a week is suspicious and likely faddish. Gradual weight loss is sustainable for life; speedy weight loss leads to yo-yo effects, when you gain back as much as you lost, if not more.

4. Is it a diet that offers enough variety so that you would feel good eating this way for life, and feeding your whole family with the foods encouraged? People on the Atkins diet, for example (see Chapter 7), have stated that they can't continue beyond a certain point, and cannot feed their children on this diet.

Rapid Weight-Loss Diets

No one with Type 2 diabetes or pre-diabetes should be on a rapid weight-loss diet unless she or he is morbidly obese, and a doctor specifically prescribes it. Any diet that causes you to lose weight rapidly (such as 2–4.5 kg [5–10 lbs] per week), in the absence of activity, is not a diet you'll be able to sustain in the long term. Even people who lose weight rapidly due to illness or depression (which frequently results in a 4.5 kg [10 lbs] weight loss) will regain their weight once they regain their health. Liquid diets, starvation diets, or taking weight-loss herbs or drugs that suppress your appetite may lead to significant weight loss that will make you feel "high" in the short term, but will not provide you with a practical, sensible, nutritious diet for life. The motivation you can gain from seeing quick results may lead some people to seek out a maintenance diet, such as Weight Watchers, in order to stay at their desired weight, but most people will find it difficult to resume normal eating habits and keep their weight off at the same time. The body adapts to rapid weight loss by going into "surviving the famine" mode in which it becomes more efficient at using calories and storing fat. Starvation or rapid weight-loss diets will simply cause the body to store calories as fat more efficiently than before the diet. Many obese people have said that they "dieted" up to the weights they are at, as discussed above.

What Balanced, Healthy Diets Encourage You to Do

1. Maximize low GI foods and minimize saturated fats.

   Low GI stands for low glycemic index foods (Chapter 7).
   Saturated fats include cheeseburgers, milkshakes, butter and
   fatty dairy products, or foods that have trans-fatty acids, such
   as anything that is hydrogenated.

2. Maximize monounsaturated fats and minimize high GI foods.

   Monounsaturated or polyunsaturated fats include olive oil,
   or omega-3 and omega-6 fatty acids, which are found in
   coldwater fish (e.g., salmon, sardines). "High GI" stands for
   high glycemic index foods (see Chapter 7), such as starch and
   refined sugar in crackers, cookies, cakes, and refined flours.

3. Minimize total fats.

   Limit total calories from any fat daily to about 30 percent. Any
   fat contains more than twice the calories of other foods, and it
   should be eaten in reduced quantities if you want to lose weight.

12

TYPE 2 DIABETES, FERTILITY, AND PREGNANCY

This chapter offers you information that is difficult to find because there is such a splintered market when it comes to pregnancy and diabetes. This chapter is designed for two specific groups of women. The first group is already diagnosed with Type 2 diabetes, has delayed having children (probably for social reasons), but nevertheless is planning a pregnancy or is already pregnant. A good many of the women in this group may also have been dealing with infertility or may be undergoing assisted reproductive technology. Many women in their mid to late forties, for example, have more options regarding pregnancy as a result of egg donation. Therefore, the old belief that women with Type 2 diabetes are too old to have babies and don't need this information is being radically revised. In fact, there has been an upsurge in post-menopausal pregnancy as a direct result of new fertility treatments. What you need to know about fertility treatments and diabetes is therefore discussed, as well as how Type 2 diabetes often affects fertility. And, of course, everything you need to know about managing Type 2 diabetes *during* pregnancy is discussed, too, under the section "Being Pregnant," on page 194.

The second group of women reading this chapter will not have been diagnosed at all with Type 2 diabetes, but instead will have been diagnosed with *gestational diabetes,* which means "diabetes during pregnancy." Gestational diabetes is not the same disease as Type 2 diabetes, even though it usually *behaves* the same way. It is a condition that occurs during pregnancy when your body is resistant to the insulin it makes, but the condition can often be managed through dietary changes and meal planning, and it often disappears after pregnancy. Gestational diabetes, however, is often a warning that unless lifestyle and dietary habits change between pregnancies or after childbirth, Type 2 diabetes may be in the cards after all. If this is the reason you're reading this chapter, go directly to the section on gestational diabetes on page 198. Finally, if you have Type 1 diabetes, this is *not* the book for you, although you may indeed find certain sections of this chapter helpful.

GETTING PREGNANT

You have Type 2 diabetes, but you still want to get pregnant. What do you need to do in order to have a healthy baby, while staying healthy yourself?

The first step is to *plan ahead!* Get your glucose levels under tight control through diet, exercise, and frequent blood sugar monitoring. If you are taking oral medication for your diabetes, you must stop; these medications cannot be taken during pregnancy. You must either discuss managing your diabetes through diet and exercise alone, or you must go on insulin during your conception phase and pregnancy. If you have to go on insulin temporarily, review Chapter 6 for some "getting started" information, as well as useful tables that will explain what kinds of insulins are available. However, be forewarned: You must be able to handle taking insulin and going through a fairly radical change in your lifestyle habits, as well as being able to handle another huge lifestyle change—having a baby! Please have a frank discussion with your partner and doctor prior to making this decision. The CDA recommends that an interdisciplinary diabetes health care team composed of diabetes nurse educators, dieticians, obstetricians, and endocrinologists be involved, which can minimize maternal and fetal risks in women with diabetes. It's also recommended that you should begin supplementing your diet with multivitamins containing 5 mg of folic acid at least three months prior to conception and continue until 12 weeks after conception. From this time and continuing throughout the pregnancy, for the first six weeks postpartum and as long as breastfeeding continues, supplementation should consist of a multivitamin with 0.4–1 mg of folic acid.

Table 12.1: Glycemic Targets before Conception and During Pregnancy

The 2008 CDA Guidelines recommend the following glycemic targets before conception and during your pregnancy:
Pre-pregnancy A1C ≤ 7.0%*
During pregnancy:
Fasting and pre-prandial PG 3.8–5.2 mmol/L
1 hour post-prandial PG 5.5–7.7 mmol/L
2 hours post-prandial PG 5.0–6.6 mmol/L
A1C ≤ 6.0% (normal)
*A1C ≤ 6.0% if this can be safely achieved. In some women, particularly those with Type 1 diabetes, higher targets may be necessary to avoid excessive hypoglycemia.
A1C = glycated hemoglobin
PG = plasma glucose

Obesity

Regardless of your diabetes, obesity may be a sign that your pregnancy will become high risk. Chapter 11 discusses obesity in more detail, but if you're pregnant, there are a vast number of potential problems for obese, diabetic women who are pregnant. Excess weight, for example, increases the risk of glucose intolerance. Even in moderately overweight pregnant women, the incidence of gestational diabetes mellitus is up to 6.5 times greater than that in normal-weight pregnant women. Other complications for obese women can include higher rates of hypertension and other pregnancy complications compared with normal-weight women. This typically means more Caesarean sections for obese women.

This is not a conspiracy. It just so happens that when you're obese *prior* to the pregnancy, the odds of a number of complications, including gestational diabetes, *during* pregnancy increase, and will be discussed further on.

Experts strongly suggest that the only way to combat this problem is to help women achieve a normal weight prior to conceiving, which would lead to a marked decrease in C-section deliveries. In fact, the current first-time Caesarean delivery rate of approximately 25 percent is blamed on obesity. If all women were of normal weight for their ages and heights, experts think that the C-section rate in the United States would drop to roughly 12 percent for first-time Caesareans and 3 percent for repeat C-sections. An obstetrician is recommended if you are obese prior to conceiving.

Having Sex

Getting pregnant means having sex—usually! But if you're a woman with diabetes, the act of having sex can interfere with blood sugar levels since it is, after all, an *activity*. Therefore, many experts recommend that you treat sexual activity as any other activity and plan for it accordingly as a physical exercise of sorts. The risk of developing low blood sugar, or hypoglycemia, is actually not uncommon with sexual activity and diabetes. You may need to eat after sex, or eat something beforehand to ward off low blood sugar.

There is also the opposite problem: *no desire* for sex. This can occur because of vaginal infections (see Chapter 16), or because of changing hormones if you are approaching menopause. Studies that looked specifically at the effect diabetes has on women and sexuality found that loss of libido was often caused by high blood sugar; vaginal infections and resulting pain or itching during intercourse; the sheer fear of pain or itching during intercourse; as well as nerve damage, which affects blood flow to the female genitalia, and hence can interfere with pleasure, sensation, and orgasm.

Many women with diabetes also report that they feel more unattractive as a result of their diabetes. They are concerned with not just their own performance, but their ability to please their partners. Fears of a low blood sugar attack in the sack are particularly common. The only way to avoid feelings of unattractiveness or fears is to be open with your partner. Discussing these issues with a sex therapist, counsellor, or your family doctor may also be a valuable experience.

Who Should Not Get Pregnant?

If your diabetes has affected your kidneys (see Chapter 19), then pregnancy is not in your best interests. You will need to weigh your desire to procreate against the risks of kidney failure. By controlling your diabetes during pregnancy, it is still possible to give birth to a healthy child even when you have kidney disease, but there are considerable health risks associated with this. These issues were dealt with in the film *Steel Magnolias*, a classic "chick flick."

Women who have only mild renal disease will likely have a successful pregnancy. The strain of pregnancy on the body, coupled with severe kidney disease, however, will likely lead to pregnancy complications. Your body will have to work extra hard to provide sustenance for both you and your baby. There are potentially serious health risks for both mother and baby associated with kidney disease. Due to extra fluid retention, pregnant women may have higher blood pressure and more waste products in their blood. A baby's growth is adversely affected when the mother has high blood pressure since the fetus will not receive enough blood through the placenta. If blood pressure gets very high, the mother is at risk of pre-eclampsia, which may result in premature delivery and brain, liver, or kidney hemorrhages in the mother. Many women should be advised by their doctor to postpone their pregnancy until their kidney disease is under control or until after they receive a kidney transplant or kidney dialysis.

Infertility and Diabetes

Then, of course, there are those of you who want to get pregnant, but cannot. This section may shed some light on a common problem affecting many women with Type 2 diabetes. It is a condition known as polycystic ovarian syndrome (PCOS), which now affects a staggering number of women. One-quarter to one-third of women of reproductive age suffer from PCOS, which frequently leads to Type 2 diabetes. The vast majority of women with PCOS also have severe insulin resistance, but may not have progressed to Type 2 diabetes. Fortunately, PCOS is manageable. The typical treatment is metformin (see Chapter 6), combined with a low glycemic index diet (see Chapter 7).

Signs and Symptoms of PCOS

The signs of PCOS range from the subtle, such as excess facial hair (clinically known as hirsutism), to the "full house syndrome." The latter can mean no periods, obesity, excess body hair, diabetes, and cardiovascular disease. It's apparent from this rainbow of symptoms that PCOS is not just an ovarian disease. PCOS affects the whole body. The underlying cause of PCOS is excess insulin in the blood, which occurs as a result of insulin resistance.

PCOS can start any time during a woman's reproductive life. Since insulin resistance rises naturally just before puberty, PCOS can even be seen in girls as young as 10 or 12 years. In fact, we now know that girls who experience early puberty (or the appearance of pubic hair and breasts at age seven or eight) have a very high risk of subsequent PCOS.

The early diagnosis and treatment of girls and women is vital. Only through early diagnosis and treatment can PCOS be prevented from progressing to the more severe "full house syndrome." If you suspect you have PCOS, speak to your doctor about testing (discussed further on in this chapter). PCOS *is* manageable. Management is rooted in lifestyle changes (such as exercise, adopting a low GI diet, and practising stress-reduction techniques), as well as taking medications for insulin resistance.

What to Look for in PCOS

The following are all classic signs of PCOS:

- Early puberty, or the appearance of pubic hair and breasts at age seven or eight

- Delayed or absent puberty
- Irregular periods, or no periods at all
- Acne, particularly if it first appears in adulthood
- Excess body hair or facial hair (also called hirsutism)
- Unexplained fatigue
- Cravings for sweets or sugar
- Hypoglycemia, or low blood sugar, occurring after or between meals
- Excess weight around the waistline
- Infertility
- Mood swings
- Hot flashes in young women (characterized by heat intolerance and excess sweating)
- Sleep disorders, particularly sleep apnea (meaning that you might stop breathing in your sleep)
- Recurrent miscarriages
- Milk leaking from the breasts (or inappropriate lactation)
- Low blood pressure noticeable when you stand up suddenly, or after exercise
- Rough, dark skin in the neck folds and armpits, known as acanthosis nigricans

Some of these signs and symptoms, such as fatigue, are a product of insulin resistance, while others can be linked to the excess production of male hormones from the ovaries and adrenal glands. Consult your doctor if you notice several of the signs and symptoms on this list.

A PCOS diagnosis is made via blood tests and ultrasound once your doctor suspects you have PCOS, based on some of the symptoms above. The diagnostic tests look for high levels of testosterone, low levels of the sex hormone-binding globulin (which is the protein that ferries testosterone and estrogen around the body), and high levels of luteinizing hormone (LH) compared to follicle-stimulating hormone (FSH). On ultrasound examination, bulky ovaries with 10 or more peripheral cysts are also an indicator of PCOS.

Insulin's Role in PCOS

Insulin resistance results in the excess production of hormones from the ovaries and adrenal glands, which accounts for the symptoms of PCOS. The ovary is the target of persistent insulin action. Insulin both directly and indirectly stimulates the growth of the ovarian tissue between the eggs, which actually comprises the bulk of the ovary. This part of the ovary makes sex hormones, and the enzymes involved in this synthesis are also turned on by insulin.

Estrogen is made in the ovary through the conversion of testosterone. In PCOS this conversion process is frequently flawed, resulting in excess testosterone. Excess testosterone causes male-patterned body changes in women. These changes can include male-patterned excess facial and body hair, abdominal weight gain, and, in some women, the development of male muscular features.

Excess insulin and testosterone also make the area at the base of the brain, known as the hypothalamus, more sensitive. As a result, the signal it sends to the pituitary gland becomes more frequent and more intense. The pulses of luteinizing hormone (LH) that the pituitary secretes periodically become larger and more frequent, causing further ovarian stimulation and creating a vicious cycle of ovarian stimulation and sex hormone oversecretion. To make matters worse, insulin is responsible for the conversation of weak male and female sex hormones to more potent forms that live in the body's fat stores. This complex and chaotic interplay between endocrine glands accounts for all of the symptoms of PCOS, which are further magnified by eating a high GI diet, not exercising, and stress.

BEING PREGNANT

When you're diagnosed with Type 2 diabetes *prior* to becoming pregnant, this section is for you. This means you have *pre-existing diabetes* (diabetes before pregnancy). If you have developed diabetes *during* pregnancy, see the separate section on page 198 on gestational diabetes (diabetes during pregnancy).

So long as your blood glucose levels are normal throughout your pregnancy and you have normal blood pressure, you can expect as normal a pregnancy as anyone else in your age group. Nevertheless, there are some concerns unique to women with Type 2 diabetes.

The 2008 CDA Guidelines offer the following recommendations for women with Type 2 diabetes who are either planning a pregnancy, who become pregnant, or who may already be pregnant:

For Women with Type 2 Diabetes Who Are Planning a Pregnancy or Become Pregnant

- Switch from an anti-hyperglycemic agent to insulin (see Chapter 6).
- This should preferably be done pre-pregnancy, except if you have PCOS, in which case metformin can be safely used to help ovulation. Metformin has not been studied in pregnant women, so its safety during pregnancy is not known.
- Discuss insulin therapy and blood glucose targets with your doctor.

For Pregnant Women with Type 1 or Type 2 Diabetes

- Strive to keep your glucose levels at these targets:
  - Fasting/pre-prandial (pre-meal): 3.8–5.2 mmol/L
  - 1 hour post-prandial (post-meal): 5.5–7.7 mmol/L
  - 2 hours post-prandial (post-meal): 5.0–6.6 mmol/L
  - Self-test your blood sugar regularly; discuss optimal times for testing with your doctor.
- Speak to a dietician about nutrition during your pregnancy.
- Avoid ketosis during pregnancy (see Chapters 5 and 7).

Staying in Control

No matter what type of diabetes you have, every diabetes book will tell you that a healthy pregnancy depends on how well *you* manage your disease. If you can keep your blood sugar levels as close to normal as possible throughout your pregnancy, then, as most books will also tell you, your chances of delivering a healthy baby are as good as a non-diabetic woman's. The only way to do this is to carefully plan your meals, exercise, and insulin requirements with your doctor if, in fact, you do require insulin during your pregnancy. If you do, your insulin requirements will continue to increase as your pregnancy progresses. Keep in mind that pregnant women's blood sugar levels will usually be lower than those in women who are not pregnant. Therefore, the values that are considered to be in the normal range for non-pregnant women will be different than what is considered normal for pregnant women. Consult your doctor about what the normal range should be for you.

When You Lose Control

If you lose control of your blood sugar levels in the first eight weeks of pregnancy, your baby is at risk for birth defects. High blood sugar levels may interfere with the formation of your baby's organs, causing heart defects or spina bifida (open spine). Once your baby's organs are formed, the risk of birth defects from high blood sugar levels disappears, but new problems surface.

High blood sugar levels will cross the placenta and feed the baby too much glucose, causing the baby to make extra fat and therefore grow too big and fat for its gestational age. This condition is called macrosomia, which is defined as birth weight greater than 4,500 g or about 10 lbs—a very large baby! If the baby is too large, delivery can be difficult. For instance, there may be problems delivering the baby's shoulders because they may be too big for the birth canal, so if your baby is too big, you will need a Caesarean section. The extra glucose that gets into the baby also causes the baby's pancreas to make extra insulin. Then, after birth, the baby's body needs time to adjust to normal glucose levels (since the placenta is gone), and this can cause the baby to suffer from hypoglycemia, or low blood glucose levels. These babies are also at higher risk for breathing problems, obesity later in life, and developing Type 2 diabetes.

Your baby may also develop jaundice after birth, which is very common for all newborns, but tends to happen more frequently in babies born to mothers with diabetes. Newborn jaundice is caused by a buildup of old or leftover red blood cells that aren't clearing out of the body fast enough. However, breastfeeding is the best cure for newborn jaundice.

Five good steps to controlling glucose levels:

1. Use a home blood glucose monitor to test your blood sugar levels. Pregnancy can mask the symptoms of low blood glucose so you cannot rely on how well you feel. The goal is to get your blood glucose levels to replicate those of a non-diabetic pregnant woman, *which would be lower than in a non-diabetic, non-pregnant woman.*

2. Ask your doctor *when* you should test your blood glucose levels. During pregnancy, it's common to test up to *eight times per day,* especially after eating.

3. Record your results in a journal you keep handy. Take the journal with you when you go out, especially to restaurants.

4. In a *separate* journal, keep track of when you're exercising and what you're eating.

5. Check with your doctor or diabetes educator before you make any changes to your diet or insulin plan whatsoever. And, no, midwives and doulas are *not* the appropriate practitioners to rely on for this information!

YOUR DIABETES PRENATAL TEAM

A healthy pregnancy also depends on a good prenatal team that can help you stay in control. In the same way that you would handpick various skill sets for a baseball team, you must do the same for this team, so here are the specialists to look for:

1. An endocrinologist or internist who specializes in diabetes and diabetic pregnancies.

2. An obstetrician who specializes in high-risk pregnancies, particularly diabetic pregnancies. You may wish to use a *perinatologist,* a doctor who specializes in high-risk pregnancies.

3. A neonatologist (a specialist for newborns) waiting in the wings, or a good pediatrician who is trained to manage babies of diabetic moms.

4. A nutritionist or registered dietitian who can help you put to-gether a realistic diet and insulin plan during your pregnancy.
5. A diabetes educator who is available to answer questions throughout your pregnancy.
6. For additional support, a midwife or doula.

GESTATIONAL DIABETES

Gestational diabetes mellitus (GDM) is diabetes that is first recognized or diagnosed at any stage during pregnancy. If you had diabetes prior to your pregnancy (Type 1 or Type 2), see the previous section. Technically, gestational diabetes means high blood sugar (hyperglycemia). In Canada, the prevalence of GDM is higher than previously thought, varying from 3.7 percent in the non-Aboriginal (but probably multiethnic) popula-tion to 8–18 percent in Aboriginal populations.

What Is GDM?

During pregnancy, hormones made by the placenta can block the in-sulin normally produced by the pancreas. This forces the pancreas to work harder and manufacture three times as much insulin as usual. In many cases, the pancreas isn't able to keep up, so blood sugar levels rise. Gestational diabetes is therefore a common pregnancy-related health problem and is in the same league as other pregnancy-related conditions that develop during the second or third trimesters, such as high blood pressure.

Since pregnancy also involves weight gain, some experts believe it is the weight gain that contributes to insulin resistance as the pancreas cannot keep up with the extra weight and the increased demand for insulin. It's akin to a small restaurant with only 10 tables that suddenly has triple the number of customers. It will be understaffed and unable to accommodate the new demand.

GDM, Type 2 diabetes, can be managed through diet and blood sugar monitoring. Getting help early with nutritional advice can be very useful. Advice from a dietician and telephone support from a health ed-ucator were the most preferred forms of health assistance in one study. Ultimately, insulin may be necessary if your GDM cannot be controlled.

GDM will usually disappear once you deliver, but it recurs in future pregnancies two out of three times. In some cases, GDM is really the unmasking of Type 2 or even Type 1 diabetes *during* pregnancy.

If you are genetically predisposed to Type 2 diabetes, you are more likely to develop Type 2 in the future if you developed gestational diabetes.

Moreover, if you have GDM, you're at greater risk for other pregnancy-related conditions, such as hypertension (high blood pressure), pre-eclampsia, and polyhydramnios (too much amniotic fluid). And if you're carrying more than one fetus, your pregnancy is even more at risk. Therefore, it's wise to seek out an obstetrician if you have GDM. In very high-risk situations, a perinatologist, an obstetrician who specializes in high-risk pregnancies, may have to be consulted.

Diagnosing GDM

The Canadian Diabetes Association suggests the Gestational Diabetes Screen (GDS), in which a woman is given a 50 g glucose load, and has her plasma glucose (PG) measured one hour later. Obviously, if you've already been diagnosed with Type 2 diabetes, you will not need to be screened for diabetes during pregnancy. Candidates for glucose screening are women who are worried about developing diabetes during pregnancy because they believe they have risk factors (see Chapter 2); they have a family history of gestational diabetes; or they have a personal history of gestational diabetes from a previous pregnancy.

Who Should Be Screened?

The symptoms of gestational diabetes are extreme thirst, hunger, or fatigue, all of which can be masked by the normal discomforts of pregnancy. The CDA Guidelines recommend that all women should be screened for GDM between 24 and 28 weeks' gestation. However, it is recommended that women with multiple risk factors should have this screening test done during the first trimester, then again during the second and third trimesters, even if the first test is negative. Screening can help to reduce further complications because the risk factors for developing GDM are as follows:

- a previous diagnosis of GDM or delivery of a macrosomic (excessive birth weight) infant
- being a member of a high-risk population, including women of Aboriginal, Hispanic, South Asian, Asian, and African descent
- being 35 years of age or older
- being obese (BMI of 30 kg/m² or higher)
- a history of polycystic ovarian syndrome (PCOS)
- acanthosis nigricans (a skin disorder characterized by the appearance of darkened patches of skin)
- use of corticosteroids

Some doctors believe it isn't necessary to screen a woman for GDM if she has no symptoms or any of the risk factors above; the attitude is that universal screening can create unnecessary anxiety. Not everyone agrees with universal screening for GDM, but the Canadian Diabetes Association now recommends this should be done for all pregnant women from 24–28 weeks' gestation. Since blood sugar levels rise steadily throughout pregnancy, it's entirely possible to have normal blood sugar levels at week 24 and high levels at week 28, which is why many physicians feel that universal screening produces more problems than it catches.

Jelly Beans versus Cola

Back in 1999, the concept of eating 18 jelly beans as an alternative to the 50 g glucose beverage as a sugar source for GDM screening was published. Many women find this preferable to the glucose beverage. Talk to your doctor about alternatives to the glucose beverage, and mention this passage! Apparently eating 18 jelly beans and having blood glucose tested an hour later can diagnose gestational diabetes just as accurately as having the drink, which many women find produces severe hyperglycemia.

Treating GDM

The treatment for GDM is controlling blood sugar levels through diet, exercise, insulin (if necessary), and blood sugar monitoring. To do this, you must be under the care of a pregnancy practitioner (obstetrician, midwife), a diabetes specialist, and a dietician! Guidelines for nutrition and weight gain during a diabetic pregnancy depend on your current health, the fetal size, and *your* weight. At least 80 percent of the time, gestational diabetes disappears after delivery. Unfortunately, it is destined to recur in subsequent pregnancies 80–90 percent of the time unless you get yourself in good physical shape between pregnancies. Women should definitely consult their physician and be screened for Type 2 diabetes when planning another pregnancy.

And experts report that each subsequent bout of gestational diabetes is more severe than the previous one.

Treating Low Blood Sugar in Pregnancy

Many women with gestational diabetes will find they have episodes of low blood sugar, which is not harmful to the fetus, but very unpleasant for the mother. The thinking is that it's better to risk low blood sugar (hypoglycemia) during pregnancy to avoid high blood sugar (hyperglycemia), which is damaging to the fetus. Treating low blood sugar is the same in pregnancy as at any other time. (See Chapter 14 for details.)

SPECIAL DELIVERY

About one in four babies is delivered by Caesarean section. A 2007 report from The Canadian Institute for Health Information notes that in 2005–2006, the Canadian estimate for the total C-section rate was 26.3 percent. A Caesarean section is a surgical procedure that is essentially abdominal delivery. The procedure, as the name suggests, dates back to Julius Caesar, who, as legend tells us, was born in this manner. Whether Caesar's truly was a Caesarean birth is hotly debated among historians, but what historians *do* know is that the abdominal delivery dates back to ancient Rome. In fact, Roman law made it legal to perform a Caesarean section *only* if the mother died in the last four weeks of pregnancy. The procedure therefore originated *only as a means to save the child*. Using the procedure to save the *mother* was not even considered until the nineteenth century, under the influence of two prominent obstetricians, Max Sanger and Eduardo Porro.

Women who have diabetes during pregnancy (pre-existing or gestational) are at a higher risk of requiring a Caesarean section than the general pregnant population because they can give birth to very large babies, who may not be able to fit through the birth canal. Prior to your due date, you need to have a frank discussion with your pregnancy health care provider (doctor or midwife), and ask him or her about which situations would warrant a Caesarean section.

Below are 12 legitimate reasons for a Caesarean section:

1. When a vaginal delivery, even with intervention, is risky *(Note: you fall into this category if your baby is large)*
2. A prolonged labour (caused by failure to dilate, lack of progress, too large a head, and several other reasons)
3. A failed induction attempt; labour induction sometimes fails, the baby is overdue, and a Caesarean is the next alternative
4. When the baby is in a breech position
5. Placental problems
6. Fetal distress
7. Health problems in the mother that prevent normal vaginal delivery
8. A history of difficult deliveries or stillbirth
9. When the baby is in a transverse lie (horizontal position)
10. When the mother has primary genital herpes or other sexually transmitted diseases, such as genital warts, chlamydia, or gonorrhea, which can be passed on to the newborn via vaginal delivery
11. When the mother is HIV-positive
12. A multiple birth

AFTER THE BABY IS BORN

The question that may be at the top of your mind after you give birth is whether your diabetes is gone. This is a valid question only for women who have had gestational diabetes. The only way to tell is to have a glucose-tolerance test when you get your first postpartum menstrual period (if you're breastfeeding) or six weeks after childbirth. If the test results are normal, then your diabetes is, indeed, gone, but should not be forgotten. It's a warning to you that you had better shape up between pregnancies, otherwise future bouts of gestational diabetes could recur, or you might develop Type 2 diabetes. Of course, there are some other issues that will surface for mothers who have (or had) diabetes.

If your test results show continuing high blood sugar, it's probably safe to assume that you have Type 2 diabetes that has just revealed itself during your pregnancy. In this case, your diabetes is a permanent health condition that was simply diagnosed during pregnancy or perhaps was even triggered by it.

Should You Breastfeed?
Yes. Next question?

Why Was I Told *Not* to Breastfeed?
Ignorant practitioners may tell you that you can't breastfeed if you've had diabetes. This is completely false! In fact, pediatric obesity-prevention guidelines stress breastfeeding in the first year, particularly if the baby was exposed to diabetes in utero. If your diabetes is well controlled and you've given birth to a healthy baby, breastfeeding is the normal way to feed your baby and does not place your baby at risk for the numerous, undisputed, and well-documented health problems associated with babies fed with cow's milk. Stick to your pregnancy rules and keep self-monitoring your blood sugar levels so you can adjust your diet and exercise routine to your new levels of hormones. Estrogen levels affect blood sugar levels. When they rise, your blood sugar rises; when they drop, which is what happens during breastfeeding as a result of the hormone prolactin, blood sugar levels may drop. That could mean you may need to eat more while breastfeeding in order to keep up your levels. If you had gestational diabetes, this natural drop in blood sugar levels is nature's way of helping you recover faster if you breastfeed. If you need to take insulin to control high blood sugar after childbirth, your baby doesn't care! Insulin cannot be ingested, so even if it crosses into the

breast milk, it will have zero effect on the baby. Remember, if insulin could be ingested, you wouldn't need to inject it in the first place!

Furthermore, several studies show that breastfed babies have lower incidences of both Type 1 diabetes and Type 2 diabetes later in life. Breastfeeding in infancy is associated with a reduced risk of Type 2 diabetes, with marginally lower insulin concentrations in later life, and with lower blood glucose and serum insulin concentrations in infancy. This helps to reduce the risk of pediatric obesity and Type 2 diabetes. (See Chapter 3.)

If you have high blood sugar in the days and/or weeks following childbirth, your milk will be much sweeter than usual. That's not dangerous to the baby, who has a functioning pancreas, which can produce the insulin she or he needs to handle the extra sugar, but the baby could begin to put on too much weight and get fat as a result of the sweet milk. There may be cases when the sweetness is a turnoff to the baby and she or he may not be as receptive to the milk, which will cause problems with your milk supply, or cause engorgement, which is painful and can put you at risk for mastitis (inflammation in the breast, usually due to bacterial infection). In general, the main danger of high blood sugar during breastfeeding is to *you*; you'll need to control your diabetes so you can be as healthy and fit as possible, but this is the case for every woman, whether she has children or not, and whether she's breastfeeding or not.

Postpartum Blues and Diabetes

Many women will find the enormous lifestyle adjustment after childbirth tiring. They may be fatigued, stressed, overwhelmed, and have all the other normal feelings that accompany the event of giving birth. Unfortunately, some women may also suffer from postpartum depression, which is characterized by a loss of interest in formerly pleasurable activities, changes in appetite, changes in sleep patterns (which happen after childbirth anyway), sadness, and a host of other emotional and physical symptoms.

Just because you have diabetes does not mean that you can't develop another condition on top of it, such as postpartum depression, but keeping your blood sugar in check after childbirth will help you to avoid a common problem of high or low blood sugar levels—and their associated mood swings—which may mask postpartum depression or vice versa. It's also recommended that you have your thyroid checked after childbirth to make sure that you are not also suffering from postpartum thyroid disease, which affects about 18 percent of the postpartum population and can be misdiagnosed as postpartum depression, too.

Diabetes never ceases to affect women in unique ways at different stages of their lives. The next chapter is the one to read after your baby graduates.

13

AGING AND TYPE 2 DIABETES

Type 2 diabetes is generally diagnosed after we turn 40. However, as we age beyond 40, other health conditions can complicate a diagnosis of Type 2 diabetes. This chapter looks at specific conditions associated with aging and Type 2 diabetes, such as menopause, osteoporosis, and Alzheimer's disease.

MENOPAUSE

When it comes to menopause, women with Type 2 diabetes have a little more to be concerned about than women without Type 2 diabetes. Estrogen loss increases *all* women's risk of heart disease, which is the major cause of death for post-menopausal women, but in post-menopausal women with diabetes, the risk of heart disease is two to three times higher than in the general female population. Furthermore, as estrogen and progesterone levels drop, women with diabetes can expect fluctuations in their blood sugar levels and possibly more episodes of low blood sugar (see Chapter 14). After menopause, women taking insulin may find that their insulin requirements have dropped by as much as 20 percent. In light of the 2002 studies on hormone-replacement therapy and heart disease, managing Type 2 diabetes after menopause presents a challenge.

Natural Menopause

When menopause occurs naturally, it tends to take place anywhere between the ages of 48 and 52, but it can occur as early as your late thirties or as late as your mid-fifties. When menopause occurs before age 45, it is technically considered early menopause, but just as menarche is genetically predetermined, so is menopause. For an average woman with an unremarkable medical history, what she eats and the activities she engages in will not influence the timing of her menopause. However, women who have had chemotherapy or who have been exposed to high levels of radiation (such as radiation therapy in their pelvic area for cancer treatment) may go into earlier menopause. In any event, the average age of menopause is 50 or 51.

Other causes that trigger early menopause include mumps (in small groups of women, the infection causing the mumps has been known to spread to the ovaries, prematurely shutting them down) and specific autoimmune diseases, such as lupus or rheumatoid arthritis (some women with these diseases find that their bodies develop antibodies to their own ovaries and attack the ovaries).

The term "perimenopause" describes a condition experienced by women who are in the thick of menopause—their cycles are wildly erratic and they experience hot flashes and vaginal dryness. This label is applicable for about four years, covering the first two years prior to the official last period to the two years following the last menstrual period. Women who are perimenopausal will be in the age groups discussed above, averaging to about 51. The term "menopause" refers to your final menstrual period. You will not be able to pinpoint your final period until you've been completely free from periods for one year. Then you count back to the last period you charted, and *that* date is the *date of your menopause*. The term "post-menopause" refers to the last third of most women's lives and describes women who have been free of menstrual periods for at least four years to women celebrating their 100th birthday.

Managing Diabetes in Menopause

As you approach menopause, you'll want to revisit your blood sugar monitoring habits. That's because menopause often masks the symptoms of low or high blood sugar, and vice versa. For example, hot flashes or sweating, moodiness and short-term memory loss are associated with menopause and with low blood sugar.

Estrogen loss will also cause vaginal changes. Since it is the production of estrogen that causes the vagina to continuously stay moist and elastic through its natural secretions, the loss of estrogen will cause the vagina to become drier, thinner, and less elastic. The vagina may shrink slightly in width and length. The reduction in vaginal secretions causes the vagina to be less acidic. This can put you at risk for more vaginal infections, particularly if you have high blood sugar.

Mood swings can be an especially tricky symptom of both menopause and fluctuating blood sugar levels. Many women with diabetes struggle with severe mood swings, which can make controlling blood sugar more difficult. While anger and depression can be symptoms of low blood sugar, anxiety and irritability can be symptoms of high blood sugar.

Many women find that because estrogen and progesterone levels are dropping, they are experiencing more frequent and severe episodes of low blood sugar. Estrogen can trigger insulin resistance; the loss of estrogen will therefore have the opposite effect, causing insulin to be taken up more quickly by the body, which could result in low blood sugar. An easy way to remember how estrogen levels affect blood sugar is to note that when estrogen is up, so is blood sugar; when estrogen is down, so is blood sugar. Therefore, high estrogen levels = high blood sugar; low estrogen levels = low blood sugar.

The only way to cope with these fluctuations is to try to eliminate other causes of blood sugar fluctuations, for example, stress or deviating from meal and exercise plans. If you're on diabetes medications (see Chapter 6), you may need to adjust your dosages around the time of menopause to compensate for the lower resistance to insulin as hormone levels drop. (Although if you go on hormone-replacement therapy, you may need to readjust your dosages again.)

Women who have persistent high blood sugar levels may find the normal menopausal symptoms, for example vaginal dryness, exacerbated. By gaining more control over blood sugar levels, they may find their menopausal symptoms are less severe.

If You're in Surgical Menopause or Premature Menopause

Surgical menopause occurs when you've had your ovaries surgically removed, or chemically shut down as a result of certain medications, such as chemotherapy for cancer. You will likely experience all the symptoms of natural menopause, but in the extreme. Most women in surgical menopause report far more severe symptoms because the process of estrogen loss has been sudden rather than gradual. Surgical menopause and premature menopause (before the age of 45) are best managed using traditional hormone therapy until the natural age of menopause; the hormone therapy (HT) replaces what your body would have been making naturally were it not for illness or premature ovarian failure. Once you reach the natural age of menopause (50–55), you can decide whether it is risky for you to continue HT, in light of heart disease risks and blood sugar control. The 2002 Women's Health Initiative study looked at the long-term use of HT in women older than 55, and found that women on HT to correct premature menopause due to surgery, chemotherapy, or other factors were not at risk.

HT and Type 2 Diabetes

The average Canadian woman will live until age 78, which means she will live one-third of her life after menopause. A survey of the general Canadian population found that 11 percent of people between the ages of 65 and 74 reported having diabetes; these numbers will soar as the first baby boomers to hit 60 began in 2006. Heart disease is a major complication of Type 2 diabetes, and women are more prone to heart disease as a result of estrogen loss after menopause. In the 1980s and 1990s, it was believed that long-term HT protected women from heart disease, so women with Type 2 diabetes were encouraged to seriously consider hormone-replacement therapy after menopause. *That's all changed.*

In July 2002, the US National Heart, Lung, and Blood Institute did a study as part of a huge research program called the Women's Health Initiative (WHI). The study suggested that HT should not be recommended for long-term use; in fact, the results were so alarming that the study was halted before its completion date. The study found that

Prempro, a combination of estrogen and progestin and a standard HT formulation for post-menopausal women, increased the risk of invasive breast cancer, heart disease, stroke, and pulmonary embolisms (blood clots). However, Prempro *did* reduce the incidence of bone fractures from osteoporosis and colon cancer. Study participants were informed in a letter that they should stop taking their pills. Among women in good health without Type 2 diabetes, taking HT to relieve menopausal symptoms is still considered a good option, and there is no evidence to suggest that short-term use of HT is harmful. The study has implications only for women on HT for long-term use, something that was recommended to millions of women over the past 20 years because of perceived protection against heart disease.

In 1998, a trial known as the Heart and Estrogen/Progestin Replacement Study (HERS) looked at whether HT might help women who already had heart disease. HT was not found to have any beneficial effect. Women who were at risk for breast cancer were never advised to go on HT; similarly, women who had suffered a stroke or were considered at risk for blood clots were also never considered good candidates for HT. It had long been known that breast cancer, stroke, and blood clots were risks of long-term HT. However, many women made the HT decision based on the perceived heart disease protection. Today, the only thing the experts can agree on is that the HT decision is highly individual and must be an informed decision, where all of the possible risks and benefits of taking or not taking HT are disclosed.

The Components of HT

Hormone therapy refers to any type of estrogen and progesterone hormone therapy, including plant-derived hormones, animal-derived hormones, or other synthesized hormones. The term "bioidentical hormones" is considered a marketing term used by those who promote and sell them, and does not mean that these hormones confer any more benefits than so-called synthesized hormones. (In the end, all hormone therapies are synthesized, even when compounded.) There are several quality-control problems in the US, for example, with compounded hormones that do not require oversight by the US Food and Drug Administration.

HT is given to prevent or even reverse the long-term consequences of estrogen loss. The only proven long-term benefit of HT is that it can help preserve bone loss and reduce the incidence of fractures. Until July 2002, it was believed that HT protected women from cardiovascular disease, but this is no longer considered true. In women who are at higher risk of breast cancer, HT was always believed to be risky; now it is believed that it may trigger breast cancer in low-risk women.

As the 2002 study suggested, women with diabetes, who are at high risk for heart disease and macrovascular complications (discussed in Part 3), face more risks if they choose HT.

Blood Sugar Levels during Menopause

Decreasing levels of estrogen and progesterone in your bloodstream lead to decreased blood sugar levels as your body's responsiveness to insulin improves. As a result, you may need to adjust your diabetes medication, or insulin regimen if you require insulin, as you experience menopause.

You may also need to adjust your meal and exercise plan because menopause slows down your metabolism. That means it will be even easier to gain weight on fewer calories. The only ways to avoid weight gain are to increase activity or to decrease your calorie intake (see chapters 7, 8, and 11).

Women who have high blood sugar levels may find that their skin is drier and more scaly, and their vaginal dryness more severe, than women with lower blood sugar levels. They may also notice that their nails are deteriorating more rapidly. Controlling blood sugar can reverse these effects.

OSTEOPOROSIS

Post-menopausal women are at highest risk of developing osteoporosis, or bone loss. Eighty percent of all osteoporosis sufferers are women, who experience the bone loss as a direct result of estrogen loss. Although osteoporosis can be disfiguring, it is a relatively silent disease: There is often no immediate pain, suffering, or other symptoms. Osteoporosis itself is not a problem; the problem is the risk of fractures. One in four women and at least one in eight men over the age of 50 have osteoporosis and it is estimated that as many as 2 million Canadians may be at risk of osteoporotic fractures during their lifetime. Osteoporosis and the fractures it causes cost the health care system in excess of $1.3 billion each year based on 1993 data, published in 2008. In fact, over 80 percent of all fractures in people over the age of 60 are osteoporosis-related. Because osteoporosis does not cause pain, often the first warning sign is a broken bone. Once an individual has broken a bone due to osteoporosis, she or he is more likely to break another one, yet fewer than 38 percent of people who fracture go on to be assessed for osteoporosis. Both vertebral (spine) and hip fractures result in an increased mortality rate. Hip fractures are the most devastating type of fracture. Up to 23 percent of women and an even higher percentage of men who suffer hip fractures will die within six months of related complications, such as pneumonia or a blood clot. Many who survive are permanently disabled and one-quarter of hip-fracture patients who survive for one year still cannot walk without assistance. Add diabetes on top of this, and many more complications can occur.

A fracture can dramatically affect your quality of life. Being bed-ridden and immobile can be debilitating. Seventy percent of all hip fractures are a direct result of osteoporosis. Twenty percent of people who suffer a hip fracture will die; half will be disabled. More women die each year as a result of osteoporosis-related fractures than from breast and ovarian cancer combined. Being bedridden with diabetes is definitely something you want to avoid. Of particular note is the risk of hip fractures. North American women have more hip fractures than other fractures. At 55, a North American woman has a 17 percent chance of sustaining a hip fracture. (Men of the same age have a 6 percent chance of fracturing a hip.) After a first fracture, a woman is four times more likely to have a second than she was to have the first fracture. Fifteen to 25 percent of people who fracture a hip are still in long-term care institutions a year after the injury. Most hip fractures occur in Caucasian or Asian women in their seventies and eighties.

Risk factors for an osteoporosis-related fracture include:

- Age 65 or older
- Vertebral compression fracture
- Fracture with minimal trauma after age 40

- Family history of osteoporotic fracture, especially if the mother had a hip fracture
- Long-term (more than three months continuously) use of gluco-corticoid therapy such as prednisone
- Medical conditions (such as celiac disease, Crohn's disease) that inhibit absorption of nutrients
- Primary hyperparathyroidism
- Tendency to fall
- Osteopenia apparent on X-ray
- Hypogonadism (low testosterone in men, loss of menstrual periods in younger women)
- Early menopause (before age 45)

There are also a number of minor risk factors, including rheumatoid arthritis, hyperthyroidism, body weight less than 57 kg (125 lbs) in women, low calcium intake, and smoking. You are especially at risk if you have low bone mineral density (BMD), have already suffered a fracture, or have used glucocorticoid therapy such as prednisone for a long time.

Increasing Calcium

Osteoporosis Canada recommends that Canadians aged 19–50, including pregnant or lactating women, receive at least 400 IU of vitamin D3 per day. Adults over 50 should receive at least 800 IU.

Age	Daily Calcium Requirement
4–8	800 mg
9–18	1,300 mg
19–50	1,000 mg
50+	1,500 mg
Pregnant or lactating women 18+	1,000 mg

Source: The Osteoporosis Society of Canada, posted to www.osteoporosis.ca, (2008).

Fractures Linked to Diabetes Drugs

As discussed in Chapter 6, the latest research yields some alarming news regarding the risk of bone loss and fracture in women who are on a type of diabetes medication known as thiazolidinediones (TZDs), which are sold as Avandia or Actos. It's believed that for every 55 women at low risk of osteoporosis or fractures who take TZDs for one year, one fracture would occur. Among women at high risk, one fracture would occur for every 21 women who take thiazolidinedione for one year. If you are on Avandia or Actos presently, discuss these risks with your doctor, and get a bone mineral density test to assess your risk. (See further on page 216.)

Preventing Osteoporosis

Preventing osteoporosis involves screening, medications that either build bone or reduce bone loss, and diet. Osteoporosis Canada recommends the following:

- All individuals age 65 or older should receive BMD testing.
- All adults between the ages of 50 and 65 should be assessed each year for their risk of osteoporosis and those with one major risk factor or two or more minor risk factors should receive bone mineral density testing.
- After beginning therapy with medications, patients should be retested in one to two years in order to assess the impact of treatment.
- For individuals who do not require therapy, repeat BMD testing is recommended in one to five years in those deemed to be at moderate risk of fracture and in five to 10 years in those deemed to be at low risk of fracture.

Bone Mineral Density (BMD) Tests

One of the critical tests all women require after age 65 is an annual bone mineral density (BMD) test. Unfortunately, access to BMD widely varies in Canada, according to a 2008 Osteoporosis Society of Canada report, which grades provinces from A to F. Table 13.1 reveals the results.

Table 13.1: Access to Bone Mineral Density (BMD) Testing

Analysis of the data on current rates of BMD testing across the country indicates that access is far from adequate; most provinces received a grade of C or lower. The results are as follows:
British Columbia: C
Alberta: B
Saskatchewan: F
Manitoba: F
Ontario: B
Quebec: D
New Brunswick: D
Nova Scotia: D
Prince Edward Island: D
Newfoundland and Labrador: D
Northwest Territories: D

Source: Osteoporosis Society of Canada, posted to www.osteoporosis.ca, (2008).

Studies and surveys show that people who have BMD testing are nine times more likely to be given treatment than those who do not. Without BMD testing, 80 percent of patients with a history of fractures are not given osteoporosis therapies. This is very alarming!

Osteoporosis Prevention Therapies

A number of medications that prevent osteoporosis are available. Osteoporosis Canada encourages osteoporosis patients to call its information line at 1-800-463-6842 (M–F, 10 a.m.–4 p.m. EST) about drug access in your province. Here's the rundown on what's available as of this writing, which may vary from province to province:

Bisphosphonates

Bisphosphonates are a family of drugs used to prevent and treat osteoporosis. Bisphosphonates bind to the surfaces of the bones and slow down the bone resorption action of the osteoclasts (bone-eroding cells). This allows the osteoblasts (bone-building cells) to work more effectively.

There are three bisphosphonates currently approved for use in Canada: alendronate (Fosamax), etidronate (Didrocal) and risedronate (Actonel). Also available are: Actonel Plus Calcium, Fosavance (Fosamax with vitamin D), and zolendric acid (Aclasta).

All three bisphosphonates increase bone density and prevent fractures of the spine (vertebral fractures). Alendronate, risedronate, and zolendric acid have also been shown to prevent hip fractures. Etidronate is the least effective of the bisphosphonate drugs.

Bisphosphonates have very specific instructions about how they must be taken. Following the directions will allow your body to absorb the drug properly and may help you avoid side effects. Because calcium interferes with the absorption of bisphosphonates, calcium supplements must be taken at other times of the day. If you are taking these medications, you should have a thorough discussion with your doctor and pharmacist about how to take the drugs, and any potential side effects and other drug interactions, particularly if you have diabetes. Depending on what you're prescribed, you may be taking your drug once a day, once a week, or once every two days, followed by a calcium supplement regimen.

Selective Estrogen Receptor Modulators (SERMs)

Although SERMs are non-hormonal, they act like the hormone estrogen in some parts of the body, such as the bones. In other parts of the body, such as the uterus and breast, they block the effects of estrogen. This is one reason why they are frequently recommended for breast cancer survivors or women at risk for breast cancer; they can protect against bone loss, as well as breast cancer. Raloxifene (Evista) is currently the SERM available in Canada, and is taken daily. Again, discuss with your doctor whether there are any drug interactions with other medications you may be on.

Parathyroid Hormone (PTH)

An analogue (or copy) of a parathyroid hormone (PTH) is available as a new class of osteoporosis treatments called bone-formation agents. Teriparatide injection (Forteo) is the first medication approved by

Health Canada in this new class. The mechanism by which bone is constantly renewed is called bone remodelling. Teriparatide injection works in a novel way on the bone-remodelling process so that new bone is generated and added to the skeleton faster than old bone is broken down. It does this by activating the osteoblast (bone-building) cells. This is reserved for people with severe osteoporosis who are at high risk of fracture or who have failed or are intolerant to previous osteoporosis therapy. This drug is taken by injection for no longer than 18 months.

Calcitonin

Calcitonin is a hormone found naturally in our bodies. It is made by the thyroid gland and controls the activity of the osteoclasts (bone-eroding cells). A synthetic form of calcitonin (Miacalcin*NS) is used in a nasal spray. Calcitonin slows down the work of the osteoclasts. This allows the osteoblasts (bone-building cells) to work more effectively. Nasal calcitonin maintains or minimally increases bone density and prevents fractures of the spine. It also reduces the pain associated with vertebral fractures. This is not a prevention drug but a treatment for people who already have severe osteoporosis. It's taken as one spray in each nostril daily.

If you have suffered some bone loss, here are some tips to "fall-proof" your home:

1. Don't leave loose wires, cords, or slippery throw rugs lying around.
2. Use a non-slip mat in the shower or bathtub.
3. Install night lights.
4. Clean up spills on the floors.
5. Install treads, rails, or rugs on wooden stairs.
6. Wear comfortable, sturdy shoes with rubber soles.
7. Avoid activity when taking medications that cause drowsiness. Cut down on alcohol.
8. Arrange a home visit from a physiotherapist or occupational therapist to "fall-proof" your home.

Risky Movements

If you have more severe bone loss, everyday movements can cause fractures. Watch out for the following:

- Lifting heavy objects (such as groceries) or excessive bending
- Forceful sneezing or coughing
- Reaching above your shoulders (for something in closets or cupboards)
- Sudden twisting or turning, for example, when driving
- Getting in and out of beds or chairs. Stiffness can be quite severe with osteoporosis; sitting or lying down in one position for too long can make the normal movements of getting up hazardous. Go slowly. To lessen stiffness, use a pillow for back support, and avoid cold drafts.

DIABETES AND "POLYPHARMACY"

Another hazard of managing diabetes as you age is the problem of "polypharmacy," meaning too many drugs from too many places, combined with other issues with natural aging, such as forgetfulness and presbyopia (old age eyes), the normal decline in our vision that makes us buy reading glasses from the drugstore! This can lead to medication compliance problems, such as taking more pills than necessary, missing pills, losing pills, or combining pills that should not be combined. Drug interactions can be serious, particularly if you have diabetes. Currently, it is estimated that at least 90 million people in the United States either have presbyopia or will develop it by 2014. This greatly complicates other vision problems resulting directly from diabetes (see Chapter 17).

Preventing Compliance Problems

Most pharmacies now have an online tracking system of all your prescriptions. Fill your prescriptions at the same pharmacy. Bring in all of the drugs you're on each time you start a new medication and specifically discuss with your pharmacist whether there are any problems with combining your various drugs. Alternatively, you can bring in a list to discuss instead, but sometimes just bringing in the bottles is easier, and then the pharmacist can see the dosage and brand you're taking.

ALZHEIMER'S DISEASE

Alzheimer's disease is a degenerative, progressive disease that affects all areas of the brain by destroying brain cells. It most often occurs in people older than 65, but can sometimes be diagnosed in people in their forties and fifties. One in 13 Canadians older than 65 has Alzheimer's disease or a related dementia.

Alzheimer's disease affects certain areas of the brain that control memory and basic functions or abilities. This results in specific symptoms or changes in behaviour, and once an ability or function is lost, it can rarely be relearned. For people with Type 2 diabetes, the loss of mental abilities can dramatically interfere with managing the disease.

In Alzheimer's disease, the ability to understand, think, remember, and communicate can be severely diminished or lost. The ability to make decisions and perform simple tasks can also be diminished or lost. The person with Alzheimer's disease becomes confused and experiences memory loss (initially short-term memory). Finally, the person may lose the ability to communicate using the right words. A person with Alzheimer's will be unable to plan meals, monitor blood sugar, and take medications or insulin correctly. These tasks must be taken over by someone else. Management goals may need to be tailored to suit the realistic quality of life of the affected person, who may have erratic eating patterns, for example. Looser control instead of tight control is often a new management target (see the section "Elder Care and Type 2 Diabetes," below). The diabetic with Alzheimer's may need to switch from medications to a long-acting insulin, for example, which would not be meal-dependent.

Behaviour may also be radically affected by Alzheimer's disease. Sometimes a person might repeat the same action or words, hide possessions, or suffer physical outbursts. All of this may make it difficult to take over the management of Type 2 diabetes. A caregiver may not be able to find medications or supplies, for example. If you suspect a loved one with Type 2 diabetes has Alzheimer's, it's crucial to involve the physician who is managing diabetes, as well as a social worker or therapist who specializes in Alzheimer's disease. Together, you can work out a realistic management plan tailored to the stage of the dementia.

The person with Alzheimer's will also experience a gradual physical decline, which will affect the ability to remain independent. Eating, bathing, and hygiene habits may become erratic. Type 2 diabetes affects all these areas, particularly in people with complications such as numbness in the feet (see Chapter 20).

Alzheimer's disease doesn't occur suddenly, but gradually; it takes place in stages. You can make caregiving decisions for yourself or another based on the predicted course of the disease, but there is no clear line between one stage and another, and stages can overlap. The type of symptoms the affected person is exhibiting is the best way to gauge the staging.

Signs of Alzheimer's Disease

1. *Forgetfulness:* Affected people seem to forget what they're doing all the time. It's more than forgetting a name or where they put the keys; they forget why they are going somewhere before they can get there. Often they cannot remember what they did yesterday or earlier in the day, and nothing seems to bring the memory back.
2. *Forgetting how to do things:* Affected people forget how to do things they have done for years, like preparing certain dishes.
3. *Language problems:* Simple words or sentences seem completely foreign. Affected people may forget the names for objects and places, and can't seem to communicate basic things.
4. *Wandering or getting lost:* Affected people get lost on the street and can't figure out where they are or how to get home.
5. *Lack of judgment:* Affected people lose the ability to judge such things as when to seek medical attention or how to dress for the weather.

6. *Loss of cognitive functioning:* Affected people can't sort out complex tasks, such as writing a cheque or making change.

7. *Misplacing objects:* Affected people may put an iron in the freezer or a wristwatch in the sugar bowl. Then they may accuse someone of stealing the object.

8. *Severe mood swings for no reason:* Affected people may be calm one minute, severely agitated or in tears the next, without any perceptible change in environment and no apparent trigger.

9. *Changes in personality:* Affected people may become suspicious, apathetic, fearful, or do things that are out of character.

10. *No initiative:* Affected people may lose all interest in doing anything. Their lack of interest will be similar to the apathy that can occur in depression, but the lack of interest really stems from not remembering why the task must be done.

Types of Alzheimer's Disease

Sporadic Alzheimer's disease and Familial Autosomal Dominant Alzheimer's disease (FAD) are the same disease with different genetic tendencies. In the first, the disease doesn't appear to run in the family; in the second, it is genetically inherited and passed on. For more information on Alzheimer's disease, contact the Alzheimer Society of Canada (www.alzheimer.ca).

ELDER CARE AND TYPE 2 DIABETES

In this book, the phrase "elder-care recipient" refers to anyone with dementia or anyone older than 65 who is dependent on caregiving from a relative or professional caregiver. Elder-care recipients may be in good physical health, but suffer from dementia (see previous section) or they may have restricted mobility due to a number of factors.

Management Goals

Ideally, the blood sugar, cholesterol, and blood sugar targets should not change with age. However, in very elderly or frail people with Type 2 diabetes, looser blood sugar control may be necessary. This is especially true when the diabetic person has a number of other diseases or conditions. The goal in the case of the frail or dependent elderly person would be to adjust blood sugar goals for a level of functioning that makes sense, given all the other health problems that person is managing. Sometimes, if there is limited life expectancy, strict blood sugar monitoring and meal planning may severely interfere with what little quality of life there is. For example, if an elderly person has hypertension and/or high cholesterol and death from a heart attack is imminent, it may make more sense to bring these conditions under control first and worry about blood sugar later.

If someone receiving elder care is in good physical health, consult with a diabetes specialist or gerontologist about appropriate management for that individual.

Medications

Elderly people (people older than 75) can manage their diabetes with exercise and diet. The use of thiazoladinediones should not be used in this population at all (see Chapter 6). Sulfonylureas (see Chapter 6) should be used with caution because the risk of hypoglycemia *increases exponentially with age*. In general, initial doses of sulfonylureas should be half those given to younger people, and doses should be increased more slowly. Gliclazide and glimepirid are the preferred sulfonylureas as they are associated with fewer incidents of hypoglycemia than is glyburide. A new, long-acting formulation of gliclazide is recommended for use by the elderly. This long-acting formulation may be preferred if the patient is confused about taking medications. (See Alzheimer's section above.) Nonsulfonylurea insulin secretagogues (repaglinide and nateglinide) may be associated with a lower frequency of hypoglycemia in the elderly and are better for people with irregular eating habits.

Acarbose (see Chapter 6) is relatively safe, although many elderly people can't tolerate its gastrointestinal side effects.

In lean elderly people with Type 2 diabetes, impaired insulin secretion is usually the main problem. Agents that stimulate insulin secretion (see Chapter 6) might be the first medication of choice. Yet in obese elderly people with Type 2 diabetes, insulin resistance is a problem, so medications that improve insulin resistance would make more sense.

Premixed insulins and pre-filled insulin pens are best. These can prevent errors (for example, incorrectly mixing insulins) and improve blood sugar control. It's best to stick with a rapid-acting insulin analogue that can be administered after meals, especially for elderly people with poor or irregular eating habits.

PART III

PREVENTING COMPLICATIONS

14

PREVENTING HYPOGLYCEMIA

When you're diagnosed with Type 2 diabetes, whether your treatment includes lifestyle modification, oral hypoglycemic therapy, or insulin therapy, you may experience an episode of low blood sugar. This is clinically known as *hypoglycemia*. Hypoglycemia can sometimes come on suddenly, particularly overnight. If left untreated, it can result in coma, brain damage, and death. Hypoglycemia is considered the official cause of death in about 5 percent of the Type 1 diabetes population. In the past, hypoglycemia was a more common problem among people with Type 1 diabetes. But since 40–50 percent of all people with Type 2 diabetes will eventually graduate to insulin therapy, the incidence of hypoglycemia has increased by 300 percent in this group. Moreover, hypoglycemia is a common side effect of oral hypoglycemic pills, the medication the majority of people with Type 2 diabetes take when they are first diagnosed.

This chapter will explain exactly what happens when you have low blood sugar, who is at risk, how to treat it, and how to avoid it.

THE LOWDOWN ON LOW BLOOD SUGAR

Any blood sugar reading below 4.0 mmol/L is considered too low. A hypoglycemic episode is characterized by two stages: the warning stage and what I call the *actual* hypoglycemic episode. The warning stage occurs when your blood sugar levels *begin* to drop. This can happen as early as a blood sugar reading of 6 mmol/L in people with typically higher than normal blood sugar levels. When your blood sugar drops to 4.0 mmol/L or less, you are *officially* hypoglycemic.

During the warning stage, your body responds by pumping adrenaline into your bloodstream. This causes symptoms such as trembling, irritability, hunger, and weakness, some of which may mimic drunkenness. The irritability can simulate the rantings of someone who is drunk, while the weakness and shakiness can lead to the lack of coordination seen in someone who is intoxicated. For this reason, it's crucial that you carry a card or wear a bracelet that indicates you have diabetes. (See "Your Diabetes ID Card" later in this chapter.) Your liver will also release any glucose it has stored for you, but if it doesn't have enough glucose to get you back to normal, there won't be enough glucose for your brain to function normally and you will feel confused, irritable, or aggressive.

Once your blood sugar is 4.0 mmol/L and falling, you'll notice a more rapid heartbeat, trembling, and sweating. As the levels become lower, your pupils will begin to dilate, you will begin to lose consciousness, and you could perhaps experience a seizure. No one with diabetes is immune to hypoglycemia; it can occur in someone with long-standing diabetes just as much as in someone newly diagnosed. The important thing is to be alert to the warning signs, be prepared, and try to avoid future episodes.

Who Is at Risk?

Since hypoglycemia can be the result of too high an insulin dose, it is often called insulin shock (or insulin reaction). This is a misleading term, however, because it implies that only people who take insulin can become hypoglycemic. For the record, all people with Type 1 or Type 2 diabetes can become hypoglycemic. If you are taking more than one insulin injection a day, you are at greater risk of developing hypoglycemia, but hypoglycemia can be triggered just as easily by:

- delaying or missing a meal or snack
- drinking alcohol (see Chapter 7)

- exercising too long or too strenuously without refuelling with extra food (see Chapter 9)
- taking too high a dose of a sulfonylureas (which can happen if you lose weight, but are not put on a lower dose of your pill)

If you're taking pills

All people taking sulfonylureas (see Chapter 6 and further in this chapter) are vulnerable to hypoglycemia because sulfonylureas stimulates the pancreas to produce insulin. It is the same as taking an insulin injection. Furthermore, if you lose weight after you begin taking sulfonylureas, but don't lower your pill dosage, you could also experience hypoglycemic episodes. That's because losing weight will make your body more responsive to insulin.

Biguanides (see Chapter 6 and further on in this chapter) do not typically cause hypoglycemic episodes since they work by preventing the liver from making glucose rather than by stimulating anything to make insulin. Similarly, acarbose does not, by itself, cause hypoglycemia. It works by delaying the breakdown of starch and sucrose into glucose. That's not to say, however, that hypoglycemia can't happen to you if you're taking biguanides or acarbose; you can still develop it if you miss meals or snacks or overexercise without compensating for it, although this is rare.

As discussed in Chapter 6, your diabetes pills may also react with other medications. For example, some of the older types of medications may work less or more effectively when combined with certain medications, including blood thinners (anticoagulants), oral contraceptives, diuretics, steroids, Aspirin, and various anticonvulsive and antihypertensive medications.

Another factor is the half-life of your oral medication. By knowing when the drug peaks in your body, you'll be able to prevent hypoglycemia from occurring. Hypoglycemia and weight gain are especially common with the insulin secretagogue glyburide. If a sulfonylurea must be used, gliclazide is associated with the lowest incidence of hypoglycemia, and glimepiride is associated with less hypoglycemia than glyburide. The likelihood of hypoglycemic episodes is higher with combination therapy than with one drug therapy for diabetes. The Canadian Diabetes Association notes that the alpha-glucosidase inhibitor acarbose (Glucobay) presents a negligible risk for hypoglycemia, and is often used in combination with other anti-hyperglycemic agents. There could be gastrointestinal (GI) side effects with it, and it is not recommended as initial therapy in people with marked hyperglycemia (A1C greater or equal to 9.0 percent).

There are also significant risks with the use of insulin. The risk of hypoglycemia is highest with regular and NPH (Humulin-N, Novolin geNPH) insulin.

Recognizing the Symptoms

If you can begin to recognize the warning signs of hypoglycemia, you may be able to stabilize your blood sugar before you lose consciousness. Watch out for the adrenaline symptoms: initial hunger and headach, then sweatiness, nervousness, and dizziness. Those who live with you or spend a lot of time with you should learn to notice sudden mood changes (usually extreme irritability, drunk-like aggression, and confusion) as a warning that your blood sugar is low. (See Table 14.1.)

Table 14.1: Symptoms of Hypoglycemia

Neurogenic (autonomic)	Neuroglycopenic
Trembling	Difficulty concentrating, confusion
Palpitations	Weakness, drowsiness, vision changes
Sweating	Difficulty speaking
Anxiety	Headache, dizziness
Hunger, nausea, tingling	

Severity of Hypoglycemia:

Mild: Autonomic symptoms are present. The individual is able to self-treat.

Moderate: Autonomic and neuroglycopenic symptoms are present. The individual is able to self-treat.

Severe: Individual requires the assistance of another person. Unconsciousness may occur. PG (plasma glucose) is typically <2.8 mmol/L.

One of the best examples of hypoglycemia symptoms on film is in the movie *Steel Magnolias,* in which Julia Roberts portrays a woman with Type 1 diabetes opposite Sally Field, who plays her mother. At the local beauty parlour, amid happy chatter over Roberts's upcoming wedding, her character suddenly becomes aggressive and begins to verbally attack her mother, shaking all the while. The other customers look alarmed. Sally Field realizes at once that Roberts's glucose is low and calmly takes over the situation. She grabs Roberts and calms people down. "It's all right, it's all right, she's just low. With all the excitement that's gone on, it's only natural. Get me some juice."

"I have a candy in my purse," pipes up a customer.

"No," insists Field. "Juice is better, juice is better." Roberts becomes even more upset. Her reaction is sheer confusion and fright. Field takes the juice and starts to feed her; Roberts, in confusion, spits it out and puts up a fight every step of the way. After Field force-feeds her a little longer, Roberts starts to drink on her own and finally utters an intelligible sentence. "Oh, she's making some sense now," coos Field. "Yes, she is. She's starting to make sense." In other words, Roberts's blood sugar is beginning to rise and the hypoglycemic symptoms that appeared out of nowhere are starting to dissipate. In this scene, Field says "juice is better" because it is a more immediate source of glucose. But in fact, juice is *not* a good idea when someone is resisting it; in this case, it is better to use glucose gel rather than risk someone aspirating or inhaling the juice when it is force-fed.

Whether you notice your own mood changes or not, you, too, will feel suddenly unwell. This is a warning that your blood sugar is low. Reach for your snack pack (see page 236). Not everyone experiences the same warning symptoms, but here are some signs to watch for:

- pounding, racing heart
- fast breathing
- skin turning white
- sweating (cold sweat in big drops)
- trembling, tremors, or shaking

- goosebumps or pale, cool skin
- extreme hunger pangs
- light-headedness (feeling dizzy or that the room is spinning)
- nervousness, extreme irritability, or a sudden mood change
- confusion
- feeling weak or faint
- headache
- vision changes (seeing double or blurry vision)

Some people will experience no symptoms at all. If you've had a hypoglycemic episode without any warning symptoms, it's important for you to eat regularly and to test your blood sugar. If you're experiencing frequent hypoglycemic episodes, it's important to find out why it keeps happening so you can adjust meal plans and activities accordingly. In some cases of long-standing diabetes and repeated hypoglycemic episodes, experts note that the warning symptoms may not always occur. It's believed that in some people, the body eventually loses its ability to detect hypoglycemia and send adrenaline. Furthermore, if you've switched from animal to human insulin, warning symptoms may not be as pronounced.

"JUICE IS BETTER"

If you start to feel symptoms of hypoglycemia, stop what you're doing (especially if it's active) and have some sugar. Next, test your blood sugar to see what it reads. Eating some regular food will usually do the trick. If your blood sugar is below 4.0 mmol/L, ingest some glucose. If you can drink and swallow, Sally Fields wasn't exactly right: Real fruit juice is certainly fine when your blood sugar is low, but any sugary drink will do. The best way to get your levels back up to normal is to ingest simple sugar; that is, sugar that gets into your bloodstream fast. Half a cup of any fruit juice or one-third of a can of a sugary soft drink is a good source of simple sugar. Artificially sweetened soft drinks are useless.

If you are experiencing the signs of a low blood glucose level, check your blood glucose immediately. If you don't have your meter with you, treat the symptoms anyway:

Eat or drink a fast-acting carbohydrate (15 g):

- 15 g of glucose in the form of glucose tablets (preferred choice)
- 15 mL (3 tsps) or three packets of table sugar dissolved in water
- 175 mL (3/4 cup) of juice or regular soft drink
- Six Life Savers (1 = 2.5 g of carbohydrate)
- 15 mL (1 tbsp) of honey

Wait 10–15 minutes, then check your blood glucose again. If it is still low, treat again.

Once you've ingested enough simple sugar, your hypoglycemic symptoms should disappear within 10–15 minutes. Test your blood sugar 10 minutes after having your sugar to see if your blood sugar levels are coming back up. If your symptoms don't go away, have more simple sugars until they do.

After a Low

If you've had a close call to the point where you experienced those adrenaline symptoms, be sure to have a snack or meal as soon as possible. If your next meal or snack is more than an hour away, eat half a sandwich or some cheese and crackers. That will ensure that your blood sugar levels don't fall again. Then check your blood sugar levels after you eat to make sure your levels are where they should be. Try to investigate the cause of your episode by asking yourself the following:

1. Did you miss a meal or eat late? (Were you at one of those dinner parties where you came on time, but everybody else arrived an hour later?)
2. Did you eat less than normal? (Are you sick or upset over something?) Did you give yourself the right amount of pills or insulin?

3. Did you do anything physically active that you hadn't planned for in the last hour or so? (For instance, did someone ask you to help move some heavy object from one side of the room to the other?)

4. Did you remember to compensate for any exercising you did with the appropriate amount of carbohydrates? (See Chapter 9.)

GLUCAGON

Most people will be able to treat their low blood sugar without becoming unconscious, but on rare occasions, it can happen. If that's the case, it's too late for juice, soft drinks, or any other kind of sugar. That's when something known as a glucagon kit comes in. Glucagon is particularly useful for people who have little or no warning symptoms of low blood sugar and have previously lost consciousness from low blood sugar.

Glucagon is a hormone injected under the skin. Like insulin, glucagon is destroyed by the digestive system when it's taken orally. Glucagon causes an increase in blood glucose concentration; it basically stimulates the body to make glucose. It does this by forcing the liver to convert all its glycogen stores into glucose almost immediately after it's injected. You'll need about 1 mg of glucagon to do the trick.

Glucagon will make you nauseous when you regain consciousness, so if glucagon is injected, it's crucial to ingest simple sugars as soon as you wake. The simple sugar will replace the glycogen your liver releases and will get rid of the nausea. Once you feel normal again, you should consume regular food. Get a prescription for a glucagon kit from your doctor, then purchase the kit at any pharmacy. One thing to keep in mind about the use of glucagon is that after the injection, the person should be turned onto his or her side to prevent choking if she or he vomits. Once the glucagon has been given, the person's doctor (and/ or diabetes health care team) should be contacted as soon as possible to discuss the episode. It is very important that all people with diabetes have a household member who knows the symptoms of low blood sugar and knows how to administer glucagon.

If you do not respond to glucagon, glucose will be administered intravenously in a hospital or ambulance.

People in states of starvation (anorexics) or who have chronic hypoglycemia will not benefit from glucagon because in those cases there will be no glycogen stores in the liver ready for conversion into glucose. Injected under the skin, glucagon takes eight to 10 minutes to work its wonders.

The Third Person

The glucagon kit is for another person to use, someone who has been shown how to administer the drug to revive you. This may be someone close to you who is likely to be with you when you lose consciousness. The kit should have all the necessary instructions regarding giving injections, but here are the instructions just in case. Photocopy these instructions and post them in a safe place:

1. Inject 1 mg of glucagon anywhere under the skin. (The abdomen or thighs are good spots.) For children five and under, .50 mg of glucagon is recommended.
2. Wait about 10 minutes for the person to regain consciousness. Call 9-1-1 if he or she does not regain consciousness in 15 minutes.
3. After the person wakes up, immediately give her or him about half a cup of fruit juice or a third of a can of a sugary soft drink. The drink must contain sugar; artificially sweetened drinks will not work.
4. Continue feeding the drink to this person until he or she feels well enough to eat regular food.

For Your Wallet

Photocopy the following and carry it in your wallet (I, the author, give you permission) as soon as you finish reading this chapter:

> To whom it may concern:
> These instructions will help you assist this person with diabetes, who has passed out because his or her blood sugar is too low.

1. Give this person a form of simple sugar (juice, candies, table sugar, honey). If this person is unconscious, go to number 2.
2. Do *not* give this person any food or drink or put anything in his or her mouth; he or she could choke.
3. Call 9-1-1 and say: "I'm with a person who has diabetes who has passed out from low blood sugar. I need someone to get here as soon as possible." Be sure to give a clear address with specific instructions about your location.

RECIPE FOR PREVENTION

The recipe for preventing hypoglycemia or low blood sugar is the same one for preventing high blood sugar: frequent blood sugar monitoring (Chapter 5), eating low glycemic foods (Chapter 7), following an exercise plan (Chapter 9), and taking your medication as prescribed (Chapter 6). Any changes in your routine, diet, exercise habits, or medication dosages should be followed by a period of very close blood sugar monitoring until your routine is more established. It is important to keep food, activity, and medications properly balanced, with the ongoing advice of your diabetes health care team.

Frequent episodes of hypoglycemia may also be a sign that your body is changing: You may be losing weight, thanks to those lifestyle changes you've made, and the dosage of pills that were prescribed to you when you weighed 86 kg (190 lbs) may be too strong now that you're down to 65 kg (145 lbs), or you may be taking too high an insulin dose.

A Snack Pack

People with Type 1 or 2 diabetes should have a snack pack with them for emergencies or for unplanned physical activity. The pack should contain all of the following:

- two or three boxes or cans of juice (in a pinch, you can substitute with two cans of a sweet soft drink, sweetened with real sugar)
- one package of dextrose tablets (alternatively, a bag of hard candies)

- some protein and carbohydrates (e.g., packaged cheese and crackers)
- extra food to cover delayed meals such as a box of cookies or crackers and fruit juice
- a card that says "I have diabetes" (see page 238)
- glucagon, if you suffer from repeat episodes
- bottled water

Wear Your Bracelet

All people with diabetes ought to wear a MedicAlert bracelet or necklace, the most recognized medical alert outerwear. The newer styles don't have that basic red lettering that announces to the world "I'm allergic or diabetic." The newer bracelets can be quite discreet, yet still have your medical information, personal ID number, and a 24-hour emergency hotline number engraved on it. This crucial jewellery is yours for a one-time, upfront registration fee of $39.00, and then your yearly membership fee is $39.00. The one-time registration fee will get you a bracelet or necklace and free updates on your information. You can reach Canadian MedicAlert Foundation at 800-668-1507, or go to their website: www.medicalert.ca.

Tell People You Have Diabetes

A crucial word about dealing with hypoglycemia: Tell people close to you, or who work closely with you, that you have diabetes. You never know when you might experience symptoms: at a family function (weddings are notorious for delayed meals), at work, and so on. If you tell people about the symptoms of hypoglycemia and instruct them on what to do, you'll have more bases covered in case you experience an episode. There are websites that will allow you to fill in your own personalized medical information to keep with you. You can visit:

http://www.medids.com/Emergency_Medical_Form.html

There is also this commercial site, which will allow you to order, for a nominal fee, special wallet cards for diabetes:

http://www.medawareid.com/wallet_cards.html

Otherwise, feel free to copy and carry the form below.

CHAPTER FOURTEEN

YOUR DIABETES ID CARD

If you don't have the following information on you already, photocopy this section and put it in an obvious place in your wallet or on your person.

I have diabetes. If I am unconscious or if my behaviour. appears unusual, it may be related to my diabetes or my treatment. I am not drunk. If I can swallow, give me sugar in the form of fruit juice, a sweet soft drink, candies, or table sugar. Phone my doctor or the hospital listed below, or phone 9-1-1 if I am unconscious.

Name:

Address:

Phone:

Chief contact:

Relationship:

My doctor's name is:

He or she can be reached at (phone number):

After hours:

My hospital:

My blood type is: ❑ A ❑ B ❑ AB ❑ O ❑ Rh+ ❑ Rh–

I wear: ❑ lens implants ❑ dentures ❑ contact lenses ❑ an artificial joint ❑ a pacemaker

I'm allergic to:

My health card/insurance number is:

My group insurance number is:

Source: Adapted from "Health Record for People with Diabetes," 1996, McNeil Consumer Products Company.

15

DIABETES, HEART, AND STROKE

The most important thing to grasp about diabetes complications is that there are two kinds of problems that can lead to similar diseases. The first kind of problem is known as a *macrovascular complication*. The prefix *macro* means "large"; the word *vascular* means "blood vessels," the veins and arteries that carry the blood back and forth throughout your body. Put it together and you have "large blood vessel complications." A plain-language interpretation of "macrovascular complications" is "*big* problems with your blood vessels."

If you think of your body as a planet, a macrovascular disease would be a disease that affects the whole planet; it is body-wide, or systemic. Cardiovascular disease is a macrovascular complication that can cause heart attack, stroke, high blood pressure, and body-wide circulation problems, clinically known as peripheral vascular disease (PVD). Peripheral vascular disease refers to "fringe" blood-flow problems and is part of the heart disease story. PVD occurs when blood flow to the limbs (arms, legs, and feet) is blocked, creating cramping, pain, or numbness. *In fact, pain and numbing in your arms or legs may be signs of heart disease or even an imminent heart attack.*

Macrovascular complications are caused not only by too much blood sugar, but also by pre-existing health problems. People with Type 2 diabetes are far more vulnerable to macrovascular complications because they usually have contributing risk factors from way back when, such as high cholesterol and high blood pressure, both of which are discussed in Chapter 2. Obesity, smoking, and inactivity can then aggravate those problems, resulting in major cardiovascular disease and leaving the individual at risk for heart attack or stroke. What people don't understand is that when the terms "heart disease" or "cardiovascular disease" are used, they refer to your risk of not just heart attack but *stroke*.

WHAT TO EXPECT WHEN YOU HAVE A HEART ATTACK

A heart attack is clinically known as a myocardial infarction (MI). Myocardium is the clinical name for "heart muscle." An MI occurs when there is not enough, or any, blood supply to the myocardium, something that happens when one of the coronary arteries is blocked. A coronary artery supplies blood to the heart muscle. Roughly 90 percent of heart attacks are due to a blood clot. A variety of symptoms can occur during a heart attack. Men experience different symptoms than women. If you're a woman reading this, please see the section "Heart Attacks in Women." If you're male, the following can be signs of a heart attack. You may experience only one of the symptoms below, or a combination:

- Feeling a crushing or compression in the chest, combined with pain. You may feel as though a heavy weight has been dropped on your chest.
- Feeling squeezed or constricted, as though a vise was gripping your chest.
- Feeling as though you're being choked or strangled, along with a sickening feeling in the chest. It may resemble a panic or anxiety attack and not feel like a heart attack.
- Burning and indigestion. This could be, in fact, heartburn, a common problem for people with diabetes. Many people believe their heartburn is a heart attack; many people also believe their heart attack is "only heartburn." Always see a doctor. If sweating, weakness, shortness of breath, and a feeling of impending doom accompany the indigestion, it's probably a heart attack.

- Tearing, gripping pain. You feel as though your chest is being ripped apart.
- Mild discomfort in the chest. Clearly, this is a mild heart attack, but it is still a sign of a heart attack.
- Tingling, numbness, or heaviness over the arm. This symptom is very common in women (see further on).
- A sharp, stabbing pain in the chest.
- Severe dizziness or weakness. This symptom may be confused with low blood sugar, but can also be a sign of heart attack.
- Nausea with chest pain. Without vomiting or diarrhea, this symptom is frequently a sign of a heart attack.
- Aching pain under the arm or breastbone.

Additional Symptoms

As you can see from this list, the pain and discomfort can vary from severe to mild discomfort. When the above heart attack symptoms are accompanied by any of the following, call an ambulance or get to an ER: profuse sweating, difficulty breathing, a feeling of impending doom (almost all heart attack survivors say they felt very anxious and fearful quite suddenly), severe and sudden weakness, dizziness or lightheadedness, nausea and vomiting, restlessness, shortness of breath, coughing, sudden drop in blood pressure (which may cause the weakness and dizziness), slower heart rate (check your pulse), and chest discomfort.

Diagnostic tests that can confirm a heart attack include a manual exam (doctor examining you with a stethoscope), an electrocardiogram, an exercise stress test, an echocardiogram, as well as myriad imaging tests that may use radioactive substances to take pictures of the heart.

Heart Attacks in Women

Heart disease is currently the number one cause of death in post-menopausal women; more women die of heart disease than of lung cancer or breast cancer. Being diabetic can complicate matters even further. Diabetes is said to travel in bad company—hypertension, dyslipidaemia, prothrombosis—and this applies particularly to women.

Diabetes increases coronary risk for both men and women, but diabetes increases the absolute rate of coronary events in women more than men. The reason for this is not clear, and may relate to biological differences, differences in treatment, or both. Essentially half of all North Americans who die from heart attacks each year are women. American Heart Association statistics for 2004 showed that for cardiovascular diseases (plus congenital heart disease), there were 410,628 deaths for males, and 459,096 for females.

One of the reasons for such high death rates from heart attacks among women is medical ignorance: Most studies looking at heart disease excluded women (see Introduction), which led to a myth that more men than women die of heart disease. The truth is, more men die of heart attacks before age 50, while more women die of heart attacks after age 50 as a direct result of estrogen loss. Moreover, women who have had oopherectomies (removal of the ovaries) prior to natural menopause increase their risk of a heart attack by *eight times*. Since more women work outside the home than ever before, a number of experts also cite stress as a huge contributing factor to increased rates of heart disease in women.

Another problem is that women have different symptoms than men when it comes to heart disease, and so the typical warning signs we know about in men—angina, or chest pains—are often never present in women. In fact, chest pains in women are almost never related to heart disease. For women, the symptoms of heart disease, and even an actual heart attack, can be much more vague, seemingly unrelated to heart problems. Signs of heart disease in women include some surprising symptoms. Some of the signs are the same as in men, but some are completely different:

- Shortness of breath and/or fatigue
- Jaw pain (often masked by arthritis and joint pain)
- Pain in the back of the neck (often masked by arthritis or joint pain)
- Pain down the right or left arm
- Back pain (often masked by arthritis and joint pain)

- Sweating (also have your thyroid checked—this is a classic sign of an overactive thyroid gland; also test your blood sugar as you may be low)
- Fainting
- Palpitations (ladies, again, have your thyroid checked, as this is also a classic symptom of an overactive thyroid)
- Bloating (after menopause, this is a sign of coronary artery blockage)
- Heartburn, belching, or other gastrointestinal pain (this is often a sign of an actual heart attack in women)
- Chest heaviness between the breasts (this is how women experience chest pain; some describe it as a "sinking feeling" or burning sensation; other describe an "aching, throbbing, or a squeezing sensation"; "hot poker stab between the chest," or feeling like your heart jumps into your throat)
- Sudden swings in blood sugar
- Vomiting
- Confusion

Clearly, there are lots of other causes for the symptoms on this list, including low blood sugar, but it's important that your doctor includes heart disease as a possible cause rather than dismissing it because your symptoms are not "male" (which your doctor may refer to as "typical"). Bear in mind that if you're suffering from nerve damage, you may not feel a lot of these symptoms. Therefore, you should take extra care to be suspicious of anything that feels out of the ordinary.

If you're diagnosed with heart disease, the "cure" is prevention through diet and exercise. Keeping your blood sugar levels in the normal range will help restore estrogen's protective properties.

Recovering from a Heart Attack

You can recover from a heart attack, but the damage resulting from the heart attack greatly depends on how long the blood supply to the heart muscle was cut off. The longer the blood supply was cut off, the more damage you will suffer. We all know that a heart attack is a major cause of death, but it can also leave you with varying degrees of disability depending upon the severity of the attack. For example, roughly half of all heart attack survivors will continue to have heart-related problems, which include reduced blood flow to the heart—called ischemia—and chest pains. As a result, the lifestyle you once enjoyed will need to change: Your diet will need to be restricted to a "heart-smart" diet (see Chapter 7), and you will need to find ways to reduce lifestyle stress and incorporate more activity into your routine. If you don't make these changes, the risk of repeated heart attacks will loom, which can greatly affect your quality of life. You may also feel more fatigued and winded after normal activities when recovering from a heart attack. Successful recovery greatly depends on the severity of the attack and lifestyle changes you make after the episode. The same medical strategies designed to prevent a first heart attack can also be used to avoid recurrent episodes.

How Can I Prevent Cardiovascular Disease?

The way to prevent heart disease and peripheral vascular disease is by modifying your lifestyle (stop smoking, eat less fat, get more exercise). Smoking, high blood pressure, high blood sugar, and high cholesterol (called the "catastrophic quartet" by one diabetes specialist) will greatly increase your risk of heart disease.

Heart Surgery

You can also reduce your risk of a heart attack or stroke by undergoing heart surgery, which ranges from minor surgical procedures such as angioplasty to major heart bypass surgery.

Angioplasty, also known as coronary balloon surgery, was developed in Zurich in 1977. This operation involves inserting a catheter through your skin into the coronary artery. The catheter has a balloon on the end, which is inflated once inside. The inflated balloon squashes the plaque that is blocking the artery, easing blood flow. The balloon also widens the artery by essentially stretching it. Several inflations may be necessary to do the trick, but it is successful about 70 percent of the time. As your blood flow improves, so does your overall health.

There is about a 5 percent risk of having a heart attack during the procedure, which you must weigh. Also, about 25 percent of the time, the artery is too narrow for the catheter to fit or too clogged for angioplasty to work.

Laser angioplasty is the same procedure as above, except a laser is passed through the catheter and dissolves the plaque. This is a good way to handle very narrowed arteries or arteries that are too hardened with plaque for balloon angioplasty to work.

The first successful coronary artery bypass surgery was performed by a heart surgeon in 1967 in Cleveland. Since then, it has become a fairly standard surgery. Here, a vein from your leg is removed and connected to the aorta as it leaves the heart; the other end is connected to the coronary artery, just before the blockage. The vein acts as a bridge between the two, enabling the blood to flow, thus fixing the blood flow problem. The risk of a heart attack during this procedure is about 10 percent higher than with angioplasty, but after five years, 70 percent of bypass patients are still enjoying an active life and are free from any symptoms of heart disease. Not everyone is a good candidate for this surgery, however. If you're considering this option, you'll need to discuss the risks of undergoing the surgery in light of your overall health.

Lower Blood Pressure
High blood pressure is discussed on page 22 in Chapter 2, along with blood pressure-lowering drugs (also called antihypertensive medications).

Lower Cholesterol
High cholesterol is discussed on page 19 in Chapter 2, along with cholesterol-lowering drugs.

Anti-platelet Therapy
Sometimes confused with anticoagulants (blood thinners), these are drugs that prevent the platelets from clumping due to stickiness. Acetylsalicylic acid (ASA) is the anti-platelet agent most commonly studied in the prevention of CV events in people with diabetes because

it is the most widely studied, and also the most economical. Many early studies on daily Aspirin therapy were done in men, and with some newer ones studying the effects of Aspirin on women, it is clear that there are differences in how a daily Aspirin works between the sexes. As far as the use of Aspirin for primary prevention goes, it is best to have a continuing discussion with your health care provider over this. As of this writing, the use of Aspirin is still an open question. So although the use of Aspirin for primary prevention of cardiovascular events in individuals with diabetes is widely recommended by existing guidelines, the evidence supporting its efficacy is surprisingly scarce. An increasing amount of evidence suggests that the efficacy of anti-platelet therapy in patients with diabetes may be lower than in individuals without diabetes. This is all the more reason to discuss the best plan of action with your health care provider. There are so many factors to take into account with Aspirin therapy, and evidently having diabetes can further complicate the matter.

Quit Smoking
This is discussed on page 28 in Chapter 2.

Reducing Stress
There's no question about it: Stress can lead to heart disease. Generally, stress is defined as a negative emotional experience associated with biological changes that allow you to adapt to it. In response to stress, your adrenal glands pump out stress hormones that speed up your body: Your heart rate increases and your blood sugar levels increase so that glucose can be diverted to your muscles in case you have to run from a threatening situation. This is known as the fight-or-flight response. These hormones are technically called the catecholamines, which are broken down into epinephrine (adrenaline) and norepinephrine.

The problem with stress hormones in the 21st century is that the fight-or-flight response isn't usually necessary since most of our stress stems from interpersonal situations rather than dangerous situations such as being chased by a predator. Occasionally, we may want to flee from a bank robber or mugger, but most of us just want to flee from our jobs or our kids! In other words, our stress hormones actually put a physical strain on our bodies and can lower our resistance to disease. Initially, stress hormones stimulate our immune systems, but after the stressful event has passed, the stress hormones can suppress the immune system, leaving us vulnerable to a wide variety of illnesses and physical symptoms.

Hans Selye, considered the father of stress management, defined stress as the "wear and tear" on the body. Once we are in a state of stress, the body adapts to the stress by depleting its resources until it becomes exhausted. The wear and tear on our bodies is mounting; we can suffer from a host of stress-related ailments that include high blood pressure, high cholesterol, and heart disease. Current statistics reveal that 43 percent of all adults suffer from health problems directly caused by stress, while 75–90 percent of all visits to primary care physicians are for stress-related complaints or disorders.

Managing your stress is no easy feat, particularly since there are different types of stress: acute stress (which can be episodic) and chronic stress. Acute stress results from an acute situation, such as a sudden, unexpected negative event, or from, for example, organizing a wedding or planning for a conference. When the event passes, the stress will pass. Acute stress is when you're feeling the pressure of a particular deadline or event, but there is an end to the stress. There are numerous symptoms of acute stress: anger or irritability, anxiety, depression, tension headaches or migraines, back pain, jaw pain, muscular tension, digestive problems, cardiovascular problems, and dizziness.

But acute stress can be what's known as "episodic," meaning that there is one stressful event after another, creating a continuous flow of acute stress. Someone who is always taking on too many projects at once is someone who suffers from *episodic* acute stress rather than simple acute stress. Workaholics and those with the so-called Type A personality are classic sufferers of episodic acute stress.

I sometimes refer to acute stress as the "good stress" because often good things come from this kind of stress, even though it feels stressful or bad in the short term. This is the kind of stress that challenges us to stretch ourselves beyond our capabilities, which is what makes us meet deadlines and invent creative solutions to our problems. Examples of "good stress" include taking on challenging projects; undergoing positive life-changing events (moving, changing jobs, or ending unhealthy relationships); or confronting fears, illness, or people who make us feel bad (this is one of those bad-in-the-short-term/good-in-the-long-term situations). Essentially, whenever a stressful event triggers emotional, intellectual, or spiritual growth, it is a "good stress." It is often not the event as much as it is your *response* to the event that determines whether it is a "good" or "bad" stress. The death of a loved one can sometimes lead to personal growth because we may see something about ourselves we did not see before—new resilience, for example, so even a death can be a "good stress," though we grieve and are sad in the short term.

What I call the "bad stress" is known as chronic stress. Chronic or bad stress results from boredom and stagnation, as well as from prolonged negative circumstances. Essentially, when no growth occurs from the stressful event, it is "bad stress." When negative events don't seem to yield anything positive in the long term, but more of the same, the stress can lead to chronic and debilitating health problems. This is not to say that we can't get sick from good stress either, but when there is nothing positive from the stress, it has a much more negative effect on our health. Some examples of bad stress include stagnant jobs or relationships, disability from terrible accidents or diseases, long-term unemployment, chronic poverty, racism, or lack of opportunities for change. These kinds of situations can lead to depression, low self-esteem, and a host of physical illnesses.

In addition to acute and chronic stress, stress can be defined in even more precise ways:

- Physical stress (physical exertion)
- Chemical stress (when we're exposed to a toxin in our environment, including substance abuse)
- Mental stress (when we take on too much responsibility and begin worrying about all that has to be done)
- Emotional stress (when our feelings stress us out, such as anger, fear, frustration, sadness, betrayal, or bereavement)

- Nutritional stress (when we're deficient in certain vitamins or nutrients, overindulged in fat or protein, or experience food allergies)
- Traumatic stress (caused by trauma to the body such as infection, injury, burns, surgery, or extreme temperatures)
- Psychospiritual stress (caused by unrest in our personal relationships or belief system, personal life goals, and so on; in general, this is what defines whether or not we are happy)

The bottom line is this: *Stress makes us sick*. Stress management is a complex topic that I can't possibly cover here, but the principles of stress management involve reorganizing your priorities so you can reduce chronic stress as well as incorporate some healing strategies to help combat acute stress. Finding ways to downshift, eat better (chapters 7 and 8), exercise (see Chapter 9), and generally care for yourself by doing simple things such as getting enough sleep, for example, can dramatically reduce your current stress and improve your overall cardiovascular health.

UNDERSTANDING STROKE

As mentioned earlier, cardiovascular disease puts you at risk for not just a heart attack, but a "brain attack" or stroke, which occurs when a blood clot (a clog in your blood vessels) travels to your brain and stops the flow of blood and oxygen carried to the nerve cells in that area. When that happens, cells may die or vital functions controlled by the brain can be temporarily or permanently damaged. Bleeding or a rupture from the affected blood vessel can lead to a very serious situation, including death. People with Type 2 diabetes are two to three times more likely to suffer from a stroke than people without diabetes. About 80 percent of strokes are caused by the blockage of an artery in the neck or brain, known as an "ischemic stroke"; the remainder are caused by a burst blood vessel in the brain that causes bleeding into or around the brain.

Since the 1960s, the death rate from strokes has dropped by 50 percent. This drop is largely due to public-awareness campaigns regarding diet and lifestyle modification (quitting smoking, eating low-fat foods, and exercising), as well as the introduction of blood pressure-lowering drugs and cholesterol-lowering drugs that have helped people maintain normal blood pressure and cholesterol levels (see pages 26 and 27).

Strokes can be mild, moderate, severe, or fatal. Mild strokes may affect speech or movement for a short period of time only; many people recover from mild strokes without any permanent damage. Moderate or severe strokes may result in loss of speech or memory, and in paralysis; many people learn to speak again and learn to function with partial paralysis. How well you recover depends on how much damage was done.

A considerable amount of research points to stress as a risk factor for stroke. The section "How Can I Prevent Cardiovascular Disease?" on page 244 suggests ways to cut down on stress.

Signs of a Stroke

If you can recognize the key warning signs of a stroke, it can make a difference in preventing a major stroke or reducing the severity of a stroke.

Call 9-1-1 or get to the emergency room of your local hospital if you *suddenly* notice one or more of the following symptoms:

- Weakness, numbness, and/or tingling in your face, arms, or legs, especially on one side of the body; this may last only a few moments
- Loss of speech or difficulty understanding somebody else's speech; this may last only a short time
- Confusion
- Severe headaches that feel different from any headache you've had before
- Feeling unsteady, falling a lot
- Trouble seeing in one or both eyes

If you have any of the signs of stroke above, it's important to get to the hospital as soon as possible. There are treatments that can reduce the severity of the damage caused by the stroke, making the difference between partial or severe disability and full recovery. For example, tPA, tissue plasminogen activator, is a thrombolytic agent (clot-busting drug) approved in the US by the FDA in 1996 (and in Canada in 1999) to treat ischemic stroke. Studies have shown that tPA and other clot-dissolving agents can help to reduce the amount of damage to the heart. The key to administering tPA is all in the timing. Generally, tPA and similar drugs should be given within the first three hours after the start of stroke symptoms. Therefore, it is very important for people to seek immediate attention if they think they are having a stroke. The latest research indicates that it is in fact safe to extend the three-hour window to four-and-a-half, based on a meta-analysis of randomized controlled trials.

Common Disabilities Caused by Stroke

There's no question that stroke is responsible for a range of functional and physical disabilities, especially in people over 45. Depending on the severity of the stroke, your general health, and the rehabilitation process involved, the following impairments may dramatically improve over time:

- Weakness or paralysis on one side of the body. The weakness or paralysis is always on the opposite side of the body from where the stroke occurred. So if the stroke affected the right side of the brain, you will experience the weakness or paralysis on the left side of your body. Paralysis may affect the face, an arm, a leg, or the entire side of the body. Walking, grasping objects, and the ability to swallow can be affected by one-sided paralysis.
- Muscle spasms or stiffness
- Problems with balance and/or coordination
- Problems understanding, speaking, and writing in your first language (called aphasia). This is a common problem, affecting about 25 percent of stroke survivors. At least one-fourth of all stroke survivors experience language impairments. These impairments can take two forms: problems comprehending others, or

problems articulating words. Stroke survivors may be able to think clearly, but are unable to make the words "come out right," resulting in disconnected gibberish when they try to speak. The most severe form of aphasia is called global aphasia, the loss of all language abilities. The person who had the stroke is not able to understand or communicate in any language. There is also a form of very mild aphasia, called anomie aphasia, where language is mostly unaffected, except for a few words that may be forgotten selectively, such as names of people or particular kinds of objects.

- Inability to respond to bodily sensations on one side of the body (a.k.a. bodily neglect). This means that the ability to feel, touch, and sense pain or temperature can be lost. There may be no recognition of the person's own limb—an arm or leg may not be noticeable any more.
- Pain, numbness, or odd sensations (called paresthesia). Pain can be the result of damage to the nervous system (neuropathic pain). Stroke survivors who have a paralyzed arm, for example, may feel as though the pain is radiating outward from the shoulder (the lack of movement causes the joint to be fixed or frozen). Physical therapy can help to alleviate this. Pain can also result from a confused signal from the damaged brain, sending out pain to the side of the body that is not affected.
- Difficulty remembering, thinking, focusing, or learning. Extremely short attention spans, combined with short-term memory loss, can make it difficult for stroke survivors to learn new tasks, make plans, or engage in a complex discussion. Often the ability to connect a thought to an action is lost.
- Unawareness of the stroke's effects. A stroke survivor may be paralyzed on one side, but not acknowledge the paralysis and have no awareness of the impairment, or the fact that a stroke has taken place.
- Difficulty swallowing (called dysphagia)
- Urinary or bowel incontinence (bladder or bowel control). The ability to sense bladder or bowel urge may be lost, or simply

the mobility required to go to the bathroom may be the obstacle. Incontinence becomes less severe with time. Physical therapists can help stroke survivors strengthen their pelvic muscles through special exercises. By following a timed voiding schedule, incontinence may be solved. In other cases, people can learn to use catheters to prevent other incontinence-related health problems from developing.

- Fatigue
- Mood swings; natural feelings of anger, anxiety, and frustration can cause extreme mood swings or even personality changes in stroke survivors. Anger is frequently taken out on loved ones, family, or friends.
- Depression; a mild depression can become a major depression when the stroke survivor loses all engagement and interest in life, doesn't maintain a healthy weight, doesn't sleep properly, and/or exhibits other physical symptoms. Sometimes intervention with anti-depressants is necessary if counselling is not effective due to language difficulties.

Recovering from Stroke

According to the National Stroke Association in the United States, 40 percent of all stroke survivors experience moderate to severe impairments that require special care, while 10 percent will need to be placed in a facility or nursing home; 25 percent of stroke survivors will recover with minor impairments, while 10 percent will survive the stroke and almost completely recover. The remaining 15 percent of stroke sufferers die shortly after the stroke.

Stroke survivors may recover in long-term care facilities within hospitals or a separate rehabilitation hospital. Many receive home care through outpatient programs or various institutions. The crucial part of stroke rehabilitation is timing: It should begin as soon as a stroke survivor is stable, which is often within 24–48 hours after a stroke. Early stroke rehabilitation doesn't imply a rigorous physical therapy program at all. Because paralysis or weakness on one side is so often the result of the stroke, it's important to get stroke survivors moving again by helping them change positions frequently while lying in bed, or having a physical therapist move stroke-impaired limbs (called passive range-of-motion exercises). Helping survivors progress to sitting up in bed or transferring them to a chair from a bed are all part of rehabilitation. Eventually, many may be able to stand, bearing their own weight, or walk with or without assistance. Early rehabilitation also includes helping stroke survivors with bathing, dressing, and using a toilet.

The Recovery Team

There are many health care providers who may become involved in stroke recovery. The recovery team can include your primary care physician, health care specialists in physical medicine and rehabilitation, neurologists, internists, geriatricians (specialists in elder care), and rehabilitation nurses, who specialize in nursing care for people with disabilities.

One of the most important steps in stroke recovery is receiving good physical therapy. Physical therapists help survivors learn to reuse their impaired limbs by teaching them how to compensate for their disabilities with other ways to move, or by preventing the impaired parts of the body from wasting away further through disuse. An occupational therapist helps stroke survivors find new ways to complete self-directed tasks, such as cleaning, cooking, gardening, dressing, and so on.

Other important recovery team members are the speech-language pathologists, who help stroke survivors relearn language or develop new ways to communicate. They coach conversations by helping survivors develop prompts or cues to remember words; they may use sign language, symbol boards, or computers as language aids. (Voice-synthesized products may be especially useful for people recovering from strokes.) Difficulties with swallowing can be improved through helping with swallowing reflexes, helping the stroke survivor manipulate food with the tongue, finding better eating positions, or encouraging different eating habits such as taking small bites and chewing slowly.

To help stroke survivors adjust to the emotional problems that may follow a stroke (such as despair or depression), social workers, psychologists, or psychiatrists may also become involved with recovery.

Quality of Life Decisions after Stroke

For many stroke survivors, quality of life decisions are a factor in long-term care. Twenty-five years ago, stroke survivors who suffered from extreme impairments leaving them with no quality of life (meaning one cannot speak, eat, understand, or move) were often kept alive through medical interventions, such as tube-feeding, force-feeding, IV, or life-saving measures when pneumonia or heart failure occurred. This is now seen as futile and an act of prolonging death rather than preserving life.

Today, when there is no quality of life, families have the option of withdrawing medical treatment. If you are at high risk for stroke, you may wish to draft an advanced directive that tells your family members your wishes should you become incapacitated by stroke and left with no quality of life. In the case of stroke, withdrawal of medical treatment means that feeding is stopped (meaning that there is no tube feeding, no IV or forced feeding), and no lifesaving interventions are introduced when breathing becomes laboured or the heart stops. Withdrawal of medical treatment is *not* the same thing as euthanasia or assisted suicide in which medical intervention is used to stop life.

Preventing Another Stroke

Preventing another stroke involves the same strategies as preventing a heart attack recurrence (see page 244).

To prevent another stroke, and to maintain good health in general, you will possibly have to take medicines for high cholesterol and/or hypertension, and also undertake lifestyle changes such as:

- Getting regular exercise
- Limiting intake of caffeine, animal fats, processed foods, sugars, and eating a wide assortment of fruits and vegetables
- Quitting smoking
- Limiting alcohol consumption

Cardiovascular disease (which leads to heart attack and/or stroke) is certainly the most common disease caused by macrovascular or large blood vessel complications. But most of the other notorious diabetes complications (eye disease, kidney problems, impotence, foot problems, etc.) result when restricted blood flow from macrovascular complications results in nerve damage, known as diabetic neuropathy, discussed in the next chapter.

16

WHEN DIABETES GETS ON YOUR NERVES

A second type of diabetes complication is known as a microvascular complication. "Micro" means "tiny," as in "microscopic." "Microvascular complications" refers to problems with the smaller blood vessels (capillaries) that connect to various body parts. A plain-language interpretation of microvascular complications would be "Houston, we've got a problem." In other words, the problem is serious, but it's not going to affect the whole planet, just the spacecraft in orbit. Nerve damage (neuropathy) is a microvascular complication that targets body parts such as feet, eyes, genitals, and skin. But unlike macrovascular complications (large blood vessel complications), microvascular complications do not cause a sudden life-threatening event such as heart attack or stroke. For example, eye disease (see Chapter 17), clinically known as retinopathy, is a microvascular complication. Blindness is a serious problem, but you won't die from it.

People with Type 1 diabetes (see Chapter 1) are more vulnerable to microvascular complications, but a good portion of people with Type 2 diabetes suffer from them, too. Microvascular complications are known as sugar-related complications. The small blood vessel damage is caused by high blood sugar levels over long periods of time. The Diabetes Control and Complications Trial showed that by keeping blood sugar levels as normal as possible, as often as possible, through frequent self-testing, microvascular complications can be prevented.

UNDERSTANDING DIABETIC NEUROPATHY

When your blood sugar levels are too high for too long, you can develop a condition known as diabetic neuropathy or nerve disease. Somehow, the cells that make up your nerves are altered in response to high blood sugar. Different groups of nerves are affected by high blood sugar; keeping your blood sugar levels as normal as possible is the best way to prevent many of the following problems. Drugs that help prevent chemical changes in your nerve cells can also be used to treat nerve damage.

Types of Neuropathy

Polyneuropathy is a disease that affects the nerves in your feet and legs. The symptoms are burning, tingling, and numbness in the legs and feet. Polyneuropathy can lead to amputations in extreme cases. Chapter 20 is devoted solely to foot problems and amputations.

Autonomic neuropathy is a disease that affects the nerves you don't notice: the nerves that control your digestive tract (see gastrointestinal tract section below), bladder, bowel, blood pressure, sweat glands, overall balance, and sexual functioning (see genitals section on page 266). Treatment varies depending on what's affected, but drugs can control individual parts of the body, such as the digestive tract.

Proximal motor neuropathy is a disease that affects the nerves that control your muscles. It can lead to weakness and burning sensations in the joints (hands, thighs, and ankles are the most common). These problems can be individually treated with physiotherapy and/or specific medication. When the nerves that control the muscles in the eyes (see Chapter 17) are affected, you may experience problems, such as double vision. Finally, nerve damage can affect the spine, causing pain and loss of sensation to the back, buttocks, and legs.

NERVE DAMAGE HEAD TO TOE

Below is an overview of the body parts most commonly affected by diabetic neuropathy, listed in order from head to toe. Keep in mind that this list is not exhaustive as there are hundreds of nerve-related problems that can occur. These are the "majors" that affect people with Type 2 diabetes.

Eyes

For details on all eye and vision problems caused by diabetes, see Chapter 17.

Gastrointestinal Tract (GI Tract)

When high blood sugar levels affect your nerve cells, the nerves that control your entire gastrointestinal tract may be affected as well. In fact, 30–50 percent of people with diabetes suffer from dysmotility, a condition in which the muscles in the digestive tract become uncoordinated, causing bloating, abdominal pain, and reflux (heartburn). This is also known as gastroparesis.

What Is Your GI Tract?

Imagine that your digestive tract is one long subway tunnel with different stops. If you were to look at the GI "subway map," the first stop is your mouth. The next stop is your pharynx, and the third stop is your esophagus. The esophagus is a major "connecting stop." This is where the train stops for a while before switching tracks and moving on to the more active parts of your gut: the stomach, which connects to your duodenum, which connects to your small intestine, which connects to the last stop on the line, your large intestine.

Swallowing your food triggers all the muscles in your digestive tract to begin contracting in wave-like motions known as peristalsis. The act of swallowing is voluntary, but once the food is down the throat, the rest of the movement through the digestive tract is involuntary, or beyond your control. Your nervous system takes over. The food goes down the throat into the pharynx and into the esophagus. The esophagus connects your throat to your stomach.

In order for your food to get from the esophagus to the stomach, it must go through a crucial tunnel known as the lower esophageal sphincter (LES). When you swallow your food, the LES relaxes to allow your food to pass from the esophagus into the stomach. This is necessary in order to prevent your digested food from backing up into the esophagus.

The stomach is an accordion-like bag of muscle and other tissue near the centre of the abdomen just below the rib cage. The bag expands to accommodate food and shrinks when it is empty. The stomach itself is a holding tank for your food until it can pass through the gastrointestinal tract.

In the same way that the larger coffee grinds stay in the filter, the larger solid particles of food go from the stomach into the duodenum for further digestion, while the mushy, nicely worked-over food remnants from the stomach will quickly pass from the duodenum into the small intestine (midgut or small bowel). The small intestine is usually called just that, but technically, it can be categorized as the duodenum, jejunum, and ileum. For simplicity, it's usually referred to as "the small intestine."

A series of tubes along your GI tract empties food particles from one into the next. This process depends on continuous movement, known as motility, which is controlled by nerves, hormones, and muscles. In fact, if you're experiencing problems with other parts of your body, the motility can be slowed down (you'll be constipated and bloated) or speeded up (you'll have diarrhea).

By the time your food gets into the small intestine, it is mushed up by the digestive secretions of your stomach, pancreas, and biliary tract. This mush stays in the small intestine for a relatively long period of time, and all the usable nutrients are absorbed through the intestinal walls. These nutrients include digested molecules of food, water, and minerals from the diet. The waste products are sent to the large intestine (colon or large bowel), where they stay for about a day or two before being expelled in the form of stools.

Diabetic nerve disease affects the GI tract north of the colon—that is, everything from the esophagus to the small intestine. A number of things can go wrong north of the colon because hundreds of nerves and secretions (hormones, enzymes, and chemicals that help break down your food into usable nutrients) go to work for you whenever you eat. If even one hormone or enzyme is off in your system, there will be consequences. There are upper GI disorders and lower GI disorders. The upper GI disorders, which can be caused by diabetic nerve disease, can include heartburn/reflux, a symptom of a larger problem of dysmotility (see below), also known as gastroesophageal reflux disease (GERD).

Diabetic nerve disease can also cause problems south of the colon, where muscles controlling the bowel become uncoordinated, causing them to open, leak stool, and allow bacteria to grow abnormally in the colon, resulting in bacterial-related diarrhea. This can be controlled with antibiotics.

Understanding Dysmotility

Dysmotility means "things not moving very well." Food travels from your esophagus into your stomach, which slowly releases it into the small intestine. There can be problems on any or all "floors" of this elevator. Things can get stuck between the esophagus and stomach, causing symptoms of heartburn and reflux (see further on). In this case, the lower esophageal sphincter relaxes when it should be taut, allowing food to come back up. Or things can get stuck between the stomach and small intestine, which causes symptoms of bloating, early fullness, and gas, so when things aren't moving very well, you can have a lot of discomfort. This is known as a motility disorder.

Dysmotility, with all of its varying symptoms, is typically a very chronic condition. Symptoms keep coming back, and by the time dysmotility is finally diagnosed, most people have had these symptoms for a long time. The only way you can stop symptoms from recurring is by changing certain lifestyle habits (losing weight, quitting smoking, and staying in control of blood sugar levels may improve your condition) or taking a motility drug as a maintenance drug. If your dysmotility goes on for a long time, it could also lead to inflammation of the esophageal lining, a condition known as esophagitis. This can lead to the narrowing of the esophagus. (When your esophagus is inflamed, it narrows, just the way your shoes are suddenly too tight when your feet expand.)

Understanding Heartburn/Reflux

As described above, your food must pass from your esophagus into your stomach through the lower esophageal sphincter, which opens and closes through a variety of involuntary muscular contractions. If you have diabetic nerve disease, the sphincter may not shut completely after dumping your ingested food particles into the stomach. So what happens? The food, now bathed in your stomach acid, can actually come back up the sphincter, causing a burning sensation in your chest and sometimes a spreading pain throughout your neck and arms, which may be mistaken for a heart attack. You can also experience nausea, belching, and regurgitation of that half-digested food. When it comes back up the sphincter, it doesn't taste as good as it did going down. Thanks to the acid and enzymes it's been exposed to, the food will taste sour and bitter in your throat. The problem will be aggravated when you bend forward or lie down. In fact, you may find that after an experience like this, you wake up with a sore throat. This problem is clinically called acid reflux, and in lay terms, it is known as heartburn or acid indigestion. For the remainder of this book, the term "heartburn/reflux" will be used.

Heartburn/reflux usually lasts about two hours. Most people find that standing up relieves the burning; that's because gravity helps. You could also take an antacid to clear acid out of the esophagus. Not everyone will experience the same degree of heartburn. Heartburn/reflux can be mild, moderate, or severe. It all depends on why it's occurring, how often it occurs, when it occurs, and how much food backup you have. But for the most part, chronic heartburn/reflux is the first sign of a more serious, underlying health problem such as dysmotility or GERD.

A number of atypical, unusual, or odd symptoms can suggest you have heartburn/reflux, too. They include:

- morning hoarseness
- drooling
- coughing spells
- waking up with a sore throat
- asthma-like symptoms (or the worsening of asthma symptoms if you are asthmatic). In these cases, you may be having heartburn/reflux at night, which is obstructing your breathing passages, causing all the strange symptoms from coughing to asthma.

Managing Diabetes-Related Dysmotility, or Diabetic Gastroparesis

Gastroparesis can occur in people with both Type 1 and Type 2 diabetes, and is a disorder in which the stomach takes too long to empty its contents.

Normally, the stomach contracts to move food down into the small intestine for digestion. The vagus nerve controls the movement of food from the stomach through the digestive tract. Gastroparesis occurs when the vagus nerve is damaged and the muscles of the stomach and intestines do not work normally. Food then moves slowly or stops moving through the digestive tract. Symptoms of diabetic gastroparesis comprise:

- heartburn
- pain in the upper abdomen
- nausea
- vomiting of undigested food, sometimes several hours after a meal
- early feeling of fullness after only a few bites of food
- weight loss due to poor absorption of nutrients or low calorie intake
- abdominal bloating
- high and low blood glucose levels
- lack of appetite
- gastroesophageal reflux
- spasms in the stomach area

Changes in your diet can help with gastroparesis. For example, by eating smaller, more frequent meals, your stomach will not become excessively full. Different drugs or combinations of drugs may be used to treat gastroparesis. These include metoclopramide, which stimulates stomach muscle contractions to help emptying and reduces nausea and vomiting; and erythromycin, an antibiotic that reportedly improves stomach emptying, but is not widely recommended by gastroenterologists.

Skin

High blood sugar levels, combined with poor circulation, put the skin on your whole body at risk for infections ranging from yeast to open wound-related infections. You may form scar tissue or develop strange yellow pimples (a sign of high fat levels in the blood), boils, or a range of localized infections. Yeast infections, which typically plague women who experience them in the form of vaginal yeast infections (see

"Genitals"), can develop not just in the vagina, but in the mouth (called thrush), under the arms, or wherever there are warm, fatty folds. And all skin, whether on the feet or elsewhere, can become dry and cracked, requiring a daily regimen of cleaning, moisturizing, and protecting.

Kidneys

Diabetic kidney disease is very serious and requires a separate chapter. For details, please see Chapter 19.

Gallbladder

The gallbladder stores bile for the liver, but you don't really need the gallbladder since the liver is large enough to store as much bile as you'd ever want or need anyway. Nevertheless, you do come equipped with this extra storage space. Bile isn't a very reliable product to store because it can form into little stones inside the gallbladder, known as gallstones (or calculi). When your gallbladder isn't emptying properly, a process controlled by nerves and one that can be impaired with diabetic nerve disease, gallstones may form. Symptoms occur when the stones become large enough to obstruct the bile ducts. And when this happens, you are said to have gallbladder disease.

The symptoms of a gallbladder attack are quite severe; you'll feel sudden, intense pain in the upper abdominal region (which may shoot into your back), often after a fatty meal, but it may not be related to meals. Vomiting frequently brings relief, although nausea is not a symptom. The pain may then subside over several minutes or hours. Many people mistake gallstone symptoms for heartburn or a heart attack.

The obstruction can become infected or even gangrenous, which is a dire emergency—you don't want gangrene in your abdominal cavity! Usually gallbladder disease presents itself as a series of gallbladder attacks in which you'll feel the pain after a meal and, if there's infection, you may experience a fever. The attacks will become progressively worse until you decide to have the darned thing removed! As a rule, any abdominal pain accompanied by a fever means there is some sort of serious infection going on in there, which is an emergency, warranting emergency medical attention.

Because of other factors, such as taking estrogen (many women take some form of estrogen product), gallbladder problems are much more common in women than men (one in five women after age 50 versus one in 20 men), and are also common in women who are on hormone-replacement therapy after menopause. Estrogen-containing oral contraceptives are also associated with gallstones.

Since the late 1980s, gastroenterologists have been able to widen the ducts with endoscopy to allow the gallstones to pass, avoiding major surgery in people who are not up to it or who do not want it. Removal of the gallbladder is called a cholecystectomy, one of the most common surgical procedures performed.

Several new approaches to gallstone treatment have been tried over the past several years, but surgical removal of the gallbladder (cholecystectomy) remains the most widely used therapy. This is partly because the newer non-surgical treatments are useful in only some gallstone patients, but surgery can be used in virtually all patients. Patients generally do well after surgery and have no difficulty with digesting food, even though the gallbladder's function is to aid digestion. Surgical options include the standard procedure, called open cholecystectomy, and a newer, less invasive procedure called laparascopic cholecystectomy ("belly-button surgery").

There are some alternatives to surgery for both stones in the gallbladder and stones in the bile duct. For example, gallbladder stones can be dissolved by a chemical (ursodiol or chenodiol), which is available in pill form. This medicine thins the bile and allows stones to dissolve. Unfortunately, only small stones composed of cholesterol dissolve rapidly and completely, and its use is therefore limited to patients with the right size and type of stones. Patients with cholesterol stones have also been treated with methyl tertbutyl ether, a chemical that can be injected into the gallbladder until the stones dissolve. This chemical is harsh and some complications have been reported. A problem with all non-surgical approaches is that gallstones return several years later in about half the patients successfully treated. Discuss all your options with your doctor, including the surgeon.

Bladder

Nerves that control the bladder can be affected, which causes you to lose your sense of bladder urge and your ability to force a bladder contraction (that is, to urinate). Ultimately this can lead to incontinence as urine will start to leak out. Women, in particular, can also suffer from repeated urinary tract infections caused by insufficient emptying of the bladder, resulting in bacteria overgrowth. Learning to go to the bathroom on a schedule (every four hours or so), instead of waiting for the urge, is one solution. Drugs can also increase the force of bladder contraction if your problem involves the inability to force bladder contraction.

Genitals

Approximately 50 percent of men with diabetes and as many as 35 percent of women with diabetes suffer from sexual dysfunction.

Men

Microvascular complications can lead to impotence or erectile dysfunction (ED) because the small blood vessels responsible for causing an erection can be damaged, or the nerves controlling sexual response could be damaged. As well, macrovascular disease can affect the flow of blood to the penis.

When nerves to the penis are damaged, blood flow is limited, preventing erection. Studies indicate that 40 percent of diabetic men older than 60 years of age have complete ED. Among the diabetic population, risk factors include increasing age, duration of diabetes, poor glycemic control, cigarette smoking, hypertension, dyslipidemia, androgren deficiency states, and cardiovascular disease. ED is defined as the persistent inability to get or maintain an erection that is satisfactory for sexual activity. Most men will experience erectile problems during their life, but if the problem lasts for three months or longer, it is clinically defined as ED. Premature ejaculation is also not considered to be ED, although it can happen when you have ED. Ejaculatory disorders are another common disorder of sexual function in men with diabetes, occurring in up to 32 percent. When a physical problem is at work, signs come on gradually. Over time, you'll notice that your penis becomes less rigid, until you are unable to obtain or sustain an erection completely.

Just because you have diabetes doesn't mean your impotence is caused by it. Therefore, to diagnose physical impotence, doctors will tell you to place a paper band around your penis before you go to sleep. Since all healthy men have erections during their sleep, if you wake up with a broken band, it means your impotence is not physical but psychological. If the band is intact upon waking, your problem is physical (although not necessarily related to diabetes—it could be hormonal).

Once it's established that you have a physical disorder, your doctor can rule out nerve damage rather than blood vessel damage by checking out both. To check nerve damage, a test involving painless electrical current can measure your penis's response.

To check blood vessel damage, a device similar to testing blood pressure in your arm can be used on your penis, or a drug that bypasses your nerves can be injected into your penis to see if you can have an erection. If you can't, blood vessel damage is indeed the problem, and it's most likely a macrovascular one. Ultrasound and a tracer dye can confirm impotence caused by macrovascular disease. This procedure allows the doctor to see whether the blood is flowing freely through the vessels into the penis.

Another physical cause of impotence is blood pressure-lowering medication, while smoking and alcohol are considered aggravating factors.

One of the most popular treatments for ED is the PDE5 inhibitors, available in Canada under the trade names Viagra, Levitra, or Cialis. These are the current mainstays of therapy, and should be offered as first-line therapy to men with diabetes with ED unless some other health problem prevents them from being used, such as heart disease. PDE5 inhibitors have been reported to have a major impact on erectile function and quality of life. These are pills that you take about an hour prior to potential sexual contact. You will get an erection only if you are aroused. Viagra should begin to take effect in about 30 minutes and lasts up to four hours. Viagra works by increasing blood flow to the penis, allowing an erection to occur naturally.

If you are unable to take a PDE5 inhibitor, or find that they do not work, there are other drugs, injections, hormone replacements, mechanical devices, implants, and surgery. All these options could be discussed with your doctor.

- *Drug injections:* Various drugs can be injected into the penis prior to intercourse; they will increase blood flow and produce an erection for at least 30 minutes. Prolonged erection, known as priapism, is a serious side effect, however. If you experience this side effect for longer than four hours, you should seek medical attention immediately.
- *Vacuum devices:* A vacuum device is used to enlarge the penis, then a tension band is placed around the penis to maintain the erection for intercourse. Bruising can occur if the rubber band is on longer than 20 minutes. Roughly 75 percent of men can achieve a functional erection using a vacuum erection device once they've been instructed properly.
- *Penile implants:* Either an inflatable or semi-rigid rod is placed inside the penis to enable you to have an erection whenever you want. There is a select group of men for whom reconstructive prosthetic surgery (placement of a penile prosthesis or implant) will restore erection, with patient satisfaction rates approaching 90 percent.
- *Blood vessel surgery:* Blood vessels that are blocking blood flow to the penis can be corrected through surgery.

Women

Nerve damage can also affect arousal for women. Special nerve fibres and blood vessels connect to the clitoris, vaginal wall, and vulva, which are necessary for achieving orgasm and lubrication. If you have sustained nerve damage, you may notice a loss of sensation in your genital area, which can be a frustrating experience. Estrogen therapy and lubricants may help, as well as trying different positions to increase arousal.

Vaginal dryness has a domino effect: The dryness itself can increase your vulnerability to yeast infections. Dry vaginas can be torn during intercourse, and the resultant wounds can become vulnerable to yeast infection. High blood sugar levels also increase the amount of sugar in the vaginal walls, which can also cause yeast infections.

Sexual dysfunction in women is also related to nerve damage to the bladder (see above). When the bladder is not emptied sufficiently, it leads to bacterial bladder infections, which makes sex uncomfortable. Since Type 2 diabetes often coincides with menopause, many women will notice a compromised libido anyway due to natural estrogen loss, which can be aggravated by nerve damage, or vice versa. Antibiotics prescribed to women for the purposes of clearing up the bladder infection can predispose them to yeast infections, too, a classic side effect that all women can experience when they take antibiotics for any reason. Yeast infections are caused by *Candida albicans*, a one-cell fungus that belongs to the plant kingdom. Under normal circumstances, *Candida* is always in your vagina, mouth, and digestive tract. It is friendly fungus. For a variety of reasons, *Candida* will overgrow and reproduce too much of itself, changing from a harmless one-cell fungus into long branches of yeast cells, called mycelia. This is known as candidiasis.

Generally, any changes to your vagina's normal acidic environment can make you vulnerable to candidiasis. The list of factors that affect your vaginal environment is quite long. High blood sugar levels increase the amount of sugar stored in the vaginal cell walls, and yeast loves sugar. In fact, women who suffer from chronic yeast infections are encouraged to be screened for diabetes since the infections are so common in women with diabetes.

Anything that interferes with the immune system will make yeast thrive, too. Antibiotics, for example, not only kill the harmful bacteria, but often the friendly bacteria that are always in the vagina and are necessary to fend off infection.

Severe itching and a curd-like or cottage-cheesy discharge are classic symptoms of candidiasis. The discharge, interestingly, may also smell like baking bread, fermenting yeast, or even brewing beer, so if the discharge is foul-smelling or fishy, you can rule out yeast. The discharge may also be thinner and mucus-like, but it is always white. Other symptoms are swelling, redness, and irritation of the outer and inner vaginal lips, painful sex, and painful urination due to an irritation of the urethra.

When yeast is in the throat, it is called thrush and usually occurs in immune-deficient women (they may be HIV-positive or undergoing cancer treatments). Thrush is unsettling because the mouth and throat are coated with a milky-white goop. It can also be present in newborns, when yeast-infected mothers give birth. Thrush is treated orally with nystatin drops. Finally, since yeast is present in the intestines, HIV-positive women can develop severe, life-threatening esophageal yeast infections.

Vaginal yeast infections are so common that over-the-counter anti-fungal agents in creams, suppositories, or pill form are available at all drugstores. A doctor will confirm yeast by taking a culture swab.

Plain yogourt, also an anti-fungal, is the best way to fend off yeast. Simply eat a small container of any kind of yogourt daily; so long as it has active bacterial culture, any brand is fine. Choose unsweetened yogourt. Alternatively, you can take *Lactobacillus acidophilus*, which is generally available in capsule form at any drugstore. If you find that you have thrush, citrus seed extract (Citricidal) and tea-tree oil can be used as a gargle.

Following an anti-yeast diet may also be helpful. Certain foods interfere with the vagina's acidity, which prevents yeast. The diet entails avoiding the following: sugar, honey, maple syrup, molasses, and any foods that contain them; alcoholic beverages; vinegars and foods containing vinegar such as pickled foods, salad dressings, mustard, ketchup, and mayonnaise; mouldy nuts, such as peanuts, pistachios, and cashews; soy sauce, miso, and other fermented products; dairy food with the exception of butter, buttermilk, and yogourt; coffee, black tea, and sweetened pop; dried fruits; processed foods.

Try to incorporate more of the following foods to compensate: whole grains such as rice, millet, barley, and buckwheat; breads, crackers, muffins that are yeast-free and preferably wheat-free; raw or cooked fresh vegetables; fish, chicken, and lean meats (organically fed and hormone- and antibiotic-free); nuts and seeds that are not mouldy; fruit in moderation (limiting sweeter fruits).

There are some other ways to avoid yeast infections:

1. *Don't wear tight clothing around your vagina:* Tight pants, panties, and nylon pantyhose prevent your vagina from breathing and make it warmer and moister for yeast. Wear looser pants that allow your vagina to breathe, switch to knee-highs or old-fashioned stockings, or wear pantyhose only for special occasions. And go "bottomless" to bed to let air into your vagina.

2. *Wear only 100 percent cotton clothing and/or natural fibres around your vagina:* Synthetic underwear and polyester pants are not good ideas. All cotton underwear, denim, wool, or rayon pants that are loose-fitting are fine.

3. *Avoid vaginal deodorants or sprays:* These products are unnecessary and disturb the vagina's natural environment, which is fully designed to self-clean.

4. *Don't douche unless it's for purely medicinal purposes:* Douching can push harmful bacteria up higher into the vagina, disturb the vagina's natural ecosystem, or interfere with a pregnancy. Always a bad idea!

5. *Watch your toilet habits:* Always wipe from front to back with toilet paper. When you do it the other way around, you can introduce fecal material and germs into your vagina. After a looser bowel movement, wet the toilet paper and clean your rectal area thoroughly so that fecal material doesn't stay on your underwear and wind up in your vagina. If you're in a less hygienic bathroom that doesn't have running water near the toilet, spit on your toilet paper and clean the rectal area. (It's better than nothing.)

6. *Don't insert anything into a dry vagina:* Whether it's a penis or a tampon, make sure your vagina is well lubricated before insertion.

7. Avoid wearing tampons.

8. *Avoid long car trips on vinyl seats:* Research indicates that vinyl seats increase a woman's risk of developing a yeast infection because the vinyl traps moisture and doesn't allow the crotch area to breathe.

The next chapter focuses on one of the most notorious microvascular (small blood vessel) complications: diabetes eye disease.

17

DIABETES EYE DISEASE

Microvascular complications (see Chapter 16) damage the small blood vessels in the eyes. High blood pressure, associated with macrovascular complications (see Chapter 2), also damages the blood vessels in the eyes. While 98 percent of people with Type 1 diabetes will experience eye disease within 15 years of being diagnosed, in Type 2 diabetes eye disease is often diagnosed *before* the diabetes; in other words, many people don't realize they have diabetes until their eye doctors ask them if they have been screened for diabetes. In fact, 20 percent of people with Type 2 diabetes already have diabetes eye disease before their diabetes is diagnosed. Because people are living longer with diabetes, it is now considered the most common cause of blindness under age 65, and the most common cause of new blindness in North America. According to 2007 statistics, diabetes eye diseases cause 600 new cases of blindness each year, and affect almost all people who have lived with diabetes for more than 30 years. As of this writing, it is estimated that approximately 2 million individuals in Canada (i.e., almost all people with diagnosed diabetes) have some form of diabetes eye disease. According to the Canadian Opthalmological Society, about one in four people with diabetes have some non-proliferative retinopathy, also called background diabetic eye disease. In this case, the blood vessels in the retina (the part of your eyeball that faces your brain, as opposed to your face) start to deteriorate, bleed, or hemorrhage (known as microaneurysms) and leak water and protein into the centre of the retina, called the macula; this condition is known as macular edema and causes vision loss, which sometimes is only temporary. However, without treatment, more permanent vision loss will occur. Although non-proliferative eye disease rarely leads to total blindness, as many as 20 percent of those with non-proliferative eye disease can become legally blind within five years.

Proliferative eye disease means "new blood vessel growth" eye disease. In this case, your retina says, "Since all my blood vessels are being damaged, I'm just going to grow *new* blood vessels!" This process is known as neovascularization. The problem is that these new blood vessels are deformed, or abnormal, which makes the problem worse, not better. These deformed blood vessels look a bit like Swiss cheese; they're full of holes and have a bad habit of suddenly bleeding, causing severe damage without warning. They can also lead to scar tissue in the retina, retinal detachments, and glaucoma, greatly increasing the risk of legal blindness.

Diabetes can also cause cataracts, a clouding of the lens inside the eye that blurs vision.

This chapter will cover signs of eye disease and failing vision, laser treatment to slow vision loss, visual aids, and coping with low vision or blindness. But first, the best step is *prevention*.

PREVENTING DIABETES EYE DISEASE

The adage "Early detection is your best protection" is true when it comes to diabetes eye disease! *It's crucial to have frequent eye exams.* The average person has an eye exam every five years. And if you're walking around with undiagnosed Type 2 diabetes, you can also be walking around with early signs of diabetes eye disease, so as soon as you're diagnosed with Type 2 diabetes, get to an eye specialist for a complete exam and make it a yearly "gig" from now on.

During an eye exam, an ophthalmologist will dilate your pupil with eye drops, then use a special instrument to check for the following:

- tiny red dots (signs of bleeding)
- a thick or milky retina, with or without yellow clumps or spots (signs of macular edema)

- a "bathtub ring" on the retina—a ring shape that surrounds a leakage site on the retina (also a sign of macular edema)
- "cottonwool spots" on the retina—small fluffy white patches in the retina (signs of new blood vessel growth, or more advanced eye disease)

Stop Smoking

Since smoking also damages blood vessels, and diabetes eye disease is a blood vessel disease, smoking will certainly aggravate the problem. Quitting smoking may help to reduce eye complications. See Chapter 2 for more details on smoking cessation.

Avoid Eye Infections

High blood sugar can predispose you to frequent bacterial infections, including conjunctivitis (pink eye). Eye infections can also affect your vision. To prevent eye infections, make sure you wash your hands before you touch your eyes, especially before you handle contact lenses.

Stay in Control

The latest studies indicate that diabetic retinopathy can be slowed by intensive glycemic and blood pressure control. Many experts and associations, including the Canadian Diabetes Association, recommend that patients with diabetes have a yearly, thorough, dilated eye exam.

SIGNS OF EYE DISEASE

It is important to remember that the longer you have diabetes, the higher your risk of having diabetic retinopathy. Most people who have had diabetes for more than 20 years have some form of retinopathy. In the early stages of diabetes eye disease, there are no symptoms. That's why you need to have a thorough eye exam every six months. As the eye damage progresses, you may notice blurred vision. The blurred vision is due to changes in the shape of the lens of the eye. During an eye exam, your ophthalmologist may notice yellow spots on your retina, signs that scar tissue has formed on the retina from bleeding. If the disease progresses to the point where new blood vessels have formed, vision problems may be quite severe as a result of spontaneous bleeding or detachment of the retina.

Vision can fail in two areas: central vision and peripheral vision. Central vision is identifying an object in focus. Peripheral vision is seeing out of the corner of your eye. When you lose your central vision, you lose the ability to focus on fine detail: print, television images, details of faces. When you lose your peripheral vision, you develop "tunnel vision" (a common sign of glaucoma, for example). This restricts you from seeing obstructions, causing you to bump into corners of chairs and doors and trip on many objects. Diabetes eye disease affects both central and peripheral vision.

Vision loss is often very gradual. It may not be something you notice suddenly. Signs of failing vision are important clues that you may have diabetes eye disease that is progressing. The following are classic signs of failing or deteriorating vision:

- You sit closer and closer to the television.
- You're squinting in order to see.
- You need a stronger prescription for your glasses or contacts.
- You have difficulty reading the newspaper.
- You're bothered by bright lights.
- You're more accident-prone, bumping into chairs or doors, tripping over curbs and steps, and knocking things over all the time.
- You can't see well in the dark or at night; night driving is difficult.

If you have signs of failing vision, any of the following eye specialists can help:
- *An ophthalmologist:* This is a medical doctor who specializes in eye conditions. You can be referred to an ophthalmologist by your family doctor or an optometrist. Ophthalmologists perform eye surgery, prescribe glasses or contacts, and recommend visual aids.
- *An optometrist:* This is not a doctor, but a professional who is trained to correct vision problems with refractions, visual exercises, and visual aids. Optometrists can diagnose and recognize eye disease and can refer you to an ophthalmologist.

- *An optician:* This is the specialist who makes lenses for glasses and who is frequently on hand at optical stores to answer questions. He or she may be your first point of contact in finding help, particularly if you think you just need stronger glasses or contacts. Opticians often recognize more serious problems with the eyes and can recommend (but not formally refer you to) an ophthalmologist.
- *Low-vision specialist:* This is a graduate of a post-secondary institution with a major in health science or vision rehabilitation, and a professional background in nursing, orthoptics, and/or ophthalmology. Low-vision specialists can provide education about your medical diagnosis, offer training in the use of optical and non-optical visual aids, and show you how to most efficiently use the residual vision you may have left. They are also able to undertake visual acuity and field-loss testing, and to refer clients to appropriate resources and organizations.

Much of the time, these specialists help you see better with what you've got. They can help you get around and complete daily tasks with visual aids (see the section in this chapter), enlarging images, assisting with lighting, and improving colour contrasts.

CAN YOU TREAT DIABETES EYE DISEASE?

The best answer is not completely, but you can greatly improve vision. Laser therapy, surgical intervention (also known as vitrectomy), and pharmacological intervention are the current treatments for diabetes eye disease. Laser therapy reduces severe visual loss and reduces legal blindness by 90 percent in people with severe non-proliferative or proliferative retinopathy.

If you have a lot of blood in the centre of your eye (vitreous gel), you may need a surgical procedure known as a vitrectomy, which is associated with a higher chance of vision recovery in people with either Type 1 or Type 2 diabetes with very severe proliferative diabetic retinopathy.

There is some current research being undertaken in treating diabetic retinopathy with various medications. There are three major classes of medications currently being studied: corticosteroids (which have well-known anti-inflammatory effects), vascular endothelial growth factor (VEGF) antagonists, and miscellaneous agents such as hyaluronidase, which, in a recent phase 3 prospective clinical trial, showed some promise. This particular agent is not yet approved by the FDA for this indication.

Tight glycemic and blood pressure control remains the cornerstone in the primary prevention of diabetic retinopathy.

After-effects of Laser Treatment

While you're healing from laser surgery, you may notice blurred vision that lasts anywhere from a few weeks to a few months. You may also notice that it takes longer for your eyes to adapt to very bright or very dark lighting (called night vision). This may or may not improve and is a common side effect of all laser eye surgery, even in people who are having it done to improve astigmatism. Finally, you may notice "floaters," which are evidence that there is bleeding inside the eye.

ALL ABOUT VISUAL AIDS

The CNIB (www.cnib.ca) offers excellent information on its website, with everything from tips on how to outfit and light your home accordingly, to tips on the types of audiovisual equipment to purchase. If your vision is deteriorating, a range of visual aids is available that can make living and working far easier than it was for many of our parents and grandparents who suffered from partial or complete vision loss. This is, in part, due to a range of technologies that can enhance images through magnification, lighting, and colour contrast. There are a number of tactile products as well as the Braille alphabet.

Visual aids are used by people with partial sight, also known as low vision, reduced vision, or impaired vision. Some people still refer to low vision as "legally blind" or partial blindness. These terms are slowly falling out of favour because of myths about what blindness means in most cases (see further on). Of the Canadians who identify themselves as visually impaired, fewer than 20 percent are totally blind—without any usable vision. When you hear that "diabetes causes blindness," it is not untrue, but it usually refers to a scenario in which you are visually impaired with *some usable vision left,* which makes you a candidate for visual aids, also called low-vision aids.

Making Things Larger

One of the most common visual aids involves products that can magnify an image. These aids are known as magnification devices. These devices can extend the image over a large enough area of the retina for it to be detected by the healthy cells at the edges, or periphery. Magnification devices typically magnify as much as 22 times the normal size. Even as I write these words now, my computer can magnify my screen so that the words I'm typing appear 500 percent larger than they actually are. Magnification aids commonly used can be telescopes, which make distant objects appear closer; binoculars, which many people can use for watching television, movies, or plays; monoculars, which can help you read distant objects such as street names, house numbers, or bus numbers; or pocket magnifiers, illuminated magnifiers, or stand-mounted magnifiers, which are frequently used for a wide assortment of tasks, from working on crafts to other leisure activities.

Some people need different visual aids for different tasks. Typically one aid will be used for fine-detail tasks, such as reading; another one for watching television; and another one for outdoor use.

You can also buy many items with large print, including books, telephones, and clocks.

High-Tech Magnification Devices

Magnification devices can be low tech (as in magnifying reading glasses) or high tech (as in software or hardware). People with diabetes have a wide variety of income levels. If you can afford it, here is a sample of some of the higher-tech magnification products you can find. Typically, high-technology products work with existing hardware you may already own, such as desktop or laptop computers, palm devices, and so on. They may be sold as software that works with your equipment, or sold as an interface, a smaller piece of hardware you connect to something like a computer, which can transform data, manipulate data, and so on.

Many computer companies offer a range of adaptive products. For example, Xerox makes a product called the Reading Edge, which is a transportable reading machine that offers magnification, scanning, speech synthesizer (if you can't read it, you can hear the data), optical character recognition (which allows you to dictate letters that come out in print), and so on. Interestingly, as the company notes on their website, in 1996, the American Foundation for the Blind recognized Xerox with its Helen Keller Award in Assistive Technology for the company's Reading Edge machine and for pioneering products that help the blind lead independent lives. Another product, called the Reading AdvantEdge, is a software program that can make your home computer do all these things (except perhaps to scan).

Large-print computer-access products allow you to select a preferred font for the computer's display of characters; change the foreground or background colours of the screen; and display large print as full-screen mode. Almost any word-processing software has some capacity to magnify, but these products, such as MAGic, can magnify the screen image from two through 20 times the normal size. A range of other options to optimize the visual image are offered with these various large-print packages.

Closed-circuit television (CCTV) can also help with magnification. This system is similar to a video camcorder device. Anything you place in front of the camera will be broadcast on your TV screen so you can see it more closely. Books, recipes, prescriptions, photographs, and so on can all be enhanced with CCTV systems. One product called Magni-Cam, for example, is a hand-held electronic magnifier that connects to any television set. The camera weighs only 198 g (7 oz) and doesn't require any focusing.

There are hundreds of high-tech visual aids available. The best way to find them is through the Internet, by purchasing a book such as the one mentioned on page 281 with all of the latest products, by going to your favourite software/hardware manufacturer's website and searching for "adaptive products," "products for the visually impaired," or "visual aids." You can also find a wealth of information on high-tech products by visiting the website of the Canadian Institute for the Blind (CNIB) (www cnib.ca).

Another website that offers excellent advice on products is the American Foundation for the Blind (www.afb.org). They offer information pages on everything from tips for computer use for people with low vision, to magnification programs for the computer screen. Also advertised on their site is the 2008 publication, now available for purchase, *AccessWorld Guide to Assistive Technology Products*. This updated 2008 edition includes detailed profiles of over 280 products for people who are blind or visually impaired, including more than 30 new products, such as special cellphones, PDAs, and GPS systems to screen readers, Braille printers, and CCTVs.

Making Things Brighter

Products that improve lighting are also visual aids. Direct light sources can dramatically improve the ability of people with low vision to complete tasks by reducing glare, improving background light, and so forth. The CNIB offers the following suggestions on how to improve lighting at home and outside the home:

- The sales staff at a lighting store or home supply store can help you determine which type of lighting (halogen, fluorescent, etc.) is best for you. Bring a newspaper or book along to help you make your choice.
- Sensor lights are a relatively inexpensive way to make sure the home's exterior entrance is always safely lit.
- Install lighting inside closets, cupboards, in staircases, or even in the shower (be sure to use a waterproof light!).
- Use task lighting for writing, sewing, or reading. Small clip-on lights are suitable, as are bendable gooseneck lamps.
- Consider buying a tiny flashlight or penlight to carry with you, which is handy for reading restaurant menus or unlocking your door at night.
- Reduce glare whenever possible. Curtains or blinds on your windows will help keep glare out of rooms and off TV and computer screens.
- Consider wearing a hat with a visor for visits to stores with overly bright lighting.

- An eye-care professional can help select a pair of tinted anti-glare sunglasses for outdoors that will eliminate glare from the sides and top, which is far better than the protection regular sunglasses provide.

Making Things Stand Out

You can make objects stand out by using colour coding, another type of visual aid. As well, you can use texture to provide contrast. The general rule is to contrast the background with the foreground; smoother textures tend to make colours appear light, while uneven surfaces tend to make colours appear darker. Here are a few suggestions:

- Countertops can be painted to contrast with dishes, cookware, and other items; hardware stores can help you find the correct paint for the task.
- Outline counter edges and electrical outlets with wide tape of a contrasting colour.
- Use light-coloured dishes on a dark tablecloth, or vice versa.
- Mark frequently used settings on the oven or other dials with a thick swipe of bright nail polish or a bumper dot, available from CNIB's Webstore or Consumer Products and Assistive Technology catalogue.
- Relabel jars and canned goods using a thick black marker and sticky labels.
- Use a liquid measure tool such as the EZ Fill Liquid Pouring Alert, available through CNIB, to help you when pouring liquids. This can help you avoid accidents with hot or cold liquids.
- Remove small throw rugs from the kitchen as they are not easily seen and may be a tripping hazard.
- Keep cupboard doors and drawers closed at all times and make sure that everything is always put away in its proper place.
- Use the clock method to identify where certain foods are located on a plate. For example, "the rice is at three o'clock and the beans at seven o'clock."

In the bathroom:

- Use illuminated and magnifying mirrors.
- Use coloured toothpaste so it shows more on the white bristles of a toothbrush.
- Use towels that contrast in colour with the bathroom decor.
- Use a rubber-backed mat in the tub.
- Float a brightly coloured sponge while running the bathwater. The sponge will indicate how high the water has risen.
- Throw out old medication and use a pill organizer to help you know which medication to take and when more easily.
- Label current medication with a thick black letter on each bottle; keep a large print list in the medicine cabinet explaining what is what (e.g., "Blood pressure pills. Take one each morning.")
- Pick up the bath mat after each use and fold it over the edge of the tub to prevent tripping.
- If treatment for your eye condition involves eye drops, consider getting an eye-drop dispenser to help you self-administer your drops easily and without spillage.

In the home, for example, as the above suggestions demonstrate, using colour contrast can make it easier to find things or identify objects. You can buy markers that are brightly coloured and that dry into a hard plastic (one example is called Hi-marks). They can be used to mark appliances, such as the stove, washer, or dryer. Nail polish or coloured tape can be used on keys or mailboxes. Brightly coloured elastic bands can be used as markers for jars or tins. You can use coloured magnets on metal surfaces, such as coloured alphabet letters. In the kitchen, dark pots against a white stove (or the reverse) can help. Otherwise, you can put coloured tape near the end of the pot handles. When you eat, colour contrast between placemats or table-cloth and dishes makes it easier to distinguish between them than using table coverings with glossy finishes or patterns. Electrical out-lets should also contrast with the surrounding walls; just buy coloured wall plates for your outlets.

A little redecorating using colour can work wonders. Colour-contrasting paint can be used around door frames or to paint cupboards.

For more information on implementing a colour-coding system, contact the CNIB.

Making Things Touchy-Feely

Tactile products are "touchy-feely." Such products are designed with Braille lettering, the raised dots system invented by Louis Braille in the nineteenth century that is still used today. Essentially, Braille is another way to read and write printed information. It is equivalent, in every way, to print. You can read or write words, numbers, music notations, and any other symbols that appear in print. It works by arranging combinations of the six dots of the Braille cell. Braille is read by touch and is therefore a tactile language. Most people use the first finger on one or both hands to read it. Braille can be used for any language, mathematics, scientific equations, and computer notations. The only people who can't use Braille are those who suffer from numbness in their fingers or hands, but most people with diabetes-related numbness will feel it in their legs or feet (see chapters 16 and 20), not their fingers.

Braille uses a system of small raised dots that are read using the fingertips and can be used to represent everything from words to math and music. For people with vision loss, Braille is also the key to literacy, leading to successful employment and independence. It provides the tools to read and write independently, and helps build skills in spelling, grammar, and punctuation. Braille can be found almost anywhere that print is found—look for it on restaurant menus, ATM keypads, business cards, textbooks, and sheet music.

You can get hundreds of Braille-adapted products, including glucose meters, pill organizers, thermometers, and so on. Braille is actually all around us in modern architecture, but the sighted population doesn't always notice. (For example, most elevators are equipped with Braille lettering on the buttons.) There are also Braille computers with Braille keyboards and a refreshable Braille screen. (Braille computers are very expensive, however, with each Braille cell retailing at roughly $55.) For lifestyle choices, there are Braille watches, games in Braille, and even Braille-embossed jewellery and clothing.

In short, the availability of tactile products is not the problem; everything you could possibly need in life either comes in Braille lettering or can probably be specially ordered (check with the CNIB).

Braille as a Second Language

The problem with tactile products has to do with people's reluctance to learn Braille. Most people equate learning Braille with being totally blind, which is truly unfortunate. Braille is just as useful for people who have partial sight, and in many situations knowing it can make life a little easier. It's like knowing a second language to enhance your communications skills. For example, learning Spanish comes in handy in all kinds of situations, from being able to communicate and make friendships with Spanish-speaking people to ordering food in a Mexican restaurant. It's the same thing with Braille: *It comes in handy* and can enhance, rather than detract from, your life.

People who lose their hearing are similarly reluctant to learn sign language (signing), but in numerous situations, signing would make a hearing-impaired person's life easier.

When you know a different language, it allows you access to a new community of people, too, which is very important when you feel isolated or alone. You already know that when you can talk to someone else who has diabetes, you immediately connect with one another because you share a common struggle. It's the same thing with vision loss; meeting someone else who is coping with vision loss helps you feel less alone and allows you to talk to someone who knows what you're going through. Imagine Braille as a bridge to new friends and a new community. It can also keep you employed as it enables you to make notes on documents, read a spreadsheet, take minutes at a meeting, file materials, read labels, and so on.

Braille also lessens your dependency on voice synthesizers (for reading or writing), audiotape recordings, magnifiers, and other print enhancers. These are great visual aids, but are not convenient in all circumstances. At home, you can also use Braille to label CDs, clothing, spices, and cans. You can also play games—cards, Scrabble, backgammon, chess.

For more information on Braille or Braille products, visit the CNIB website (www.cnib.ca).

Making Things Talk

An obvious visual aid is a product that talks. Before the popularity of voice synthesizers, audio-taped books were about the only talking product available. Today, voice synthesizers can be used with almost any information product, including small things such as thermometers. With scanners, you can scan printed material into a voice-synthesized computer that can tell you what something says, including labels or fine print. One danger is an overreliance on voice-synthesized products, however.

COPING WITH LOW VISION OR BLINDNESS

The hardest part of losing some or all of your vision is coping with it. This has a lot to do with misconceptions about what "blindness" means. "Blindness" is defined as total loss of sight. That said, more than 80 percent of people who are considered blind can usually make out the outlines of objects, identify the sources of light, ascertain the direction of light, and distinguish light from dark.

Registered Blind

The degrees of blindness go from low or impaired vision to profound vision loss. All these degrees can be classified as "registered blind," a category that allows you to be eligible for income tax and other government benefits. You are considered registered blind or, as the American Optometric Association refers to, as "legally blind." A person with 20/20 vision can clearly identify a row of 9 mm (.35 in) letters from 6 m (20 ft). A legally blind person with vision 20/200 has to be as close as 6 m (20 ft) to identify objects that people with normal vision can spot from 60 m (200 ft). So a legally blind person needs a distance of .6 m (2 ft) to spot the letters on a standard eye chart that is 6 m (20 ft) away. That means that you can see at 6 m (20 ft) what someone with perfect vision can see at 60 m (200 ft). (Visual acuity refers to the sharpness and clarity of "near vision"—close-up objects.) You can also be registered blind if your visual field (peripheral vision) results in a narrowing of your central vision to 20 degrees or less (you may be able to read, but walking around is hazardous because you can't see what's around you).

So that means that most people who are registered blind see *something*. A lot of people who appear sighted in public and who seem to get around just fine with some visual aids are registered blind.

Rehabilitation Services

You have access to a range of rehabilitation services through the CNIB (you can request a CNIB rehabilitation teacher) and other organizations, which can help you improve your mobility with daily living—cooking, banking, grooming, and getting around town.

Trained individuals (volunteers or professionals) are on hand through these organizations to take you out and get you used to walking around and travelling by yourself, with perhaps the aid of a cane. These individuals can help you find the right visual aids (see previous section) to enhance your usable vision; they can also help you find mobility aids, guide dogs, and canes. All types of white canes require special training from an orientation and mobility instructor, who demonstrates proper techniques, way-finding, and safety. In order to find an instructor in your area, you can contact the CNIB directly.

The white cane is often perceived as an announcement to the world that you are visually impaired, *but that's not necessarily a bad thing*. One of the cane's chief purposes is to get people to be considerate and *move out of your way* when you are trying to get around. It also gives permission for people to approach you to offer their assistance. There are three types of white canes available. Generally they are used to check for objects in a person's path, changes in the walking surface (from cement to grass, for example) and to check for dangers like steps and curbs. A secondary function is identification: recognized around the world, the white cane clearly tells other pedestrians and drivers that the user is a person with vision loss.

The three types of canes are:

1. *Identification cane:* Is lightweight, can be folded or collapsed to fit in a bag when not in use, and is handy for depth perception and for finding curbs or steps.

2. *Support cane:* Is designed to safely support the person's weight. Perfect for a user who is elderly or who may have a physical disability, it can be either rigid or collapsible, depending on the person's preference.
3. *Long canes:* Are used as probes, and are usually the choice when a person is travelling in an unfamiliar area to provide an extra measure of security and safety.

A Word about Denial

Coping with vision loss often involves overcoming denial that you are losing your sight. This is a normal reaction, but it can also foster behaviours that are not helpful in the long run. It can lead to a lesser quality of life because those in denial often refuse help with visual aids or from the CNIB. Some people may also become overly dependent on others, which can foster a range of unhealthy relationships with friends or family members. You may rely on family members to cook, clean, shop for you, and so on. Vision loss does *not* have to mean loss of mobility, and with the right visual aids and training, you can do lots of things on your own and regain your independence.

Distinguishing Your Medications

People with perfect vision can make all kinds of mistakes when it comes to medications; they can confuse pills, misread labels, and so forth. Keeping track of your medications is especially challenging if you're visually impaired. The following tips from the CNIB may help. You're also encouraged to contact the CNIB and arrange for a CNIB rehabilitation teacher to work with you on designing a system for keeping track of all your medications. In the meantime, try some or all of the following:

- Get a pill organizer with different sections. (These come with Braille lettering, too.)
- Arrange your medications alphabetically on the shelf.
- Get some large-print labels, coloured labels, or Braille labels to identify them.

- Put personal markings on the lids, and keep your personal marked lid for refills.
- Try to use different sizes or shapes of bottles for your medications.
- Use elastic bands to indicate the number of doses per bottle you need to take. (A bottle with two bands around it means you take it twice a day, and so on.) Remove a band as you take your dose and replace it the next day.

Staying Physically Active

As you know from Chapter 8, staying physically active is an important way to manage your diabetes and help stabilize blood sugar. Visual impairment does not mean you need to be inactive. Swimming, golfing, skiing, curling, tandem bicycling, and walking are just a few of the many activities you can enjoy with a few adaptations. For example, you can utilize a sighted guide to help you with some of these activities. You can incorporate brightly coloured guide wires in swimming pools; you can find a sighted partner for tandem cycling (it may be a sighted friend who needs to get active, too, and could use a partner). You can find beeping balls for ball sports or tactile markers for bowling. The range of visual aids or adaptations is endless, and you're encouraged to contact the CNIB to discuss how to use adaptations to accommodate your activities.

Coping with Blind Ignorance

The most disabling part of vision loss is the ignorance you encounter from the general public. You may want to pass on the following tips to friends and family members (who, in turn, can tell a few more people), which can make life a little easier for everyone.

- When speaking to someone with vision loss, face them and speak clearly in a moderate tone. Don't shout. Vision loss does not mean the person is hearing impaired, too.
- Anyone can act as a sighted guide. Just offer your arm and say, "My name is X. Here's my arm if you need some assistance." Then

allow the person to take it. Never just grab someone's arm without permission. When acting as a sighted guide, walk at a normal pace. You can hesitate slightly before stepping up or down.

- Don't pat a guiding dog, please. And speak to the person, not the dog!
- If you're giving directions, use phrases such as "on your left" or "right behind you" instead of "over there" or "over here."
- At social gatherings, describe who is in a large group; don't just leave someone alone in the middle of the room with no sense of who's in it. Identify yourself when you approach a visually impaired guest so she or he knows who's talking.
- When dining with a visually impaired person, describe what's on the table to elicit a mental image of the food and help enhance appetite.
- Describe what's on the plate clockwise to make it easier.
- Assist with cutting meat if it's requested.
- Use extra-large napkins if possible.

Hopefully this chapter has helped to alleviate some of your fears about maintaining independence with vision loss. As you can see, vision loss is certainly not the end of the world, but it is a preventable problem. By staying in control of your diabetes and keeping your blood sugar levels as normal as possible as much as possible, you may be able to avoid severe vision loss and the eye problems that so many people with diabetes develop. But did you know that the same strategy can help you avoid losing your teeth? Gum disease and tooth decay are other diabetes complications that are a growing problem mainly because of a lack of awareness about the relationship between diabetes and tooth decay. The next chapter will benefit everyone, diabetic or not. Losing your teeth can be a very uncomfortable experience (as anyone with dentures will tell you) that you ought to avoid if you can.

18

BRUSHING UP ON
TOOTH DECAY

High blood sugar levels get into your saliva and feed the bacteria in your mouth. The bacteria, in turn, break down the starches and sugars to form acids that eventually break down your tooth enamel. This is how cavities are formed.

Moreover, damage to the small blood vessels in your gums can lead to periodontal problems, while blood sugar levels naturally rise when you're fighting a gum infection (known as a periodontal infection), such as an abscess. Preventing dental problems means the usual regimen (see "Combatting Gum Disease"). You're also advised to have your teeth cleaned and examined at least every six months or more frequently depending on your periodontal health, and to avoid sugary foods (which you should be doing anyway). Unfortunately, this is just not enough information for most people with diabetes, especially if they already have gum disease.

GUM DISEASE AND HEART DISEASE

Here is some news you don't want, but must have: Gum disease increases your risk of heart disease. According to the American Academy of Periodontology, there are several theories that explain the link between periodontal (gum) disease and heart disease. One theory is that oral bacteria can affect the heart when they enter the bloodstream, attaching to fatty plaques in the coronary arteries (heart blood vessels) and contributing to clot formation. Blood clots can obstruct normal blood flow, restricting the amount of nutrients and oxygen required for the heart to function properly. This may lead to heart attacks. Studies show that people with periodontal disease are almost twice as likely to suffer from coronary artery disease as those without periodontal disease. There is a similar relationship between periodontal disease and stroke.

Although this link has been known for years, very few people are aware of it. Since people with Type 2 diabetes are already at high risk for heart disease and stroke (see Chapter 15), this means that Type 2 diabetes, combined with gum disease, puts you at extreme risk for heart disease. Treating or preventing gum disease can have a positive effect on your cardiovascular health! For more information about heart disease and stroke, see Chapter 15.

Diabetes-Related Gum Disease

Gum disease, also called periodontitis, is often not noticeable until it's serious. It's caused by bacteria that are normally in the mouth, which can vary in aggressiveness. The bacteria settle around and under the gum line, where the gums and teeth meet; this is called plaque. Brushing and flossing can remove the plaque, preventing it from hardening into tartar (also called calculus). Bacterial infections can develop from tartar. At this stage, it's called gingivitis, but as the bacterial infection worsens, you're looking at full-blown gum disease or periodontitis.

Healthy gums go around the tooth the way a cuff goes around your wrist. When the gums fit more loosely, the bacteria get high up, alongside the tooth, near the bone, where no toothbrush or floss can go (but a periodontist can with special cleaning instruments). The bacteria can cause an inflammatory reaction that erodes the bone supporting the teeth, making them loose. Eventually, you may have to have your teeth pulled and wear dentures.

Roughly 90 percent of all Canadians have gum disease at some point in their lives. Because people with diabetes have more frequent infections and are slower to heal due to inefficient white blood cells, this can also affect the gums. Remember, any kind of infection, such as a urinary tract infection, or even a cold or a flu, will increase blood sugar levels, so when your gums become infected, there may be serious consequences for your overall health. Damage to small vessels (microvascular complication) can also affect the support tissues in the gums.

Two things are going on with diabetes-related gum disease: High blood sugar can make you vulnerable to gum disease, and gum disease can increase your blood sugar levels even more because it is an active infection. (Of course, the same can be said for any infection, but many of us don't think of gum disease as an active infection.) High blood glucose helps bacteria flourish, which can lead to red, sore, and swollen gums that bleed when you brush your teeth. People with diabetes can have tooth and gum problems more often if their blood glucose stays high. High blood glucose can make tooth and gum problems worse. You can even lose your teeth.

Red, sore, and bleeding gums are the first sign of gum disease. These problems can lead to periodontitis, an infection in the gums and the bone that holds the teeth in place. If the infection gets worse, your gums may pull away from your teeth, making your teeth look long.

THE SMOKING GUM

If you've read other chapters in this book, you know what a bad combination smoking and diabetes is. Unfortunately, smoking can predispose you to gum disease, making your already high risk from diabetes higher still. More smokers than non-smokers have gum disease; at least half of all cases of gum disease are directly linked to smoking. Tobacco reduces blood flow to the gums, depriving them of oxygen and nutrients that allow gums to stay healthy, and leaving them vulnerable to bacterial infection.

If you quit smoking, you can reduce the likelihood of developing gum disease; the longer you've not smoked, the greater the chances you will not suffer from gum disease.

Smokers have the highest risk of gum disease, ex-smokers have the next highest, and non-smokers have the lowest risk. But diabetes is another significant risk factor, which means if you smoke and have diabetes, you're at highest risk of developing serious gum disease.

Furthermore, if you do develop diabetes and gum disease concurrently, controlling your blood sugar levels becomes increasingly more difficult, and can lead to serious complications. See Chapter 2 for information on smoking cessation. Quitting smoking will make it easier for you to treat your gum disease, too. Quitting will also reduce your risk of oral cancers and bone and tooth loss, keeping teeth whiter, and allowing sores to heal and disappear.

COMBATTING GUM DISEASE

The strategy is to try to prevent gum disease, if possible, by employing all of those boring dentist rules (see "Doing the Right Thing the Right Way") that have been drilled (no pun intended) into you since you can remember: brushing after eating, flossing, using rubber-tip massages, using fluoride rinses, and, most of all, having frequent dental check-ups. Going for regular cleaning by your dentist or dental hygienist to remove built-up tartar is considered a first-line prevention strategy; however, it is what you do at home that can really make the difference. Ask your dentist or hygienist to show you how to brush and floss properly; it's amazing how many of us were taught the wrong way by our parents or dentists of yesteryear, and these poor habits contribute to dental problems. We also should not be using hard brushes, but soft only.

If you have diabetes, consider going for routine dental cleanings every three months instead of every six months, too. Extra cleaning can really help reduce plaque, which is the building block of gum disease.

Bottled Water and Lack of Fluoride

The bottled water industry has experienced phenomenal growth in the last decade. According to statistics from the Beverage Marketing Corporation and the International Bottled Water Association, per capita consumption of bottled water in the United States grew from 51 L (13.5 gal.) in 1997 to 111 L (29.3 gal.) in 2007. This has also led to an increase in cavities in children. Many medical professionals, including dentists, agree that with the move away from drinking tap water, children, in particular, are missing out on fluoride, an established preventive that is important for tooth decay. It is not the actual bottled water itself that is causing tooth decay, but rather the lack of fluoride.

If your main source of drinking water is bottled, it is important to realize that you could be missing the tooth decay-preventive benefits of fluoride. Generally speaking, however, tap water is safe, and offers good protection for your teeth via the fluoridation.

Doing the Right Thing the Right Way

Whether you want to prevent gum disease or are being treated for gum disease, brushing and flossing are "doing the right thing," but many of us are doing the right thing *the wrong way!* The first thing most people do when their gums start to bleed from brushing or flossing is stop. This is the worst response. Keep at it; the bleeding should stop after a few days as you strengthen the gums. Sometimes people use the wrong brushes. Use soft bristles; hard bristles can damage the gums, and you can brush off gum tissue, which can lead to recession and root exposure.

Next, people buy the wrong floss and then assume that flossing doesn't work for them. If you're finding that your floss is shredding or breaking, get another brand. If your teeth are very close together, finer, unwaxed floss is better. If shredding is a problem, a thicker, waxed floss is better.

I'm all for recycling, but *please* don't recycle your floss. Use a clean piece for each tooth. Take a long piece of floss and inch your way to the end with each tooth. If the plaque you remove is foul-smelling, by the way, that is a sign you have bad breath. You can recheck for the smell when you floss next; if the smell improves, so has your breath, and you can rest assured that it was a plaque problem and not a chronic, unsolvable problem.

Brushing your teeth for five seconds is better than nothing, but the Canadian Dental Association recommends you need to brush every 24 hours at least, for about three minutes. Again, use soft instead of hard brushes. With soft brushes, you can also massage your gums and loosen plaque that is high up. Ask your dentist to show you how to do this and for a sample of a special brush you can use for hard-to-reach places, one that can brush behind your front teeth, for example, an area often missed, or behind your side teeth.

Research from the late 1990s suggested that gum disease may be passed from parents to children and between a couple. Bacteria that cause gum disease can pass through saliva; the common contact of saliva in families puts children and couples at risk for contracting the disease of another family member. Based on this research, most oral health professionals recommend that all family members see a dental professional for screening, but this research is far from conclusive and needs more study.

Tongue Scrapers

There has been some fairly recent research into the efficacy of tongue scrapers to prevent bad breath, or halitosis, which could be a by-product of poor periodontal health. A 2006 study in the journal *General Dentistry* looked at the effects of using a tongue scraper rather than a toothbrush to brush the tongue. The data revealed that the tongue scraper showed a big difference in reducing volatile sulfur compounds, which are produced when bacteria and amino acids interact to produce halitosis. Tongue scrapers also cut down on plaque.

A Gum-Smart Diet

A gum-smart diet can start with the right chewing gum! If you don't have the opportunity to brush after eating, chew some dental gum, a new product that has exploded onto the shelves "in the toothpaste section," as one commercial tells us. A 2008 study concluded that chewing gum containing dental-protective substances, particularly xylitol, can reduce tooth decay. Dozens of chewing gum manufacturers have introduced dental gums. These gums may have tartar-fighting or whitening agents, are sugar-free, and so on. When you chew a sugar-free gum after eating, you activate the saliva, which can wash away bacteria that form plaque.

All that stuff you tell your kids about sugar and cavities still applies! Use the same rules for yourself. Avoid sticky sweets and sugary snacks—something you need to do anyway (see Chapter 7). Ask your dietitian about gum-smart snacks (nuts, seeds, raw fruits, and vegetables).

If you plan to eat something sweet, have it with a meal so your saliva can wash it down. After meals, if you can't brush, rinse your mouth with water and chew some sugar-free or dental gum.

A Word about Whitening

Tooth-whitening products have grown in popularity in the last number of years. There are many home kits available on the market now, whereas in the past a tooth whitening (or bleaching) procedure would likely have taken place in your dentist's office. There are a few different ways to apply the whitening, including a strip, paint-on, or tray kit. Both Health Canada (www.hc-sc.gc.ca) and the American Dental Association (www.ada.org) offer excellent information on these procedures on their websites. According to Health Canada, if you are pregnant, have mouth or gum disease, or have teeth stained by medication, you should not use tooth whiteners. Depending on whether or not you perform it at home or at a dentist's office, there are varying levels of active ingredients involved in tooth whitening, and it's best for diabetic patients to consult a medical professional, especially if you do have any type of oral health issues, such as gum disease.

SIGNS OF GUM DISEASE

Any of the following are signs that you already have gum disease:

- *Bleeding gums:* This is often the first sign of gum disease. You may notice bleeding when you brush your teeth or floss. If your gums are bleeding, it's always a sign of gum disease, but you can also have gum disease and not have bleeding gums.
- *Receding gums:* This occurs when the gum is not covering as much tooth as it should, sometimes exposing the roots.
- *New spaces between teeth:* This is called migration and refers to two teeth that used to touch but that no longer do.
- *Chronic bad breath (halitosis):* Bad breath can be caused by poor digestion, or by insufficient cleaning and a buildup of plaque. And, of course, there are many foods that cause bad breath. But if bad breath persists after proper cleanings and a good oral hygiene

routine (including brushing the tongue), gum disease is probably the reason, where pus and bleeding are contributing to the bad breath problem.

- *Red gums:* Healthy gums should be the colour of salmon or coral, not blood. If you breathe through your mouth, red gums are more common, too.
- Loose teeth.
- *Less tapered gum coverage around the teeth:* The gum should meet the tooth at a knife-edge margin. If this margin is rolled and swollen, it's a sign of gum disease.
- *Shiny gums:* Gums should have some "stippling" to them (little dots) so they don't shine; shiny red gums are not a good thing.

When you notice any of these signs of gum disease, see your dentist. Your dentist will look for a host of things you can't see yourself, such as root cavities, pockets in the gums, or tooth decay under the gum line.

WHAT TO DO IF YOU HAVE GUM DISEASE: SEE A GUM SPECIALIST

If gum disease has progressed beyond the early-stage gingivitis, you'll be referred to a periodontist. This is a dentist who has done a three-year residency in treating gum problems and gum disease. Periodontists can restore gum tissue or regenerate it. At your first visit, the periodontist will use a special probe that can measure gaps between the gums and teeth, as well as look for exposed roots, which need special care, too. Gaps between the gum and teeth are called pockets and normally shouldn't be deeper than 1–3 mm. Pockets deeper than this can be a sign of serious gum disease.

Periodontists may also do special cleanings called root planing, where the gum tissues are usually anaesthetized, and the roots of the teeth (these may be exposed or still covered by gums) are cleaned. The goal is to get rid of as much plaque and tartar as possible to prevent bacterial infections from developing or progressing once they have developed. Root planing may also involve using antibiotics to help kill off the bacteria high inside the gums. Gum surgery involves restoring the gum line to a more readily cleanable state by reducing the pockets and removing the diseased state.

If you have gum disease, it must be treated. Doing so will lower your blood sugar levels and can improve your overall health and ability to control your diabetes. If gum disease has progressed to the point where your teeth are loose, or keep becoming infected (forming root infections or abscesses), dentures or dental implants may be the next step. Compared to losing your eyesight (see Chapter 17) or a kidney (see Chapter 19) or a foot (see Chapter 20), dentures are certainly not the end of the world, but each set of dentures comes with its own set of problems. For more information on dentures and other options, speak to your dentist directly, contact the Canadian Dental Association, or go to their website (www.cda-adc.ca). Although based in the US, another website to visit is for the American Academy of Periodontology (www.perio.org). They have excellent general information on gum disease and treatments that will of value to people in Canada, as well. If you still have your teeth, the information in this chapter can help you keep them.

The road to complications doesn't stop at the mouth. It keeps on going. What you put in your mouth can help prevent kidney failure if you're showing signs of diabetes-related kidney disease, discussed next.

19

KEEPING YOUR KIDNEYS

Diabetic kidney disease, also known as diabetic nephropathy, is what happens when macrovascular complications *and* microvascular complications converge. The high blood pressure caused by macrovascular complications, combined with the small blood vessel damage caused by microvascular complications, together can cause kidney failure, something you *can* die from unless you have dialysis (filtering out the body's waste products through a machine) or a kidney transplant. About 15 percent of people with Type 2 diabetes will develop kidney disease, which often goes by the term "renal disease" or "nephropathy." Once the kidneys are functioning at less than 10–20 percent of their normal rate, either dialysis or transplantation will be needed to keep you alive. This period is called *end-stage renal disease* or ESRD. Your doctor will tell you when you need to start treatment based on your specific medical condition and blood tests. Chronic kidney disease (CKD) is one of the most common and potentially devastating complications of diabetes. Fifty percent of people with diabetes have CKD, and CKD associated with diabetes is the leading cause of kidney failure in Canada. People with CKD are among those at highest risk for dying from cardiovascular disease (see Chapter 15). Certain population groups, such as Aboriginal Canadians (in the United States Aboriginal groups include American Indians, Native Hawaiians, and Alaskan Natives) and people of African or Hispanic descent, are more at risk for kidney failure than Caucasians. The good news is that the risk of developing chronic kidney disease decreases with the length of time you've had diabetes, so by getting your diabetes under control early in the game, you may be able to prevent kidney disease or kidney failure.

WHAT DO YOUR KIDNEYS DO ALL DAY?

Kidneys are the public servants of the body; they're busy little bees! If they go on strike, you lose your water service, garbage pickup, and a few other services you don't even appreciate. Kidneys regulate your body's water levels; when you have too much water, your kidneys remove it by dumping it into a large storage tank, your bladder. The excess water stays there until you're ready to "pee it out." If you don't have enough water in your body (or if you're dehydrated), your kidneys will retain the water for you to keep you balanced.

Kidneys also act as your body's sewage-filtration plant. They filter out all the garbage and waste that your body doesn't need and dump it into the bladder; this waste is then excreted into your urine. The two waste products your kidneys regularly dump are *urea* (the waste product of protein) and *creatinine* (waste products produced by the muscles). In people with high blood sugar levels, excess sugar will get sent to the kidneys, and the kidneys will dump it into the bladder, too, causing sugar to appear in the urine.

Kidneys also balance calcium and phosphate in the body, both of which are needed to build bones. Kidneys operate a little side business on top of all this. They make two hormones. One hormone, called renin, helps to regulate blood pressure. Another hormone, called erythropoietin, helps bone marrow make red blood cells.

What Affects Your Kidneys?
The Macro Thing

When you suffer from cardiovascular disease, you probably have high blood pressure. High blood pressure damages blood vessels in the kidneys, which interferes with their job performance. As a result, they won't be as efficient at removing waste or excess water from your body. And if you are experiencing poor circulation, which can also cause water retention, the problem is further aggravated.

Poor circulation may cause your kidneys to secrete too much renin, which is normally designed to regulate blood pressure, but in this case increases it. All the extra fluid and the high blood pressure place a heavy burden on your heart—and your kidneys. If this situation isn't brought under control, you'd likely suffer from a heart attack before kidney failure, but kidney failure is inevitable.

The Micro Thing

When high blood sugar levels affect the small blood vessels, which includes the small blood vessels in the kidneys' filters (called the nephrons), it's called "diabetic nephropathy." In the early stages of nephropathy, good, usable protein is secreted in the urine. That's a sign that the kidneys were unable to distribute usable protein to the body's tissues. (Normally, they would excrete only the waste product of protein—urea—into the urine.)

Another microvascular problem affects the kidneys: nerve damage. The nerves you use to control your bladder can be affected, causing a sort of sewage backup in your body. The first place that sewage hits is your kidneys. Old urine floating around your kidneys isn't a healthy thing. The kidneys can become damaged as a result, aggravating all the conditions discussed so far in this section.

The Infection Thing

There's a third problem at work here. If you recall, frequent urination (urinating more often that what is usual for you) is a sign of high blood sugar. That's because your kidneys help rid the body of too much sugar by dumping it into the bladder. Well, guess what? You're not the only one who likes sugar; bacteria such as *E. coli* (the "hamburger bacteria") like it, too. In fact, they thrive on it, so all that sugary urine sitting around in your bladder and passing through your ureters and urethra can cause these bacteria to overgrow, resulting in a urinary tract infection (UTI) such as cystitis (inflammation of the bladder lining). The longer your urethra, the more protection you have from UTIs. Men have long urethras; women have very short urethras, however, and at the best of times are prone to these infections, especially after a lot of sexual activity, which explains the term "honeymoon cystitis." Sexual inter-course can introduce even more bacteria (from the vagina or rectum) into a woman's urethra due to the close space the vagina and urethra share. Women who wipe from back to front after a bowel movement can also introduce fecal matter into the urethra, causing a UTI.

Any bacterial infection in your bladder area can travel back up to your kidneys, causing infection, inflammation, and a big general mess, aggravating all the other problems!

The Smoking Thing

In the same way that smoking contributes to eye problems (see Chapter 17), it can also aggravate kidney problems. Smoking causes small vessel damage throughout your body. I hate to be a nag, but review Chapter 2 on smoking cessation.

SIGNS OF DIABETIC KIDNEY DISEASE

Obviously, there are a lot of different problems going on when it comes to diabetes and kidney disease. If you have any of the following early warning signs of kidney disease, see your doctor as soon as possible:

- Bad taste in the mouth (a sign of toxins building up; see also Chapter 18 on tooth decay)
- Blood or pus in the urine (a sign of a kidney infection)
- Burning or difficulty urinating (a sign of a urinary tract infection)
- Fever, chills, or vomiting (a sign of *any* infection)
- Foamy urine (a sign of kidney infection)
- Foul-smelling or cloudy urine (a sign of a urinary tract infection)
- Frequent urination (a sign of high blood sugar and/or urinary tract infection)
- High blood pressure (see Chapter 2)
- Itching
- Leg swelling or leg cramps (a sign of fluid retention)
- Less need for insulin or oral diabetes medications
- Morning sickness, nausea, and vomiting
- Pain in the lower abdomen (a sign of a urinary tract infection)

- Protein in the urine (a sign of microvascular problems)
- Puffiness around eyes or swelling of hands and feet (a sign of edema, or fluid retention)
- Weakness (a sign of anemia)

In the early stages of kidney disease, there are often no symptoms at all. Many of the symptoms above are signs that your kidney function has deteriorated to the point where toxins and wastes have built up, causing, for example, nausea and vomiting, fluid retention, even chronic hiccups. Heart failure (not to be confused with a heart attack, discussed in Chapter 15) and fluid in the lungs are characteristic of very late stages of kidney failure.

When you experience any of these symptoms, it's crucial to have a blood test that looks for creatinine levels. Again, creatinine is a waste product removed from the blood by healthy kidneys. A creatinine blood test greater than 1.2 for women and 1.4 for men is a sign of kidney disease. Another test that is usually ordered along with the creatinine blood test is the blood urea nitrogen (BUN) test, which is also important because when the BUN rises, so to speak, it's a sign of kidney disease, too. Other more sensitive tests that detect the level of kidney function include creatinine clearance, glomerular filtration rate (GFR), and urine albumin.

TREATING KIDNEY DISEASE

If you have high blood pressure, getting it under control through diet, exercise, or blood pressure-lowering medication will help save your kidneys. If you have high blood sugar, treating any UTI as quickly as possible with antibiotics is the best way to avert kidney infection, while drugs known as ACE inhibitors can help control small blood vessel damage caused by microvascular complications. In general, slowing the progression of kidney disease can be done by:

- controlling high blood pressure (see Chapter 2)
- controlling blood sugar levels (see Chapter 5)
- adopting a kidney-smart diet (see below)

- avoiding medications that may damage the kidneys (sit down with your pharmacist or doctor to find substitutes for medications that can affect the kidneys; there are many substitutes for commonly prescribed medications)
- treating urinary tract infections (see Chapter 16 on neuropathy)
- exercise and weight loss (see Chapter 11 on obesity and Chapter 9 on active living)

The Kidney-Smart Diet

To prolong the life of your kidneys when you experience signs of kidney disease or are in the early stages and perhaps have been alerted through blood test results, you can adjust your diet to cut down on the work your kidneys normally do as well as meet nutritional needs, such as increasing iron intake, which may be lower due to anemia. Diet can even control the buildup of food wastes and reduce fatigue, nausea, itching, and a bad taste in the mouth, which can occur when toxins build up in the body. And, of course, diet will help control high blood sugar. When you think about a kidney-smart diet, remember "3PS," a term I've coined to remember protein, potassium, phosphorus, and sodium. The diet involves *cutting down on 3PS*. A dietitian or nutritionist can help you make the cuts necessary to save your kidneys, but keep you as healthy as possible.

Energy Foods

Energy foods provide the fuel (calories) you need to do your daily activities and help you maintain a healthy body weight. When you are controlling your protein intake, it is important to get the energy you need from other food sources. Energy is found in most foods, particularly starches, sugars, grains, fruits, vegetables, fats, and oils. Following the guidance of chapters 7 and 8 on low glycemic eating and the right fats (good fats) should help you maintain energy, although you will need to cut down on fish (due its protein content—see next).

Protein

Protein is a good thing normally; it builds, repairs, and maintains your body tissues, and also helps you fight infections or heal wounds, but as protein breaks down in the body, it forms urea, which is a waste product. The kidney normally flushes out urea. When it can't, urea builds up in the blood, so cutting down on protein is necessary. If you have too much urea in the blood, it may cause fatigue, nausea, headaches, and a bad taste in your mouth. You need to eat enough for health, however. Meat, fish, poultry, eggs, tofu, and dairy products are high in protein.

Potassium

Your nerves and muscles normally rely on the mineral potassium to work well, but without the filtering process of your kidneys, too much potassium can build up in your blood, which can affect your heart. If the potassium level in your blood is too high or too low, it can affect your heartbeat. A very high level can cause the heart to actually stop beating. Normally your kidneys get rid of potassium excess, so most of us never think about it. But when your kidneys aren't functioning well, you can cut down on potassium-rich foods, such as potatoes, squash, bananas, oranges, tomatoes, dried peas, and beans.

Phosphorus (Phosphate)

Your bones normally rely on the mineral phosphorus to stay healthy and strong. When phosphorus levels rise, usually the kidneys just filter out excess phosphorus and you feel fine. But when the kidneys aren't working well, phosphorus levels rise until you get itchy skin or painful joints. Therefore, you may need to limit certain foods which contain even a moderate amount of phosphorus. These include milk, cheese, and other milk products, and protein foods such as meat, fish, and poultry. These foods include anything with protein (see "Protein"), seeds, nuts, dried peas, beans, and processed bran cereals. You'll need some phosphorus-containing foods for health. When you ingest them, you can also take a phosphate binder, a medication that binds with the phosphorus in your intestine so it can pass in your stool. Ask your doctor about prescribing the binder.

Sodium

Sodium affects your body fluids and blood pressure. As a general rule, you need to control your salt intake and try to avoid foods with a high sodium content. Reducing sodium means cutting down on salt and packaged or canned products with sodium (canned soups are notorious). Start reading labels and stop salting your foods. Processed foods, such as deli meats, fast foods, salty snacks, and anything with salty seasonings, are high in sodium. There are many herbs you can use instead; lemon and vinegar are terrific substitutes, too.

A Word about Fluids

Kidneys produce urine, which eliminates many of your wastes. When kidneys are not functioning well, not as much urine is produced, and this can cause fluid retention—swelling in hands, legs, and feet. Limiting your fluid intake may help, but it isn't necessary in all cases. Fluids include water, soup, juice, milk, popsicles, and gelatin; you and your doctor should discuss how to limit your fluid intake.

FROM KIDNEY DISEASE TO KIDNEY FAILURE

Kidney failure is also known as chronic renal insufficiency (CRI); this term means your kidneys are operating at 50 percent or less than normal capacity. By this point, your kidneys are working with "half the staff" and are not able to remove the bodily wastes as efficiently. Chronic renal insufficiency usually occurs over a number of years as the internal structures of the kidney are slowly damaged. In the early stages, there may be no symptoms. The progression of CRI may actually be so slow that symptoms do not occur until kidney function is less than one-tenth of normal. As the disease progresses, and as the kidneys continue to fail, more waste products build up, and you'll begin to feel sick. Because your kidneys stop making enough of the crucial hormone erythropoietin (EPO), you can suffer from low iron levels or anemia, as well as weakness. When the kidneys are functioning at less than 10 percent of their capacity, you'll need to consider dialysis or even a kidney transplant, if possible. By this point, you've progressed to end-stage renal disease.

Initial symptoms may include the following:

- Fatigue
- Frequent hiccups

- General ill feeling
- Generalized itching (pruritus)
- Headache
- Nausea, vomiting
- Unintentional weight loss

Later symptoms may include the following:
- Blood in the vomit or in stools
- Decreased alertness, including drowsiness, confusion, delirium, or coma
- Decreased sensation in the hands, feet, or other areas
- Easy bruising or bleeding
- Increased or decreased urine output
- Muscle twitching or cramps
- Seizures
- White crystals in and on the skin (uremic frost)

Additional symptoms that may be associated with this disease:
- Abnormally dark or light skin
- Agitation
- Breath odour
- Excessive nighttime urination (going more often than what is normal for you)
- Excessive thirst
- High blood pressure
- Loss of appetite
- Nail abnormalities
- Paleness

When You Need Dialysis

The word "dialysis" comes from the root word "dissolution," which means "to set free." It is a life-saving treatment that replaces many of your kidney's functions, such as removing waste, salt, and extra water to prevent them from building up in the body; it keeps levels of potassium, sodium, and bicarbonate in check, and helps control your blood pressure. Dialysis has been available since the mid-1940s and began to be used as a regular treatment for people with kidney failure in the 1960s. Dialysis allows people with kidney failure to live a long time, often as long as someone with functioning kidneys. There are two types of dialysis: hemodialysis ("hemo" means blood) and peritoneal dialysis ("peritoneal" means abdominal). Recent statistics from the Kidney Foundation show that among the 19,721 patients on dialysis at year-end 2005, 81 percent were on hemodialysis, and 19 percent were on peritoneal dialysis. In Canada, the cost of dialysis is covered by the provinces. In the United States, many people simply die because they don't have health insurance coverage for dialysis and can't afford it. However, the need for dialysis in Canada is putting a strain on our resources. While there are dialysis units across Canada, you need to plan your treatments several months in advance due to limited staff and space. This may mean you have to travel great distances and pay for many expenses yourself, such as accommodation, travel costs, and so on. Your local Kidney Foundation office (find an office via www.kidney. ca) has information about the nearest dialysis units in your area and can give you some advice about making suitable arrangements for accommodations. Dialysis can be done at home, but it requires supervision with a trained health care professional. You still need to be "retrofitted" for home dialysis, get the equipment, and make other arrangements. Your health care team will assist you in making the best decision regarding your dialysis treatment.

Hemodialysis

Hemodialysis involves cleaning your blood through an artificial kidney machine (dialyzer). The blood flows into the machine and goes back into your body nice and clean, free of waste products and excess build-up from chemicals and fluid.

You are connected to the artificial kidney through a blood vessel in your arm or leg. If there are problems finding a healthy blood vessel, a bridge can be created through a graft or catheter, a narrow plastic tube. The connection process can be uncomfortable, depending on how it's done.

The length of time a hemodialysis treatment lasts depends on the functioning capacity of your kidneys, how much waste has built up, how much fluid builds up between treatments, your overall size, and the type of artificial kidney used.

Each hemodialysis treatment normally takes four to five hours, and usually three treatments a week are needed. More frequent, shorter treatments or longer treatments may be indicated for certain patients. Only a small amount of your blood is out of the body at one time, so your blood must circulate through the machine many times before it is cleaned. Hemodialysis can be done in a variety of settings, including a hospital dialysis unit, in a clinic away from the hospital, in a self-care centre (with some assistance from the staff), or at home. Furthermore, special training is needed for self-care or home hemodialysis. These days, home hemodialysis is much improved from even a few years ago, but it's critical to be trained properly by a health professional who can visit the home and help you handle the machine and equipment.

Peritoneal Dialysis

Peritoneal dialysis uses a filtration process similar to hemodialysis, but the blood is cleaned inside your body rather than in a machine. There are three types of peritoneal dialysis.

Continuous ambulatory peritoneal dialysis (CAPD): In CAPD, you carry about 2.0–2.5 L of dialysis fluid in your peritoneal cavity all the time. An exchange is usually done four times a day by draining out the old fluid and refilling your peritoneal cavity with fresh fluid. The exchanges are often done early in the morning, lunchtime, late in the afternoon, and at bedtime. Each exchange takes about 30–45 minutes.

Assisted continuous ambulatory peritoneal dialysis (ACAPD): Assisted CAPD involves the use of simple equipment so that an extra exchange can be done while you sleep.

Automated or cycler peritoneal dialysis (APD): In APD (previously called continued cycling peritoneal dialysis), a machine called an automatic cycler performs exchanges every night while you sleep. In the morning, when you come off the machine, about 2 L of dialysis fluid are left in your peritoneal cavity for the day. In the evening, you drain out this fluid when you connect yourself to the automatic cycler for the night. While APD allows you to do dialysis at home with no interruptions to your day, it does require that you be attached to the machine every night for eight to 10 hours. Some people may also do an additional exchange during the day to provide adequate removal of waste products.

A special test called a PET test will help your health care team decide which method of peritoneal dialysis is best for you.

Lifestyle Adjustments for Dialysis

Dialysis treatments, unlike some other treatments such as chemotherapy, do not leave you feeling sick or weak afterwards; they leave you feeling healthier. But during the procedure, you may feel muscle cramps, nausea, or dizziness because the waste products are removed more abruptly than they are when kidneys are functioning. Low blood pressure can also occur, causing dizziness, headaches, and even vomiting. As you have more treatments, these side effects should pass.

Dialysis also means you have to stay on your 3PS diet (see above), cutting down on protein, potassium, phosphorus, and sodium. A good meal plan can help improve both your dialysis outcome and your health in general.

You can travel while on dialysis; you just have to contact the closest dialysis centre to your place of destination and make arrangements for a treatment. If you're using CAPD, don't worry about it. Just pack your equipment and luggage and go. There are dialysis units across Canada and in many parts of the world. They have suitable facilities for visitors who need hemodialysis treatment. However, it is necessary to plan several months in advance due to limited space and staff. Your dialysis unit and local Kidney Foundation office can provide more information and advise you about travel costs and arrangements.

You can also continue to work if you're on dialysis; you just need to arrange your work schedule around your dialysis treatments. Physical jobs involving heavy lifting, digging, and so on do not mix well with kidney failure. You can't do hard labour when you're on dialysis.

Stopping Dialysis

Dialysis is a medical treatment that keeps you alive. As discussed in the chapter about stroke (Chapter 15), when someone has no quality of life, life-saving medical interventions can be withdrawn. This decision is ethical and legal and is not in any way the same thing as euthanasia, which means you use medical intervention to stop a life. In the film *Whose Life Is It Anyway?* Richard Dreyfus plays a quadriplegic who is dependent on dialysis (as most people with spinal cord injury are). Because he cannot move on his own, he feels his life does not have quality or value, and he asks for withdrawal of all medical treatment, including dialysis.

Stopping dialysis may be a decision you make yourself, or it may be a decision your surrogate makes (this is the person, such as a spouse, other family member, or friend you appoint to make decisions on your behalf when you're not conscious or are incapacitated).

There may be other health problems behind this choice; you may be experiencing failing health as a result of stroke or cancer, for example. In these cases, you may decide to stop your dialysis treatment.

You may also decide that being on dialysis is not allowing you the quality of life you want; if this is the case, you may be a candidate for a kidney transplant (see further on), but that may involve dialysis until a donor comes forward. Depending on your age, level of mobility, and other circumstances in your life, you may decide to refuse dialysis treatment and die a natural death of kidney failure. These are all choices that are yours to make and no one else's. You may also decide to state the conditions under which dialysis should be stopped, such as in the event of a coma or stroke that leaves you with no quality of life. This is called an advance directive. In an advance directive (also called a living will), you can stipulate that you do not want to be resuscitated if you die of a heart attack. You can also stipulate that dialysis should be stopped in such an event.

Palliative Care for Kidney Failure

If your kidneys fail and you do not choose dialysis, and you are not a candidate for a kidney transplant, you can die a peaceful death from kidney failure and be made comfortable with palliative care. As the toxins build up in your body, fluid will fill your lungs and can cause shortness of breath. The fluid can be removed manually or through diuretics, which will make you comfortable. You can also be pain-free through medications, but usually kidney failure is not painful; the discomfort comes from breathing difficulties as fluids build up in the lungs. Dying from kidney failure is more like drowning and slipping away rather than experiencing agony and pain.

WHEN YOU WANT A KIDNEY TRANSPLANT

The good news is that you can get a new kidney when the one you have stops working. Kidney transplants are an option for people with kidney failure. That's because we have two kidneys, but can live with only one. As long as people are healthy, they can give away a kidney to someone who needs it. (In fact, kidney donation is so doable that medical ethicists are worried that some people are selling their kidneys as a way to make money, creating a scenario where the rich buy kidneys from the poor!)

Living Donors

In the film *Steel Magnolias* (which I mentioned earlier), Sally Field plays mother to Julia Roberts, whose character has Type 1 diabetes. When Julia Roberts's kidneys fail, Sally Field donates one kidney to her. The general rule is this: If you've got a donor, you've got a new kidney! The person donating the kidney is called a living donor. Kidney donation is similar to bone marrow donation, in that the blood type and tissues should match as closely as possible to avoid your body's rejection of the kidney as foreign. Relatives are always good bets, but you can use anybody's kidney if the match is there. Living donor transplants have a 90–95 percent success rate. That means that after one year, 90–95 of every 100 transplanted kidneys are still working. Most importantly, living donor kidneys tend to function longer and last 15–20 years on average. Of the 1,202 kidney transplants performed in 2006, 40 percent were from living donors.

Transplant Waiting Lists

There are many Canadians on waiting lists for transplants of various kinds. Of the 4,240 Canadians on the waiting list for a transplant (as of

December 2006), 3,075 were awaiting a kidney transplant. If you don't know anyone willing to give you a kidney, you have to wait for a kidney from someone who has filled out a donor card on a driver's licence, which could take a while, depending on where you live in the country. Many people die each day in car accidents and other types of accidents, but unless they specify that they *want* to donate their organs, they cannot be donors. People who donate organs after they die are known as deceased donors. The success rates with deceased donors are not as high as those with living donors, but it's still about 80 percent successful for the first year.

Without a living donor, you have to be on a transplant waiting list, and the wait can be long when you factor in the blood and tissue matching. When you don't have a donor, you receive kidneys according to need, rather than "first come, first serve," but your overall health is also weighed. For example, if your kidneys are failing because you're in terrible health as a result of out-of-control diabetes and a host of other complications, a new kidney may not fare very well in your body and may eventually fail, too. Someone in better health may get a kidney faster than you because he or she has a greater chance of being a successful recipient.

Generally, to be considered for a transplant from either a live or posthumous donor, you must be healthy enough to have the surgery and be free from infection or other diseases, such as cancer. You must also be willing to take anti-rejection drugs, which can have side effects.

Preparing for a Transplant

Obviously you don't just bring your sister to a hospital and say, "Give me her kidney." Preparing for a transplant is rather involved. First, you will need to meet with a transplant surgeon or a team of transplant specialists to find out whether the risks of the transplant surgery and anti-rejection medications outweigh the inconveniences of dialysis. In other words, is a new kidney going to give you a better quality of life than the one you have now? In many cases, the answer is *yes,* but in a significant number of cases, the answer is *no* because of health complications. There are also risks to the donor, and to date, we have done an insufficient job of tracking how living donors are doing in the long term.

In most transplant units, you're provided with some names of recipients you can talk to about the process. You then have to prepare for major surgery, which can be planned in advance if you have a living donor. Numerous tests and workups determine your fitness for undergoing a transplant surgery. In a nutshell, if you're a good candidate for a kidney transplant and you can find a donor, you may have a better quality of life than you do on dialysis, provided the rejection drugs used for the transplant don't cause worse side effects.

Complications run head to toe and, unfortunately, do not bypass the kidneys, as you can see. If you are successful in either saving your kidneys by preventing kidney disease or kidney failure, or finding success through treatments such as transplant or dialysis, don't put on your dancing shoes until you read the next chapter. You can be a "walking complication" and not even know it.

20

FOOT NOTES

Foot complications related to diabetes were dramatized in the mid-1980s film *Nothing in Common,* in which Jackie Gleason plays the ne'er-do-well diabetic father, and Tom Hanks plays the son who cannot accept him. In a heartbreaking scene, Tom Hanks is shocked to discover how ill his father really is when he finally sees his feet. They are swollen, purple, and badly infected. Ultimately, the story ends with the father and son coming to terms as Gleason must undergo surgical amputation.

I share this example with you because many of us are used to ignoring and abusing our feet. We wear uncomfortable shoes, we pick at our calluses and blisters, we don't wear socks with our shoes, and so on. You can't do this any more. Your feet are the targets of both macrovascular (large blood vessel) complications and microvascular (small blood vessel) complications. In the first case, peripheral vascular disease affects blood circulation to your feet. In the second case, the nerve cells to your feet, which control sensation, can be altered through microvascular complications. Nerve damage can also affect your feet's muscles and tendons, causing weakness and changes to your feet's shape.

WHAT CAN HAPPEN TO YOUR FEET

The combination of poor circulation and numbness in your feet means that you can sustain an injury to your feet and not know it. For example, you might step on a piece of glass or badly stub your toe and not realize it. If an open wound becomes infected, and you have poor circulation, the wound will not heal properly, and infection could spread to the bone or gangrene could develop. In this situation, amputation may be the only treatment. Or, without sensation or proper circulation, your feet could be far more vulnerable to frostbite or exposure than they would be otherwise. Diabetes can also cause your feet to thicken as a result of poor circulation. The skin on the foot becomes very thin and blood vessels are visible through the skin, which has a shiny appearance and looks red. Thinner skin can be more easily pierced and infected.

As if this weren't enough for your feet, they can also be damaged from bone loss: osteoporosis of the feet! Diabetes can cause your body to take more calcium from bones. Because there are 26 bones in your foot alone, bone loss in the foot can weaken it, and it can break more easily or become deformed with bigger arches and a claw-like toe. All of this can cause calluses that can get infected, leading to gangrene and amputation, too.

Diabetes accounts for approximately half of all non-emergency amputations, but all experts agree that doing a foot self-exam every day (see below) can prevent most foot complications from becoming severe. As of 2008, it was noted that foot complications are a major reason for admission to the hospital for people with diabetes, accounting for approximately 20 percent of all diabetes-related admissions in the North American population. Aboriginal Canadians seem to be particularly vulnerable to the problems; in Manitoba, it's predicted that by 2016, there will have been a 10-fold increase in foot *amputations* since 1996.

Signs of Foot Problems

The most common symptoms of foot complications are burning, tingling, or pain in your feet or legs. These are all signs of nerve damage. Numbness is another symptom that could mean nerve damage or circulation problems. If you do experience pain from nerve damage, it usually gets worse with time (as new nerves and blood vessels grow), and many people find that it's worse at night. Bed linens can increase discomfort. Some people notice foot symptoms only after exercising or a short walk. But many people don't notice immediate symptoms until they've lost feeling in their feet.

Other symptoms people notice are frequent infections (caused by blood vessel damage), hair loss on the toes or lower legs, or shiny skin on the lower legs and feet. Foot deformity or open wounds on the feet are also signs.

When You Knock Your Socks Off

When you take off your socks at the end of the day, get in the habit of doing a foot self-exam. This is the only way you can do damage control on your feet. You're looking for signs of infection or potential infection triggers. If you can avoid infection at all costs, you will be able to keep your feet. Look for the following signs:

- Reddened, discoloured, or swollen areas (blue, bright red, or white areas mean that circulation is cut off)
- Pus
- Temperature changes in the feet or "hot spots"
- Corns, calluses, and warts (potential infections could be hiding under calluses; do not remove these yourself—see a podiatrist, a foot specialist)
- Toenails that are too long (your toenail could cut you if it's too long)
- Redness where your shoes or socks are rubbing due to a poor fit. (When your sock is scrunched inside your shoe, the folds could rub against the skin and cause a blister)
- Toenail fungus (under the nail)
- Fungus between the toes (this is athlete's foot, common if you've been walking around barefoot in a public place)
- Breaks in the skin (especially between your toes), or cracks, such as in calluses on the heels, which open the door for bacteria

If you find an infection, wash your feet carefully with soap and water; *don't use alcohol.* Then see your doctor or a podiatrist as soon as possible. If your foot is irritated but not yet infected (redness, for example, from poor-fitting shoes but no blister yet), simply avoid the irritant—the shoes—and it should clear up. If not, see your doctor. If you're overweight and have trouble inspecting your feet, get somebody else to check them for the signs listed above. In addition to doing a self-exam, see your doctor to have the circulation and reflexes in your feet checked four times a year.

By following these foot steps, you can help to prevent diabetes foot complications:

DO:
- Wear socks at night if your feet get cold.
- Elevate your feet when you are sitting.
- Wiggle your toes and move your ankles around for a few minutes several times a day to improve blood flow in your feet and legs.
- Inspect your feet daily and in particular feel for skin temperature differences between your feet.
- Walk a little bit every day; this is a good way to improve blood flow and get a little exercise!
- Check your shoes before you put them on: shake them out in case something such as your (grand)child's Lego piece, a piece of dry cat food, or a pebble is in there.
- Trim your toenails straight across to avoid ingrown nails. Don't pick off your nails. Use only a nail clipper, and be sure not to cut into the corners of the nails. Use a nail file or emery board to smooth or round rough edges.
- Place your feet flat on the floor when sitting down. Sitting cross-legged or in cross-legged variations can cut off your circulation, and frequently does in people without diabetes.
- Wear comfortable, proper-fitting footwear. See the box on page 322 for tips about shoe shopping.
- Avoid heat. Extreme heat, such as heating pads, very hot water, and even hot sun, can cause swelling or burn your feet.

DON'T:
- Cross your legs for long periods of time.
- Walk around barefoot. Instead, wear proper-fitting, clean cotton socks with your shoes daily, and get in the habit of wearing slippers around the house and shoes at the beach. If you're swimming, wear some sort of shoe (plastic "jellies" or canvas running shoes). If it's cold out, wear woollen socks.

- Perform "bathroom surgery" on your feet, which may include puncturing blisters with needles or tweezers, shaving your calluses, and the hundreds of crazy things people do to their feet (but never disclose to their spouses).
- Wear clothing that restricts blood flow to your legs and feet, including girdles, garters, tight pantyhose, or socks that cut off the circulation.
- Remain overweight. Lose some weight; less weight puts less pressure on your feet.
- Use over-the-counter medications to treat corns and warts. These can be dangerous for people with diabetes.
- Soak your feet.
- Take very hot baths.
- Use lotion between your toes.
- Wear tight socks, garters or elastics, or knee-highs.
- Wear over-the-counter insoles; they can cause blisters if they're not right for your feet.
- Sit for long periods of time; check with your doctor if you have to take a long flight.
- Have pedicures by non-health care professionals.
- Smoke.

The Foot Self-Exam (FSE)

Examine and care for your feet daily. Start by assembling a foot-care kit containing nail clippers, nail file, lotion, a pumice stone, and a non-breakable hand mirror.

1. Wash your feet in warm (not hot) water, using a mild soap. Don't soak your feet as this can dry your skin.
2. While your feet are still wet, use a pumice stone to keep calluses under control.
3. Dry your feet carefully, especially between your toes.
4. Thoroughly check your feet and between your toes to make sure there are no cuts, cracks, ingrown toenails, blisters, etc. Use a

hand mirror to see the bottom of your feet, or ask someone else to check them for you.

5. Clean cuts or scratches with mild soap and water, and cover with a dry dressing suitable for sensitive skin.

6. Trim your toenails straight across and file any sharp edges. Don't cut the nails too short.

7. Apply an unscented lotion to your heels and soles. Wipe off excess lotion that is not absorbed. Don't put lotion between your toes as the excessive moisture can promote infection.

8. Wear fresh clean socks and well-fitting shoes every day. Whenever possible, wear white socks—if you have a cut or sore, the drainage will be easy to see.

If you have any swelling, warmth, redness, or pain in your legs or feet, see your doctor right away. If you have any corns (thick or hard skin on toes), calluses (thick skin on bottom of feet), in-grown toenails, warts, or slivers, have them treated by your doctor or a foot care specialist (such as a podiatrist, chiropodist, or experienced foot-care nurse). Do not try to treat them yourself. In addition, have your bare feet checked by your doctor at least once a year. Also, ask your doctor to screen you for neuropathy and loss of circulation at least once a year. Remove your socks at every diabetes-related visit to your doctor and ask him or her to inspect your feet.

To save your feet, you may not be able to save on your next pair of shoes. These are new shoe-shopping rules:

- Shoe shop at the time of day when your feet are most swollen (such as afternoons). That way, you'll purchase a shoe that fits you in "bad times" as well as good times.
- Don't even think about high heels or any type of shoe that is not comfortable or that doesn't fit properly. Say goodbye to thongs. That strip between your toes can cause too much irritation.
- Buy leather; avoid shoes with the terms "man-made upper" or "man-made materials" on the label. Such shoes are made

of synthetic materials, and your foot will not breathe. Cotton
or canvas shoes are fine as long as the insole is cotton, too.
Synthetic materials on the very bottom of the shoe are fine
as long as the upper—the part of the shoe that touches your
foot—is leather, cotton, canvas, or something breathable.
- Remember that leather does, indeed, stretch. When that
  happens, the shoe could become loose and cause blisters. On
  the other hand, if the shoe is too tight and the salesperson tells
  you the shoe will stretch, forget it. The shoe will destroy you in
  the first few hours of wear, which sort of "defeets" the purpose.
- If you lose all sensation and cannot feel whether the shoe is
  fitting, make sure you have a shoe salesperson fit you.
- Avoid shoes that have been on display. A variety of people try
  these shoes on; you never know what bacteria and fungi these
  previously tried-on shoes harbour.

WHEN YOU HAVE AN OPEN WOUND OR FOOT ULCER

Open wounds on the feet are also called "foot ulcers" and affect roughly
200,000 Canadians with diabetes; about 20 percent of diabetes-related foot ulcers don't heal, leading to amputation to prevent gangrene.
Any tear in the skin can lead to an open wound that becomes infected.
Blisters, cracks in the feet from dryness, and stepping on something
sharp (see above) are the most common causes of open wounds.

Healing Open Wounds

The first order of business is removing the source of irritation that
caused the sore, such as bad shoes or poor hygiene (see "Foot Steps"
above). In many cases antibiotics can heal the wounds, as well as dressing the wound well (cleaning it, using proper bandages, and so on).
Keeping pressure off the feet can also help them heal. Often healing a
foot ulcer requires home care; you may need to have a nurse or home
health care worker come into your home and dress your wounds.

When wounds are open and not healing well, an unpleasant odour can develop. Waiting for your daily dressing while you heal your foot sore can be pretty isolating and depressing for many people. One experience with this is often enough for you to take prevention steps seriously (see above).

When Wounds Don't Heal

Not all open wounds heal. To heal cuts, sores, or any open wound, your body normally manufactures macrophages, special white blood cells that fight infection, as well as special repair cells, called fibroblasts. These "ambulance cells" need oxygen to live. If you have poor circulation, it's akin to an ambulance not making it to an accident scene in time because it gets caught in a long traffic jam.

When wounds don't heal, gangrene infections can set in. Until recently, amputating the infected limb was the only way to deal with gangrene, but a new therapy is available at several hospitals throughout Canada called hyperbaric oxygen therapy (HBO). The procedure involves placing you in an oxygen chamber or tank and feeding you triple the amount of oxygen you'd find in the normal atmosphere. To heal gangrene on the feet, you'd need about 30 treatments (several per day for a week or so). The result is that your tissues become saturated with oxygen, enabling your body to heal itself. HBO may be useful in addition to systemic antibiotics for people with deep, long-standing, non-healing foot infections.

There are also two wound-healing products available as well. One is "replaceable skin" called Dermagraft, which is made of skin cells that are grown in a lab. Dermagraft is applied once a week to the wound and actually replenishes the skin. Another product, Regranex, contains natural growth factors in our skin cells and comes in a gel applied once a day to jump-start healing. These products don't always work, but are a good option for wounds that won't heal. Your doctor may suggest other therapies as well, but these biological products are not a substitute for good wound care and pressure reduction, and should be selected only after a professional consultation.

WHEN YOU REQUIRE AN AMPUTATION

Many people are amputees, including former Quebec premier Lucien Bouchard. When you require an amputation to stop a gangrene infection, there are a few ways you can maximize your health prior to surgery; they'll also help you heal after surgery.

Quit smoking. (See Chapter 2 for more details on smoking-cessation programs.) Smoking restricts your blood vessels as I've said many times in this book. You need your blood vessels to be as healthy as possible prior to surgery and after.

Next, compile a list of questions for your surgeon, anaesthesiologist, or other health care professionals. Here's a list to get you started, courtesy of the Amputee Coalition.

Questions for Your Surgeon

1. Is amputation the best solution?
2. What experience do you have in this type of surgery?
3. How long is the procedure?
4. What are the major risks of the surgery? What steps will you take to minimize those risks?
5. What kind of pain will I have after the surgery and for how long?
6. How will my pain be managed immediately following the surgery?
7. How will long-term pain be managed?
8. How long will I have to remain in bed?
9. Will I have drains? If so, when will they be removed?
10. How long will you supervise my care after surgery?
11. When will I be fitted with my first prosthesis?
12. Will I be able to meet with a prosthetist before the surgery?
13. Should I be able to use a prosthesis? How much functional ability will the prosthesis provide?
14. If I want to talk with someone who has been through a similar amputation, could you refer me?
15. Could you refer me to a support group?

Questions for Your Nurse and Anaesthesiologist

1. How long will I be in the recovery room?
2. When will I be able to visit with my family?
3. What kind of anaesthesia will be used during surgery? What measures will be taken to reduce reactions to the anaesthesia?
4. When will stitches be removed?

For a support structure, you can reach out across the border, too. For example, the Amputee Coalition of America networks with thousands of amputees across the United States. They can be reached at 888-267-5669, or via their website (www.amputee-coalition.org), which has excellent and current Fact Sheets on a wide variety of topics.

Getting an Artificial Limb

Artificial limbs are also called prosthetic limbs, or simply a prosthesis. In Canada, some of the costs for the prosthesis (usually about 70 percent) are covered by the province. If you have private health insurance, through your job, for example, it will cover the rest of the costs. You can also look into non-profit agencies for help.

Doctors do not have prosthetic limbs you can purchase. You have to go to a special artisan, known as an orthotist or prosthetist, a person who is trained in making artificial limbs and understands amputees' needs. In Canada, the Canadian Board for Certification of Prosthetists and Orthotists (CBCPO) is the regulatory body for the prosthetic and orthotic profession within the country (www.cbcpo.ca). By going to their website, you can find a certified professional in your area.

The orthotist or prosthetist must have a doctor's prescription before they make the limb. Some prosthetic companies have catalogues, allowing you to order direct and bypass the prescription, but it's best to be fitted for a limb in person and to work directly with a prosthetist. Ordering from the Internet or a catalogue is akin to ordering a breast implant from a catalogue: You should be fitted. Amputees recommend shopping around for an orthotist or prosthetist; the limb prices vary wildly from manufacturer to manufacturer and prosthetist to prosthetist.

Most prosthetists are willing to work with you and answer the many questions you may have about how the limb is made, durability, ranges of motions, and so on.

The Amputee Coalition of America (www.amputee-coalition.org) has put together this informative page on their website outlining some of the things to consider as a new amputee needing a prosthesis. These are some answers to questions new amputees frequently ask:

Q: **What happens after the amputation? Are bionic limbs available that can make me just like I was before?**

A: A prosthesis is not bionic. It is an artificial replacement for a missing limb or part of a limb. Although a prosthesis is never as natural as your own limb, it can help you to do many things quite effectively if you are willing to combine your energy and willpower into learning how to use it. The most important aspect of success is working with your doctor, prosthetist, and therapist to address all of your concerns, and then to work with them on the processes of design, fitting, and training, which are required to be a successful user.

Q: **What does a prosthesis look like? How will it stay on?**

A: Depending on the level of your amputation, physical ability, and functional needs, each prosthesis will be somewhat different. If you desire a "cosmetic look," prosthetic supplements are available. But, for most standard prostheses, they are comprised of conventional component parts attached to a socket that fits over your residual limb.

Q: **How does a prosthesis work? Will I be able to do all the things I did before I lost my limb?**

A: The majority of people who lose a limb can get back to a normal mode of functioning within a few to several months, depending on the location of the amputation as well as physical ability. How well they function depends primarily on their goals along with timely, comfortable prosthetic fitting, good follow-up care, and a "can do" attitude from themselves as well as their medical team.

Q: When will I get a prosthesis?

A: Generally, you should be ready for prosthetic measurements and fitting a few weeks after surgery, when the wound is healed and the tissue swelling is decreased. Then you will be ready for prosthetic measurements and fitting. This process can be easily attained with exercise and rehabilitation. During this stage, your medical team also will be concerned with maintaining proper shape of the residual limb, as well as increasing overall strength and function. Fitting is usually stress-free and involves several steps to create a unique prosthesis for you.

Q: What if the prosthesis doesn't fit right?

A: Follow-up is as important as the initial fitting. You will need to make several visits for adjustments with the prosthetist as well as training with a therapist. They can help you ease pressure areas, adjust alignment, work out any problems, and regain the skills you need to adapt to life after limb loss. Tell your prosthetist if the manufactured limb is uncomfortable, too loose, or too tight. Ask questions about things you need or want to do. Communicate honestly about your needs. The more you communicate with your prosthetist and therapist, the better you will be able to succeed with a prosthesis.

Q: How long will it last?

A: Depending on your age, activity level, and growth, the prosthesis can last anywhere from several months to several years. In the early stages after limb loss, many changes occur in the residual limb that can lead to shrinking of the limb. This may require socket changes, the addition of liners, or even a different device. Later on, increased activity level and desire for additional function can necessitate a change in the prosthesis or its parts. Once you are comfortably adjusted and functioning at the desired level of activity, the prosthesis needs only minor repairs or maintenance and can last for an average of three years.

Q: Is it difficult learning to use a prosthesis?

A: Learning to use a prosthesis is a tough job. It takes time, great effort, strength, patience, and perseverance. You will do best to work with a therapist while learning how to handle the new device. Much like learning how to operate a car, you will need guidance on how to:

- take care of the prosthesis
- put on (don) and take off (doff) the prosthesis
- walk on different types of surfaces, including stairs and uneven terrain
- handle emergencies safely, including falling down and getting up again
- perform daily activities at home, at work, and even in a car
- investigate new things you may be uncertain of, including sports and recreational activities

Q: What can I do to prepare myself for a prosthesis?

A: There is a lot you can and must do to be able to use a prosthesis and use it well. The top priorities are:

- working through the feelings about losing a limb and deciding how to rebuild your life after amputation
- exercising to build the muscles needed for balance and ambulation
- preparing and taking care of your residual limb to attain a proper, sound shape for the prosthesis
- learning proper body positioning and strengthening to maintain tone and prevent contractures

Q: Will I need to use a wheelchair or crutches?

A: Some people elect not to use a prosthesis, relying exclusively on mobility devices. However, with a prosthesis, the use of crutches or a wheelchair depends on several factors, including level of amputation, whether you have a single or bilateral amputation, and your respective level of balance and strength. Most amputees have a pair of crutches for times when the limb is off, including nighttime trips to the bathroom, showering, participating in certain sports, and to help if problems arise that may require leaving the prosthesis off for any length of time.

If you are a person who has lost both legs, you will probably use a wheelchair at least some of the time. Unilateral amputees may find it helpful to use a cane or crutches for balance and support in the early stages of walking or just to have a break from the prosthesis. This is an individual decision based on factors such as age, balance, strength, and sense of security.

Q: **Once I have been fitted and feel comfortable in its function, what will happen next?**

A: Plan on making follow-up visits to your prosthetist a normal part of your life. Proper fit of the socket and good alignment will insure that the prosthesis is useful to you. Prostheses, like cars, need regular maintenance and repair to continue efficient functioning. Small adjustments can make a big difference.

Q: **Can the limb break down?**

A: Yes, things can happen that will require repair or replacement, so it's a good idea to know about warranties and what to expect from your prosthetist. Get small problems with your prosthesis taken care of promptly. There is no benefit to waiting until something falls apart or causes you serious skin breakdown. If you wear a prosthesis too long when it needs repairs or replacement, you can do harm, not only to your residual limb, but also to other parts of your body. Strain on other muscles, especially in your back and shoulders, will affect posture in addition to performance of the device and energy needed to use it. Early prevention is more valuable than long-term treatment.

Source: "Prosthetic FAQs for the New Amputee," September 2008. Posted at: http://www.amputee-coalition.org/fact_sheets/prosfaq.html

APPENDIX 1
A BRIEF HISTORY OF DIABETES

1552 B.C.: Earliest known record of diabetes appears on third-dynasty Egyptian papyrus by physician Hesy-Ra; he mentions polyuria (frequent urination) as a symptom.

First Century A.D.: Diabetes is described by Arateus as "the melting down of flesh and limbs into urine."

A.D. 164: Greek physician Galen of Pergamum mistakenly diagnoses diabetes as an ailment of the kidneys.

Up to 11th Century: Diabetes is commonly diagnosed by "water tasters," who drank the urine of people suspected of having diabetes; the urine of people with diabetes is thought to be sweet-tasting. *Mellitus,* the Latin word for honey (referring to its sweetness) is added to the term diabetes as a result.

1500s: Swiss-born alchemist and physician Paracelsus identifies diabetes as a serious general disorder.

Early 1800s: First chemical tests are developed to indicate and measure the presence of sugar in urine.

1800s: French researcher Claude Bernard studies the workings of the pancreas and the glycogen metabolism of the liver.

1800s: Czech researcher I.V. Pavlov discovers the links between the nervous system and gastric secretion, making an important contribution to science's knowledge of the physiology of the digestive system.

Late 1800s: Italian diabetes specialist Catoni isolates his patients under lock and key to get them to follow their diets.

Late 1850s: French physician Priorry advises diabetes patients to eat extra-large quantities of sugar as a treatment.

1869: Paul Langerhans, a German medical student, announces in a dissertation that the pancreas contains two systems of cells. One set secretes normal pancreatic juice; the function of the other is unknown. Several years later, these cells are identified as the islets of Langerhans.

1870s: French physician Bouchardat notices the disappearance of glycosuria in his diabetes patients during the rationing of food in Paris while under siege by Germany during the Franco-Prussian War; formulates idea of individualized diets for his diabetes patients.

1889: Oskar Minkowski and Joseph von Mering at the University of Strasbourg, Austria, first remove the pancreas from a dog to determine the effect of an absent pancreas on digestion. They prove that without its pancreas a dog becomes severely diabetic. They also show through experiments with duct ligation (surgically tying off different parts of tissue) that the pancreas indeed has two secretions: the *external* (which feeds directly into the bloodstream and regulates carbohydrate metabolism) and a mysterious *internal* secretion, which appears to be the "missing secretion" in diabetics. This connection between diabetes and the pancreas results in a series of early experiments using pancreatic extracts to treat animals and humans. But unfortunately, these experiments don't work, and serve to challenge the entire hypothesis of this internal secretion.

November 14, 1891: Frederick Banting is born near Alliston, Ontario. His parents, devout Methodists, try to pressure their son into joining the ministry; however, Banting enrols in medical school at the University of Toronto in 1912 instead.

February 28, 1899: Charles Best is born in West Pembroke, Maine.

1900–1915: "Fad" diabetes diets include the "oat-cure" (in which the majority of the diet was made up of oatmeal), the milk diet, the rice cure, "potato therapy," and even the use of opium.

1906: German scientist Georg Zuelzer makes some interesting progress on June 21, 1906. He injects pancreatic extract under the skin of a comatose 50-year-old diabetic. The man is momentarily revived, reinforcing the connection between pancreatic extract (pancreatic secretion) and diabetes. Zuelzer obtains funding from the Schering drug company to produce a viable extract for therapy. By 1907, he produces what appears to be a workable pancreatic extract, but the Schering company decides that the results of his work don't justify their costs and pulls funding. This is a shame, considering that Zuelzer's formula is the first pancreatic extract to suppress *glycosuria* (sugary urine). Unfortunately, Zuelzer's extract also causes many toxic side effects— what we know today as insulin shock. What should have been a major breakthrough in research is viewed by pancreatic researchers as a setback. Caution rules, and the risks of these "toxic side effects" interfere with many pancreatic extract experiments.

1910–1920: Frederick Madison Allen and Elliot P. Joslin emerge as the two leading diabetes specialists in the United States. Joslin believes diabetes to be "the best of the chronic diseases" because it is "clean, seldom unsightly, not contagious, often painless and susceptible to treatment."

1913: After three years of diabetes study, Frederick Allen publishes *Studies Concerning Glycosuria and Diabetes*, a book that is significant for the revolution in diabetes therapy that developed from it. J.J.R. Macleod, a professor of medicine at the University of Toronto, publishes a book called *Diabetes: Its Pathological Physiology*. Library records show that Frederick Banting borrows Macleod's book for his research in 1920.

1919: Frederick Allen publishes *Total Dietary Regulation in the Treatment of Diabetes*, citing exhaustive case records of 76 of the 100 diabetes patients he observed, and becomes the director of diabetes research at the Rockefeller Institute.

1919–1920: Frederick Allen establishes the first treatment clinic in the United States, the Physiatric Institute in New Jersey, to treat patients with diabetes, high blood pressure, and Bright's disease; wealthy and desperate patients flock to it.

July 1, 1920: Dr. Banting opens his first office in London, Ontario; he receives his first patient on July 29; total earnings for his first month of work are $4.

October 30, 1920: Dr. Banting conceives of the idea of insulin after reading Moses Barron's "The Relation of the Islets of Langerhans to Diabetes with Special Reference to Cases of Pancreatic Lithiasis" in the November issue of *Surgery, Gynecology and Obstetrics*. In fact, Banting's notebook from that night is fully preserved at the Academy of Medicine in Toronto. In it he writes, "Diabetus. Ligate pancreatic ducts of dogs. Keep dogs alive till acini degenerate leaving Islets. Try to isolate the internal secretion of these to relieve glycosurea."

November 1920: Banting approaches Dr. J.J.R. Macleod with his idea. In that meeting, Macleod apparently brings Banting up to date on a variety of research attempts in the area of pancreatic extract. Macleod concedes that no one thought about the fact that the digestive agents of the pancreas may be responsible for destroying the secretion made by the islets of Langerhans. Banting proposes to Macleod that by using duct-ligated pancreases to make an extract, which will destroy the digestive secretions, they can find a treatment for diabetes. (Macleod is apparently irritated by Banting's clear lack of knowledge in the area of diabetes. Nevertheless, it is a damned good idea! Macleod, it would appear, is sorry the idea never occurred to him.) For the next year, with the assistance of Charles H. Best, J.B. Collip, and J.J.R. Macleod, Dr. Banting continues his research using a variety of different extracts on de-pancreatized dogs.

December 30, 1921: Dr. Banting presents a paper entitled "The Beneficial Influences of Certain Pancreatic Extracts on Pancreatic Diabetes," summarizing his work to this point at a session of the American Physiological Society at Yale University. Among the attendees are Frederick Allen and Elliot Joslin. Little praise or congratulation is received.

January 23, 1922: One of Banting's insulin extracts is first tested on a human being, a 14-year-old boy named Leonard Thompson, in Toronto; treatment is considered a success by the end of the following February.

May 21, 1922: James Havens becomes the first American successfully treated with insulin.

May 30, 1922: Pharmaceutical manufacturer Eli Lilly and Company and the University of Toronto collaborate on the mass production of insulin in North America.

October 25, 1923: Dr. Banting and Dr. Macleod are awarded the Nobel Prize for Medicine; Banting shares his award with Best; Macleod then shares his award with Collip. (History would not remember Macleod's nor Collip's role in the discovery of insulin. While Banting, Best, Collip, and Macleod would privately acknowledge they were a team, they could never admit it to each other. For Banting's obituary tribute, Collip wrote that his own contribution to insulin was trivial compared to Banting's. Banting apparently admitted in his later years that he and Best wouldn't have "achieved a damned thing" without Collip.*)

1934: Dr. Banting is knighted and becomes Sir Frederick Banting.

February 21, 1941: Sir Frederick Banting is killed in an airplane crash over Newfoundland while en route to England.

1971: 50th anniversary of the discovery of insulin celebrated worldwide.

1996: 75th anniversary of the discovery of insulin celebrated.**

* In 1978, Banting's first biographer, Lloyd Stevenson, published an article that contained Macleod's personal account of the insulin discovery. Although Macleod died in 1935, the University of Toronto did not want to reopen old wounds and for many years prevented the publication

of that account. Macleod's account was bitter. He left the University of Toronto in 1928 and returned to Scotland as Regius Professor at the University of Aberdeen; it is believed that he moved away from Toronto because he couldn't stand living in the shadow of Banting's idea.

Charles Best replaced Macleod as professor of physiology at the University of Toronto when he was just 29 years old. He went on to enjoy a long, distinguished career and many awards and honours until he died in 1978. Best continued Macleod's work on the properties of insulin and received delayed credit for insulin's discovery after Banting's death in 1941. The Best Institute was erected next door to the Banting Institute in 1953.

J.B. Collip attempted to invent another version of insulin he called *gluclokinin*, and then abandoned it. He is also known for pioneering work on parathyroid hormone. Collip received his M.D. and eventually became Chair of Biochemistry at McGill University. He became a world-renowned endocrinologist in Canada, and in 1947 was made Dean of Medicine at the very university that triggered Banting's idea: the University of Western Ontario. Collip enjoyed a great career and died in 1965 at the age of 72.

** New evidence challenges whether Canadians have the right to claim complete ownership of the insulin discovery at all. Romanian scientist Nicolas Paulesco, who was concentrating on measuring the impact of *his* pancreatic extract (called "pancreine") on blood sugar, likely would have been the discoverer of insulin had we Canadians not beaten him to human testing. In 1971, on the 50th anniversary of the discovery of insulin, a campaign was launched by Bucharest medical students to honour Paulesco's work and give him due credit.

SOURCES

Bliss, Michael. "Rewriting Medical History," *Journal of History of Medicine and Allied Sciences, Inc.,* 1993, Vol. 48: 253–74.

_____. *Banting: A Biography.* Toronto: McClelland & Stewart, 1984.

_____. *The Discovery of Insulin.* Toronto: McClelland & Stewart, 1982.

Canadian Diabetes Association. *Diabetes Timeline.* Toronto: The Canadian Diabetes Association, 1997.

Williams, Michael J. "J.J.R. Macleod: The Co-discoverer of Insulin." *Proceedings of the Royal College of Physicians of Edinburgh,* July 1993, Vol. 23, No. 3.

APPENDIX 2
WHERE TO GO ONLINE: YOUR GOOGLE STARTER KIT

This list is not exhaustive, but is meant as a "get started" list if you want to search online for more information.

DENTAL HEALTH
American Academy of Periodontology: www.perio.org
American Dental Association: www.ada.org
Canadian Dental Association: www.cda-adc.ca
Canadian Dental Hygienists Association: www.cdha.ca

DIABETES ORGANIZATIONS
American Association of Diabetes Educators:
   www.diabeteseducator.org
American Diabetes Association: www.ada.org
Canadian Diabetes Association: www.diabetes.ca
Canadian Diabetes Education Certification Board: www.cdecb.ca
Diabetes Exercise and Sports Association: www.diabetes-exercise.org
International Diabetes Federation: www.idf.org
Juvenile Diabetes Research Foundation Canada: www.jdrf.ca
National Institute of Diabetes and Digestive and Kidney Diseases:
   http://diabetes.niddk.nih.gov

DIETITIANS
American Dietetic Association: www.eatright.org
Dietitians of Canada: www.dietitians.ca

FOOT HEALTH

Canadian Podiatric Medical Association: www.podiatrycanada.org

HEART HEALTH

American Heart Association: www.americanheart.org
Heart and Stroke Foundation of Canada: www.heartandstroke.ca

KIDNEY

Kidney Foundation of Canada: www.kidney.ca

MEDIC ALERT

MedicAlert Canada: www.medicalert.ca

PODIATRISTS

Canadian Podiatric Medical Association: www.podiatrycanada.org

VISUALLY IMPAIRED/BLIND REHABILITATION

American Foundation for the Blind: www.afb.org
American Optometric Association: www.aoa.org
Canadian National Institute for the Blind: www.cnib.ca
Canadian Ophthalmological Society: www.eyesite.ca

WOMEN'S HEALTH

American College of Obstetricians and Gynecologists: www.acog.org
Osteoporosis Society of Canada: www.osteoporosis.ca
Society of Obstetricians and Gynaecologists of Canada:
   www.sogc.org

OTHER

American Gastroenterological Association: www.gastro.org
American Urological Association: www.auafoundation.org
Amputee Coalition of America: www.amputee-coalition.org
Canadian Board for Certification of Prosthetists and Orthotists:
   www.cbcpo.ca
Canadian Society for Exercise Physiology: www.csep.ca
Health Canada: www.hc-sc.gc.ca

BIBLIOGRAPHY

SELECTED SOURCES FOR FIRST AND SECOND EDITIONS

"Ad Hoc Technical Committee Working Group on Development of Management Principles and Guidelines for Subsistence Catches of Whales by Indigenous (Aboriginal) Peoples." *International Whaling Commission and Aboriginal/Subsistence Whaling: April 1979 to July 1981*, Special Issue 4. Cambridge, England, International Whaling Commission.

Allsop, Karen F., and Janette Brand Miller. "Honey Revisited: A Reappraisal of Honey in Preindustrial Diets." *British Journal of Nutrition*, vol. 75 (1996):513–520.

American Diabetes Association. *2003 Clinical Practice Recommendations in Diabetes Care*, vol. 27, supp. 1 (January 2004).

"Standards of Medical Care for Patients with Diabetes Mellitus." *Diabetes Care*, vol. 21, supp. 1 (1998), Clinical Practice Recommendations.

"The United Kingdom Prospective Diabetes Study (UKPDS) for Type 2 Diabetes: What You Need to Know about the Results of a Long-Term Study." Posted to www.diabetes.org, January 1999.

Amputation Prevention Global Resource Center. *Prevent Foot Ulcers and Amputations*. Booklet. Retrieved online July 2001 from www.diabetesrousource.com.

Antonucci, T., et al. "Impaired Glucose Tolerance Is Normalized by Treatment with the Thiazoladinedione Troglitazone." *Diabetes Care*, vol. 20, issue 2 (February 1997):188–193.

Appavoo, Donna, Rayanne Waboose, and Stuart Harris. ACPM Dialogue, "Sioux Lookout Diabetes Program." *Diabetes Dialogue*, vol. 41, no. 3 (Fall 1994):19–20.

Armstrong, David G., Lawrence A. Lavery, and Lawrence B. Harkless. "Treatment-Based Classification System for Assessment and Care of Diabetic Feet." *Journal of the American Podiatric Medical Association*, vol. 87, no. 7 (July 1996):303–308.

Augustine, Freda. "Helping My People." *Diabetes Dialogue*, vol. 41, no. 3 (Fall 1994):42–43.

Barnie, Annette. "At Risk in Northern Ontario: Looking for Answers in the Sioux Lookout Zone." *Diabetes Dialogue*, vol. 41, no. 3 (Fall 1994):18–20.

Barwise, Kim, and Danielle Sota. "Two Views." *Diabetes Dialogue*, vol. 43, no. 3 (Fall 1996):42–43.

Bell, S.J., and R.A. Forse. "Nutritional Management of Hypoglycemia." *Diabetes Education*, vol. 25, no. 1 (January–February 1999):41–47.

Bliss, Michael. "Rewriting Medical History." *Journal of History of Medicine and Allied Sciences*, vol. 48 (1993):253–274.

———. *Banting: A Biography*. Toronto: McClelland & Stewart, 1984.

———. *The Discovery of Insulin*. Toronto: McClelland & Stewart, 1982.

Boctor, M.A., et al. "Gestational Diabetes Debate: Controversies in Screening and Management." *Canadian Diabetes*, vol. 10, no. 2 (June 1997):5–7.

Bril, Vera. "Diabetic Neuropathy—Can It Be Treated?" *Diabetes Dialogue*, vol. 41, no. 4 (Winter 1994):8–9.

Brubaker, Patricia L. "Glucagon-Like Peptide-1." *Diabetes Dialogue*, vol. 41, no. 4 (Winter 1994):17–18.

Canadian Diabetes Association. "2003 Clinical Practice Guidelines for the Prevention and Management of Diabetes in Canada." *Canadian Journal of Diabetes,* vol. 27, supp. 2 (2003).

Canadian Institute of Child Health. "Aboriginal Children." In *The Health of Canada's Children: A CICH Profile*, 2nd ed., 131–148. Ottawa: Canadian Institute of Child Health, 1994.

Canadian Medical Association. "CMA's Submission to the Royal Commission on Aboriginal Peoples." In *Canadian Medical Association*

Bridging the Gap: Promoting Health and Healing for Aboriginal Peoples in Canada, 9–17. Ottawa: Canadian Medical Association, 1994.

Canadian Medical Association Journal and the Canadian Diabetes Association. 1998 Clinical Practice Guidelines for the Management of Diabetes in Canada. *Canadian Medical Association Journal*, vol. 159, no. 8, supp. (1998):s1–s27.

Canadian Pharmacists Association. *Compendium of Pharmaceuticals and Specialties*, 35th ed. Toronto: Webcom Ltd., 2000.

———. "Blood-Glucose Testing: Keep Up with the Trend." *Canadian Pharmacy Journal* (September 1996):17.

"Complications: The Long-Term Picture." *Equilibrium*, Issue 1 (1996): 8–10. Canadian Diabetes Association.

"Corn and the Environment—Historical Perspectives." Ontario Corn Producers Association (OCPA) Corn and Environment Index Homepage, 1997.

Cox, Bruce Alan, ed. *Native People, Native Lands: Canadian Indians, Inuit, and Métis*. Ottawa: Carleton University Press, 1988.

Creighton, Donald. *The Forked Road: Canada 1939–1957*. Toronto: McClelland & Stewart, 1976.

The Expert Committee on the Diagnosis and Classification of Diabetes Mellitus. *Report of the Expert Committee on the Diagnosis and Classification of Diabetes Mellitus*. American Diabetes Association, January 1, 1998.

Feig, Denice S. "The Fourth International Workshop Conference on Gestational Diabetes Mellitus." *Canadian Diabetes*, vol. 10, no. 2 (June 1997):2.

Fox, Mary Lou. "Zeesbakadapenewin: Words of an Elder Grandmother about the Sugar Disease." *Diabetes Dialogue*, vol. 41, no. 3 (Fall 1994):22–24.

Foxman, Stuart. Adapted from "Human vs. Beef/Pork Insulin." In *The Report of the Ad Hoc Committee on Beef-Pork Insulins* by Nahla Aris-Jilwan, et al. Canadian Diabetes Association, June 6, 1996.

Mulvad, Gerth and Henning Sloth Pedersen. "Orsoq—Eat Meat and Blubber from Sea Mammals and Avoid Cardiovascular Disease." *Inuit Whaling*, Special Issue (June 1992); published by the Inuit Circumpolar Conference.

Gordon, Dennis. "Acarbose: When It Works/When It Doesn't." *Diabetes Forecast* (February 1997):25–28.

"The Gum Disease Project." Retrieved online July 2001 from www.periodiabetes.com.

"Health and Healing: Inroads of Chronic Disease." *Final Report on Royal Commission on Aboriginal Peoples*, vol. 3, Ch. 3. Posted to the Internet at www.libraxus.com.

Heart and Stroke Foundation of Canada. *The Canadian Family Guide to Stroke: Prevention, Treatment, Recovery.* Toronto: Random House, 1996.

"Heart Attack No Stranger to Canadians." Retrieved online July 2001 from the Heart and Stroke Foundation of Canada www. na.heartandstroke.ca.

"Heart Attack Picture in Canada Receives Mixed Grade." Retrieved online February 7, 2001 from the Heart and Stroke Foundation of Canada www.na.heartandstroke.ca.

"Heart Attack Survival in Canada." Retrieved online July 2001 from the Heart and Stroke Foundation of Canada www.na.heartandstroke.ca.

"Hemodialysis." Retrieved online July 2001 from the Kidney Foundation of Canada www.kidney.ca.

Houlden, Robyn. "Health Beliefs in Two Ontario First Nations Populations." *Diabetes Dialogue*, vol. 41, no. 4 (Winter 1994): 24–25.

"Increased Awareness of Stroke Symptoms Could Dramatically Reduce Stroke Disability—New NIH Public Education Campaign Says Bystanders Can Play Key Role." Retrieved online May 8, 2001 from the American Heart Association www.americanheart.org.

"The Importance of Braille Literacy." Retrieved online July 2001 from the Blindness and Visual Impairment Centre, Canadian National Institute for the Blind www.cnib.ca.

International Food Information Council. *IFIC Review: Uses and Nutritional Impact of Fat Reduction Ingredients.* Washington: International Food Information Council, 1995.

———. *Sorting out the Facts about Fat.* Washington: International Food Information Council, 1997.

"A Jelly Bean Glucose Test." *American Baby* (April 1996):6.

"Jelly Beans Offer Sweet Relief." *Diabetes Dialogue*, vol. 44, no. 2 (Summer 1997):52–53.

Jovanovic-Peterson, Lois, June Biermann, and Barbara Toohey. *The Diabetic Woman: All Your Questions Answered.* New York: G.P. Putnam & Sons, 1996.

Kenshole, Anne. "To Be or Not to Be Pregnant." *Diabetes Dialogue*, vol. 44, no. 2 (Summer 1997):6–8.

Kra, J. Siegfried. *What Every Woman Must Know about Heart Disease.* New York: Warner Books, 1996.

Kuczmarski, R.J., et al. "Increasing Prevalence of Overweight among US Adults: The National Health and Nutrition Examination Surveys, 1960 to 1991." *Journal of the American Medical Association*, vol. 272 (1994):205–211.

Kumar, S., et al. "Troglitazone, an Insulin Action Enhancer, Improves Metabolic Control in NIDDM Patients." *Diabetologia*, vol. 30, issue 6 (June 1996):701–709.

Lebovitz, Harold E. "Acarbose, an Alpha-glucosidase Inhibitor in the Treatment of NIDDM." *Diabetes Care*, vol. 19, supp. 1 (1996):554–561.

Lichtenstein, A.H., et al. "Hydrogenation Impairs the Hypolipidemic Effect of Corn Oil in Humans." *Arteriosclerosis and Thrombosis*, 13 (1993):154–161.

Liebman, Bonnie. "Syndrome X: The Risks of High Insulin." *Nutrition Action*, vol. 27, no. 2 (March 2000):3–8.

Linden, Ron. "Hyperbaric Medicine." *Diabetes Dialogue*, vol. 43, no. 4 (Fall 1996):24–26.

Lindesay, J.E. "Multiple Pain Complaints in Amputees." *Journal of Rehabilitation and Social Medicine*, vol. 78 (1985):452–455.

Ludwig, Sora. "Gestational Diabetes." *Canadian Diabetes*, vol. 10, no. 2 (June 1997):1, 8.

Macdonald, Jeanette. "The Facts about Menopause." *Diabetes Dialogue*, vol. 44, no. 2 (Summer 1997):24–26.

MacMillan, Harriet L., et al. "Aboriginal Health." *Canadian Medical Association Journal*, vol. 155 (1996):1569–1578.

Marshall, M., E. Helmes, and A.B. Deathe. "A Comparison of Psychosocial Functioning and Personality in Amputee and Chronic Pain Patients." *Clinical Journal of Pain* 8 (1992):351–357.

McCarten, James. "Toxic or Not, Inuit Stand by Whale Meat." *The Edmonton Journal* (December 28, 1995).

Morrison, Bruce R., and C. Roderick Williams. *Native Peoples Canadian Experience*. Toronto: McClelland & Stewart, 1986.

End Stage Renal Disease in the United States. Booklet. Retrieved online July 2001 from www.kidney.org.

"Microalbuninuria in Diabetic Kidney Disease." Retrieved online July 2001 from www.kidney.org.

"Preventing Diabetic Kidney Disease." Retrieved online July 2001 from www.kidney.org.

"Olestra: Yes or No? Excerpt from The University of California at Berkeley Wellness Letter." *Diabetes Dialogue*, vol. 43, no. 3 (Fall 1996):44.

"Some Limitations of a Left Critique and Deep Dilemmas in Environmental–First Nations Relationships." Learned Societies Conference, "The Environment and the Relations with First Nations," co-sponsored by the Society for Socialist Studies and the Environmental Studies Association of Canada, Montreal, June 5, 1995.

Poirier, Laurinda M., and Katharine M. Coburn. *Women and Diabetes: Life Planning for Health and Wellness*. New York: American Diabetes Association and Bantam Books, 1997.

"Position of the American Dietetic Association: Use of Nutritive and Nonnutritive Sweeteners." *Journal of the American Dietetic Association*, vol. 93 (1993):816–822.

Postl, B., et al. "Background Paper on the Health of Aboriginal Peoples in Canada." In *Bridging the Gap: Promoting Health and Healing for Aboriginal Peoples in Canada*, 19–56. Ottawa: The Canadian Medical Association, 1994.

"Prevention and Treatment of Obesity: Application to Type 2 Diabetes (Technical Review)." *Diabetes Care*, vol. 20 (1997):1744–1766.

"Report on the Second International Conference on Diabetes and Native Peoples." Prepared by the First Nations Health Commission, Assembly of First Nations, November 1993.

———. *The Gynecological Sourcebook*, 4th ed. Chicago: McGraw-Hill, 2003.

———— *The Pregnancy Sourcebook*, 3rd ed. Chicago: McGraw-Hill, 1999.

———— *The Skinny on Fat*. Toronto: McClelland & Stewart, 2004.

Rowlands, Liz, and Denis Peter. "Diabetes—Yukon Style." *Diabetes Dialogue*, vol. 41, no. 3 (Fall 1994).

Rubin, Alan L. *Diabetes for Dummies*. Chicago: IDG Books, 1999.

Schwartz, Carol. "An Eye-Opener." *Diabetes Dialogue*, vol. 43, no. 4 (Winter 1996):20–22.

———— "Complications: Your Eyes and Diabetic Retinopathy." Retrieved online July 2001 from the Canadian Diabetes Association www.diabetes.ca.

Society of Obstetricians and Gynecologists of Canada. *A Guide for Health Care Professionals Working with Aboriginal Peoples: A Policy Statement*, 1–15. Booklet, April 2001.

Spicer, Kay. "Traditional Foods of Aboriginal Canadians." *Diabetes Dialogue*, vol. 41, no. 3 (Fall 1994).

"Spring at Last!" *The Diabetes News*, prepared by the LifeScan Education Institute, Spring 1996.

Stehlin, Dori. "A Little Lite Reading." Posted to FDA website www.fda.gov/fdac/foodlabel/diabetes.html.

Tetley, Deborah. "Fish Farmer Hopes to Tame Diabetes on Akwesasne." *The Toronto Star* (April 12, 1997).

Tookenay, Vincent F. "Improving the Health Status of Aboriginal People in Canada: New Directions, New Responsibilities." *Canadian Medical Association Journal*, vol. 155 (1996):1581–1583.

"Trapped by Furs." Presentation at the Symposium of Conflicting Interests of Animal Welfare and Indigenous Peoples. Erasmus University, Rotterdam, Finn Lynge, January 17, 1997.

White, John R., Jr. "The Pharmacologic Management of Patients with Type II Diabetes Mellitus in the Era of New Oral Agents and Insulin Analogs." *Diabetes Spectrum*, vol. 9, no. 4 (1996):227–234.

Willett, W.C., et al. "Intake of Trans Fatty Acids and Risk of Coronary Heart Disease among Women." *Lancet*, vol. 341 (1993):581–585.

Williams, Michael. "Macleod: The Co-discoverer of Insulin." *Proceedings of the Royal College of Physicians of Edinburgh*, vol. 23, no. 3 (July 1993).

Williamson, G.M., et al. "Social and Psychological Factors in Adjustment to Limb Amputation." *Journal of Social Behavior and Personality*, vol. 9 (1994):249–268.

Williamson, Gail M. "Perceived Impact of Limb Amputation on Sexual Activity: A Study of Adult Amputees." *The Journal of Sex Research*, vol. 33, no. 3 (1996):221–230.

Wormworth, Janice. "Toxins and Tradition: The Impact of Food-Chain Contamination on the Inuit of Northern Quebec." *Canadian Medical Association Journal*, vol. 152, no. 8 (April 15, 1995).

Zinman, Bernard. "Insulin Analogues." *Diabetes Dialogue*, vol. 43, no. 4 (Winter 1996):14–15.

SELECTED SOURCES FOR THIRD EDITION

Asikainen, S., S. Chen, S. Alaluusua, and J. Slots. "Can One Acquire Periodontal Bacteria and Periodontitis from a Family Member?" *Journal of the American Dental Association*, vol. 128, no. 9 (September 1997):1263–1271.

Cali, A.M.G., and S. Caprio. "Prediabetes and Type 2 Diabetes in Youth: An Emerging Epidemic Disease?" *Current Opinion in Endocrinology, Diabetes, and Obesity*, vol. 15 (2008):123–127.

Canadian Diabetes Association. "Canadian Diabetes Association 2008 Clinical Practice Guidelines for the Prevention and Management of Diabetes in Canada." *Canadian Journal of Diabetes*, vol. 32, supp. 1 (September 2008).

Canadian Institute for Health Information. *Giving Birth in Canada: Regional Trends from 2001–2002 to 2005–2006.* Ottawa: Canadian Institute for Health Institute, 2007.

Davidson, J.A., T.A. Ciulla, J.B. McGill, K.A. Kles, and P.W. Anderson. "How the Diabetic Eye Loses Vision." *Endocrine*, vol. 32, no. 1 (August 2007): 107–116.

Farid, N.R., and N. Gilletz. *The PCOS Diet Cookbook.* Victoria: Trafford Publishing/Your Health Press.

Farshchi, H., A. Rane, A. Love, and R.L. Kennedy. "Diet and Nutrition in Polycystic Ovary Syndrome (PCOS): Pointers for Nutritional Management." *Journal of Obstetrics and Gynaecology*, vol. 27, no. 8 (November 2007): 762–773.

Galtier, F., I. Raingeard, E. Renard, P. Boulot, and J. Bringer. "Optimizing the Outcome of Pregnancy in Obese Women: From Pregestational to Long-Term Management." *Diabetes Metabolism,* vol. 34, no. 1 (February 2008): 19–25.

Gill, J.S., and Alberta Kidney Disease Network. "Residence Location and Likelihood of Kidney Transplantation." *Canadian Medical Association Journal,* vol. 175, no. 5 (August 2006): 478–482.

Glueck, C.J., N. Goldenberg, L. Sieve, and P. Wang. "An Observational Study of Reduction of Insulin Resistance and Prevention of Development of Type 2 Diabetes Mellitus in Women with Polycystic Ovary Syndrome Treated with Metformin and Diet." *Metabolism,* vol. 57, no. 7 (July 2008):954–960.

Gottschalk, M, T. Dannee, A. Vlanjnic, and J.F. Cara. "Glimepiride versus Metformin as Monotherapy in Pediatric Patients with Type 2 Diabetes." *Diabetes Care,* vol. 30, no. 4 (2007):790–794.

Hawley, C.M., J. Jeffries, J. Nearhos, and C. Van Eps. "Complications of Home Hemodialysis." *Hemodialysis International,* vol. 12, supp. 1 (July 2008):S21–25.

Herriot, A.M., S. Whitcroft, and Y. Jeanes. "A Retrospective Audit of Patients with Polycystic Ovary Syndrome: The Effects of a Reduced Glycaemic Load Diet." *Journal of Human Nutrition and Dietetics,* vol. 21, no. 4 (August 2008):337–345.

Hollander, M.H., K.M. Paarlberg, and A.J. Huisjes. "Gestational Diabetes: A Review of the Current Literature and Guidelines." *Obstetrics and Gynecological Survey,* vol. 62, no. 2 (February 2007):125–136.

Horn, O.K., et al. "Incidence and Prevalence of Type 2 Diabetes in the First Nation Community of Kahnawá:ke, Quebec, Canada, 1986–2003." *Canadian Journal of Public Health,* vol. 98, no. 6 (2007):438–443.

Kane, M.P., A. Abu-Baker, and R.S. Busch. "The Utility of Oral Diabetes Medications in Type 2 Diabetes of the Young." *Current Diabetes Review,* vol. 1, no. 1 (February 2005):83–92.

Wahlgren, N, et al. "Thrombolysis with Alteplase 3-4.5 h after Acute Ischaemic Stroke (SITS-ISTR): An Observational Study." *Lancet,* vol. 372, no. 9646 (October 11, 2008):1303–1309.

Lamar, M.E., T.J. Kuehl, A.T. Cooney, L.J. Gayle, S. Holleman, and S.R. Allen. "Jelly Beans as an Alternative to a Fifty-Gram Glucose Beverage for Gestational Diabetes Screening." *American Journal of Obstetrics and Gynecology*, vol. 181, pt. 1 (November 1999):1154–1157.

Lee, J.M. "Why Young Adults Hold the Key to Assessing the Obesity Epidemic in Children." *Archives of Pediatric and Adolescent Medicine*, vol. 162 (2008):682–687.

Lipscombe, L.L. "Thiazolidinediones: Do Harms Outweigh Benefits?" *Canadian Medical Association Journal*, vol. 180, no. 1 (January 2009):16–17.

Loke, Y.K., S. Singh, and C.D. Furberg. "Long-Term Use of Thiazolidinediones and Fractures in Type 2 Diabetes: A Meta Analysis." *Canadian Medical Association Journal*, vol. 180, no. 1 (January 2009):32–39.

Ly, K.A., P. Milgrom, and M. Rothen. "The Potential of Dental-Protective Chewing Gum in Oral Health Interventions." *Journal of the American Dental Association*, vol. 139, no. 5 (May 2008):553–563.

Ma, Y., B.C. Olendzki, P.A. Merriam, D.E. Chiriboga, A.L. Culver, W. Li, J.R. Hébert, I.S. Ockene, J.A. Griffith, and S.L. Pagoto. "A Randomized Clinical Trial Comparing Low-Glycemic Index versus ADA Dietary Education among Individuals with Type 2 Diabetes." *Nutrition*, vol. 24, no. 1 (January 2008):45–56.

Meeuwisse-Pasterkamp, S.H., M.M. van der Klauw, and B.H. Wolffenbuttel. "Type 2 Diabetes Mellitus: Prevention of Macrovascular Complications." *Expert Reviews in Cardiovascular Therapy*, vol. 6, no. 3 (March 2008):323–341.

Mohamed, Q., M.C. Gillies, and T.Y. Wong. "Management of Diabetic Retinopathy: A Systematic Review." *Journal of the American Medical Association*, vol. 298, no. 8 (August 2007):902–916.

Nadeau, J.O., S. Shi, J. Fang, M.K. Kapral, J.A. Richards, F.L. Silver, M.D. Hill, and Investigators for the Registry of the Canadian Stroke Network. "TPA Use for Stroke in the Registry of the Canadian Stroke Network." *Can J Neurol Sci*, vol. 32, no. 4 (November 2005):433–439.

Nicolucci, A. "Aspirin for Primary Prevention of Cardiovascular Events in Diabetes: Still an Open Question." *Journal of the American Medical Association*, vol. 300, no. 18 (November 2008):2180–2181.

Ogawa, H., M. Nakayama, T. Morimoto, S. Uemura, M. Kanauchi, N. Doi, H. Jinnouchi, S. Sugiyama, and Y. Saito for the Japanese Primary Prevention of Atherosclerosis with Aspirin for Diabetes (JPAD) Trial Investigation. "Low-Dose Aspirin for Primary Prevention of Atherosclerotic Events in Patients with Type 2 Diabetes: A Randomized Controlled Trial." *Journal of the American Medical Association*, vol. 300, no. 18 (November 2008):2134–2141.

Outhouse, T.L., Z. Fedorowicz, J.V. Keenan, and R. Al-Alawi. "A Cochrane Systematic Review Finds Tongue Scrapers Have Short-Term Efficacy in Controlling Halitosis." *General Dentistry*, vol. 54, no. 5 (September–October 2006):352–359; 360, 367–368.

Owen, C.G., R.M. Martin, P.H. Whincup, G.D. Smith, and D.G. Cook. "Does Breastfeeding Influence Risk of Type 2 Diabetes in Later Life? A Quantitative Analysis of Published Evidence." *American Journal of Clinical Nutrition*, vol. 84, no. 5 (November 2006):1043–1054.

Pedrazzi, V., S. Sato, de Mattos, G. Mda, E.H. Lara, and H. Panzeri. "Tongue-Cleaning Methods: A Comparative Clinical Trial Employing a Toothbrush and a Tongue Scraper." *Journal of Periodontology*, vol. 75, no. 7 (July 2004):1009–1012.

Phillips, P.J. "Women, Coronary Artery Disease, and Diabetes." *Australian Family Physician*, vol. 37, no. 6 (June 2008):441–442.

Prentice, A.M., B.J. Hennig, and A.J. Fulford. "Evolutionary Origins of the Obesity Epidemic: Natural Selection of Thrifty Genes or Genetic Drift following Predation Release?" *International Journal of Obesity* London, vol. 32, no. 11 (November 2008):1607–1610.

Puhl, R.M., and J.D. Latner. "Stigma, Obesity, and the Health of the Nation's Children." *Psychology Bulletin*, vol. 133, no. 4 (2007):557–580.

Rosenthal, M.S. "Ethical Problems with Bioidentical Hormone Therapy." In *Journal of Impotence Research*, vol. 20 (2008):45–52.

———. *The Canadian Type 2 Diabetes Sourcebook*, 2nd ed. Toronto: John Wiley & Sons Canada, 2004.

———. *The Skinny on Fat*. Toronto: McClelland & Stewart, 2004.

———. *Stopping Cancer at the Source*, 2nd ed. Victoria: Trafford Publishing/Your Health Press, 2008.

"Rosiglitazone No Longer Recommended." *Lancet*, vol. 372, no. 9649 (November 2008):1520.

Satpathy, H.K., A. Fleming, D. Frey, M. Barsoom, C. Satpathy, and J. Khandalavala. "Maternal Obesity and Pregnancy." *Postgraduate Medicine*, vol. 120, no. 3 (September 15, 2008):E01–E09.

Scheen, A.J. "Exenatide Once Weekly in Type 2 Diabetes." *Lancet* (September 7, 2008).

Schwartz, S.G., and H.W. Flynn, Jr. "Pharmacotherapies for Diabetic Retinopathy: Present and Future." *Experimental Diabetes Research*, (2007):524–587.

Sellers, E.A.C., and H.J. Dean. "Screening for Type 2 Diabetes in High-Risk Pediatric Population: Capillary vs. Venous Fasting Plasma Glucose." *Canadian Journal of Diabetes*, vol. 29, no. 4 (2005):393–396.

Speakman, J.R. "Thrifty Genes for Obesity and the Metabolic Syndrome—Time to Call Off the Search?" *Diabetes and Vascular Disease Research*, vol. 3, no. 1 (May 2006):7–11.

Tonelli, M., S. Klarenbach, B. Manns, B. Culleton, B. Hemmelgarn, S. Bertazzon, N. Wiebe, J.S. Gill, and Alberta Kidney Disease Network. "Residence Location and Likelihood of Kidney Transplantation." *Canadian Medical Association Journal*, vol. 175, no. 5 (August 29, 2006):478–482.

Unger, J. "Current Strategies for Evaluating, Monitoring, and Treating Type 2 Diabetes Mellitus." *American Journal of Medicine*, vol. 121, supp. 6 (June 2008):S3–S8.

Van Winkelhoff, A.J., and K. Boutaga. "Transmission of Periodontal Bacteria and Models of Infection." *Journal of Clinical Periodontology*, vol. 32, supp. 6 (2005):16–27.

Vrolix, R., L.E. van Meijl, and R.P. Mensink. "The Metabolic Syndrome in Relation with the Glycemic Index and the Glycemic Load." *Physiology and Behavior*, vol. 94, no. 2 (May 2008):293–299.

Wahlgren, N., N. Ahmed, A. Dávalos, W. Hacke, M. Millán, K. Muir, R.O. Roine, D. Toni, R. Lees Weiss, and F.R. Kaufman. "Metabolic Complications of Childhood Obesity." *Diabetes Care*, vol. 31 (2008):S310–S316.

Wolever, T.M., C. Mehling, J.L. Chiasson, R.G. Josse, L.A. Leiter, P. Maheux, R. Rabasa-Lhoret, N.W. Rodger, and E.A. Ryan. "Low Glycaemic

Index Diet and Disposition Index in Type 2 Diabetes (the Canadian Trial of Carbohydrates in Diabetes): A Randomised Controlled Trial." *Diabetologia*, vol. 51, no. 9 (September 2008):1607–1615.

Yaggi, H.K., A.B. Araujo, and J.B. McKinlay. "Sleep Duration as a Risk Factor for the Development of Type 2 Diabetes." *Diabetes Care*, vol. 29, no. 3 (March 2006):657–661.

Zaltzman, J.S. "Kidney Transplantation in Canada: Unequal Access." *Canadian Medical Association Journal*, vol. 175, no. 5 (August 2006):489–490.

Zehle, K., B.J. Smith, T. Chey, M. McLean, A.E. Bauman, and N.W. Cheung. "Psychosocial Factors Related to Diet among Women with Recent Gestational Diabetes: Opportunities for Intervention." *Diabetes Education*, vol. 34, no. 5 (September–October 2008):807–814.

INTERNET SOURCES USED IN THIRD EDITION

Alberta Centre for Active Living: www.centre4activeliving.ca

American Academy of Periodontology: www.perio.org

American College of Obstetricians and Gynecologists: www.acog.org

American Dental Association: www.ada.org

American Diabetes Association: www.diabetes.org

American Foundation for the Blind: www.afb.org

American Gastroenterological Association: www.gastro.org

American Heart Association: www.americanheart.org

American Optometric Association: www.aoa.org

American Urological Association: www.auafoundation.org

Amputee Coalition of America: www.amputee-coalition.org

Canadian Board for Certification of Prosthetists and Orthotists: www.cbcpo.ca

Canadian Dental Association: www.cda-adc.ca

Canadian Dental Hygienists Association: www.cdha.ca

Canadian Diabetes Association: www.diabetes.ca

Canadian Diabetes Education Certification Board: www.cdecb.ca

Canadian MedicAlert Foundation: www.medicalert.ca

Canadian National Institute for the Blind: www.cnib.ca

Canadian Ophthalmological Society: www.eyesite.ca

Canadian Society for Exercise Physiology: www.csep.ca

Certified Professional Trainers Network: www.cptn.com

Decision Resources: www.decisionresources.com

Health Canada: www.hc-sc.gc.ca

International Bottled Water Association: www.bottledwater.org

Kidney Foundation of Canada: www.kidney.ca

National Institute of Diabetes and Digestive and Kidney Diseases: www.diabetes.niddk.nih.gov

Osteoporosis Society of Canada: www.osteoporosis.ca

Toronto Public Health: www.toronto.ca/health

World Health Organization: www.who.int

INDEX